The Medical Secretary's and Receptionist's Handbook

including Hospital Office Practice

The Medical Secretary's and Receptionist's Handbook

including Hospital Office Practice

Michael Drury
OBE, PRCGP, MB, ChB
Professor of General Practice
University of Birmingham
President of the
Royal College of General Practitioners

Marion Collin
Lecturer in Office Arts
West Kent College of Further Education
Tonbridge, Kent

FIFTH EDITION

Baillière Tindall London Philadelphia
Toronto Sydney Tokyo

Baillière Tindall 24-28 Oval Road,
London NW1 7DX

W.B. Saunders The Curtis Center
Independence Square West
Philadelphia, PA 19106-3399, USA

1 Goldthorne Avenue
Toronto, Ontario M8Z 5T9, Canada

Harcourt Brace Jovanovich Group (Australia)
Pty Ltd, 32-52 Smidmore Street, Marrickville,
NSW 2204, Australia

Harcourt Brace Jovanovich (Japan) Inc.
Ichibancho Central Building, 22-1 Ichibancho
Chiyoda-ku, Tokyo 102, Japan

Drury—The Medical Secretary's and Receptionist's Handbook
First published 1965
Third edition 1975
Reprinted 1979
Fourth edition 1981
Reprinted 1982, 1984

Collin—Hospital Office Practice
First published 1981

Combined edition
First published 1986
Reprinted 1989

Typset by Scribe Design, Gillingham, Kent
Printed and bound in Great Britain by T.J. Press (Padstow) Ltd,
Padstow, Cornwall

British Library Cataloguing in Publication Data

Drury, Michael
  The medical secretary's and receptionist's
  handbook : (including Hospital office
  practice)—5th ed.
  1. Medical secretaries
  I. Title   II. Collin, Marion   III. Collin,
  Marion. Hospital office practice
  651.3'741   R728.8

ISBN 0 7020 1172 X

Contents

Preface

The first edition of this book appeared twenty-one years ago and coincided with the establishment of full-time training courses for medical secretaries and receptionists leading to recognized qualifications. In the intervening period the subsequent editions have reflected the changing structure of health services, the altered role of health care personnel and the increasing recognition that improving the care of patients depends as much on the quality of administrative service as on the quality of medical care.

This new edition continues in this direction but it has been thought appropriate to bring under one cover and one title two established books, *The Medical Secretary's and Receptionist's Handbook* and *Hospital Office Practice*.

The two authors have thus combined in an attempt to make it a thoroughly comprehensive book covering the many areas in which people may work.

Changes in the organization of the health service, and in particular hospital services, have been incorporated. The sections relating to the introduction of the electronic office have been much expanded and the general practice section now reflects more closely the importance of managerial skills and communication skills.

February 1986

Michael Drury
Marion Collin

Acknowledgements

Once again it is a pleasure to acknowledge the support and assistance of so many people without which this work would not have been possible. Ms Lyn Shields has carefully prepared the manuscript and advised on some matters of fact. Many practice managers have made helpful comments.

Michael Drury

With acknowledgements to the Tunbridge Wells Health District for permission to reproduce their hospital forms, the Association of Medical Secretaries, Practice Managers and Receptionists for permission to use questions from the Office Practice section of their Diploma examination papers, and to those firms who have been kind enough to provide photographs: Roy Bulmer Ltd, Nuplana, Tonbridge, Kent; Granard Communications, 4 Babmaes Street, London SW1Y 6HD; Communications Librarian, IBM UK Ltd; LSI Computers Ltd, Copse Road, St John's, Woking, Surrey; Vydec (UK) Ltd, Borax House, Carlisle Place, London SW1P 1HT.

Marion Collin

1

Patients

Medical secretaries and receptionists usually do their job because they want to help people. In whatever field of medical practice they work they will meet people and patients and will find this the most compelling and absorbing part of the job. In this introduction we have explained some of the factors that make people become patients, i.e. seek help for their symptoms, and some of the ways in which becoming a patient may affect their behaviour. The medical secretary, receptionist, medical records officer or practice manager will find that an understanding of this assists her in the development of attitudes to the people that present and in the application of the knowledge she learns and the skills she possesses.

Despite the fact that large numbers of people consult doctors every day most people when they feel something is wrong with them do not consult. Three out of four people treat themselves or seek advice from a friend, a relative or the local pharmacist. Indeed, if we take the World Health Organization's definition of health as 'a state of perfect physical, psychological and social well-being' we find that only five out of every hundred people in the United Kingdom believe they fit this definition at any particular moment and very few of them consult doctors.

BECOMING A PATIENT

When people consult a health professional, a doctor or a nurse about symptoms they convert themselves from a 'person' into a 'patient'. This conversion is a very significant step and is done in a different way by different people at different times. There is a well-known diagram (Figure 1.1) showing the squares in which people with symptoms can be placed. There are three squares in the diagram. Square A includes those who consult the doctor about non-significant symptoms. It is the area where health education might help most. Square B includes those who report significant symptoms and those in Square C are patients who fail to report with significant symptoms.

What makes people move from one square into another? Some of the answers to this question will be obvious. For example, a person with pain in the chest may believe that this is serious, represents a possibility of heart disease, and so will consult a doctor early. Even in this case it is not quite so simple because when they consult will depend upon their knowledge and their previous experience. In a young man, for example, the pain is much less likely to be due to heart disease than in a middle-aged man, so the younger man may be more likely to attribute it to muscle strain and thus delay consultation. (A common, more serious example of this is the belief that cancer is painful and

1

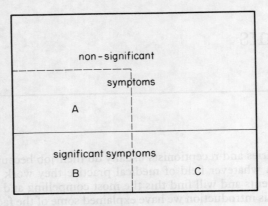

Fig. 1.1 Differing responses to symptoms.

this frequently leads women with painless lumps in the breast to delay seeking help for a disease that later turns out to be cancer.) However, if the young man with pain in the chest had noted that several colleagues in the factory where he works had had heart attacks recently this might make him more ready to become a patient with any symptom that he attributed to his heart. I use the word 'attribute' because many interviews have shown that although most people know the heart to be in the middle of the chest a surprisingly large number of adults place organs of their body in quite strange positions.

The severity of the symptom. This may be the factor causing a person to become a patient. Very bad pain makes it more likely, of course, that a person will consult. Some people, however, tolerate pain much more than others. This may be due to cultural reasons; some races of people are more demonstrative than others who are accustomed to endure their pain stoically. It may be due to training in early life: an example from parents or schools. It may be due to biochemical causes, or it may be the circumstances surrounding the pain; pain when you're worried, pain in the night, pain that you cannot explain is often worse than pain in the daytime, pain that you know the cause of and so on.

Appropriateness of seeking help. If people believe effective treatment to be available and important they will seek help. The consultations of some people about coughs and colds are influenced by their belief that cough mixtures and linctuses are important and effective treatments, which they very rarely are, and this belief can be strengthened by the fact that the doctor prescribes them, which 'medicalizes' the disease. This becomes a way in which doctors influence the change from a person to a patient. If the doctors treat a condition it should be apparent to patients that they have consulted appropriately. Today it seems quite appropriate for people to consult doctors about such matters as marital disturbances, sexual problems and worries about work and finances, whereas twenty years ago this was much less common. Even now it does not seem appropriate to all people to do this but it does for some and if doctors interest themselves in such topics then these topics become 'medicalized'.

The availability of the source of help. In our society women tend to consult general practitioners (GPs) more frequently than men do and, although there are a number of complex reasons for this, one factor is that the doctor has become more accessible to women. The times at which the surgery is open, and the fact that women bring their children to the doctor (which enables them to consult 'by the way') makes professional advice more readily available to women than men.

There are, of course, another group of forces working the other way across this dividing line between people and patients. Fear of finding out what is wrong with them keeps some people away; people do not want to present a lump to the doctor for fear of being told that it is cancer. Fear of the consequences of treatment, treatment that takes up their time, treatment that is painful, and treatment that removes a person from their home may also prevent people consulting and so occasionally may the social stigmata consequent upon the potential consultation that relates to, say, contraception or abortion. It will be seen from this list of some of the factors that the medical and psychological reasons for becoming a patient are quite complex, and this is made even more confusing by social factors which are concerned in adopting what we call the 'sick role'.

THE SICK ROLE

Once a person has decided that he is going to become a patient he will usually adopt certain patterns of behaviour that society expects a sick person to have. Firstly, he will want to get better. If he does not obviously 'want' to get better he may be labelled as a hypochondriac, and expressions like 'pull yourself together' or 'snap out of it' may be used. Some people may not want to get better though; they may use the sick role as a useful protection against the problems and responsibilities of life. Secondly, patients are expected to seek help and follow advice. There are many reasons why people do not do so, but usually they are criticized by society for failing.

In our society being in the sick role exempts us from a lot of normal social responsibilities; sick people do not work and sick children do not go to school. Sometimes sick people come to a doctor first to gain this exemption by 'getting a note'; however society frowns on people who are not ill but claim this exemption, and labels them malingerers.

We see why patients report sick and what society expects of them but how do they behave when they are sick? An understanding is important because it explains the behaviour of patients in many other areas.

Sickness nearly always causes anxiety. Most patients do not like going to a doctor and would rather keep away. They may be afraid of hearing the truth, afraid of the investigations that might be ordered, afraid of being stopped doing something they enjoy, such as smoking, drinking or eating, or they may be afraid of having to talk about private or embarrassing things. This fear may make it difficult for them to talk properly and difficult to remember simple things. They may appear stupid and cause irritation to receptionists and doctors and this irritation may make them more frightened. Sometimes they conceal their fear by bravado or by aggression and this too has to be understood so that they can be sympathetically dealt with.

The aggressive patient is not always afraid. Sometimes aggression is a reflection of previous experience. If the patient has just had a battle with a parking attendant the consequent emotion may carry over into the doctor's surgery or hospital clinic. Sometimes they have had to battle in life with post-offices, shops and banks, or even previous doctors and receptionists, so they may feel they have to battle to achieve their expectations.

Similarly, the stupidity may not always be a mask for fear. The patient may not be very intelligent, may be deaf, may be confused or may not speak the same language; it is clearly important to recognize this so that patients receive sensitive handling.

Patients need to be treated as equals, but they will have the same anxieties and behavioural patterns as any of us in their situation. They need to be cared for as well as cured by all those who are privileged to be in a position to help. The skills required to deal with the great variety of patients' problems and personalities are many but the attitudes can be more simply expressed. The patients should be aware that the receptionist or secretary is there to help them and this must be conveyed at every level of their work. No discussion about the skills and efficiency in later chapters should be allowed to conceal this most essential point.

I

The Development of
the Health Service

1

The Development of
the Health Service

2

The History of Medicine

THE BIRTH OF MEDICINE

The earliest medical records known to exist are six books written by *Thot*, an Egyptian, in the year 4500 BC. This date is of interest to the medical secretary because during all her working life she will be concerned with handling medical records. These early records are of importance because they tell us how doctors worked and thought in days gone by and because the medical reports of one generation are the foundations upon which are built the advances in treatment and diagnosis made by the next generation. The common theme which will be seen to run throughout this book is the constant attention to care and accuracy when dealing with these records. Memory is a frail and unreliable thing and the written word endures.

Myth and magic

At the time when Thot wrote his books medical treatment was based entirely on a cult of myth and magic. This superstition was not confined to method only, for the Egyptians deified their royal physician, *Imhotep*. He was, in fact, a historical person and writings on papyrus have been found which are attributed to him. These consist of descriptions of surgical cases and the operations that he performed. We know from the writings of Persia, Babylon and ancient India that medicine in these civilizations was based on belief in the power of the stars and the casting out of devils. The Minoan people who occupied all the eastern end of the Mediterranean and the island of Crete from about 3000 BC to 1000 BC used the symbol of the serpent in their religion and their primitive medicine. About 1000 BC the Minoan people were over-run by tribes from the North who occupied their lands and enslaved them. As a race the Minoans were not exterminated but were absorbed by the conquerors who settled on their lands. In just the same way many of their beliefs and superstitions were absorbed, and this complex and mixed people with roots and origins from many countries became the Ancient Greeks. Their medicine was drawn from many sources: from Egypt on their southern boundaries and from Babylon in the east as well as from the Minoans they had conquered, and to all these the Greeks applied a system of rational thought which enables us to label them as the founders of scientific medicine.

The Ancient Greeks also deified one of their first physicians, *Aesculapius*, who is depicted as a benign old man leaning upon a staff around which entwines a serpent—perhaps the serpent of Minoan religion. This staff and serpent are still used today as a medical badge and symbol all over the world.

Greek medicine

The Greek method was to observe and analyse and from these observations to make deductions. Using these methods they developed centres of learning where they taught a system of calmness, wisdom and dignity far removed from the primitive savageries and dark ways of the medicine that had gone before. The finest example of this system is the work of *Hippocrates* which still sets a standard twenty-three centuries after his death. He is known as the 'Father of Medicine' and a collection of about a hundred books has been gathered together under his name, although it is not known for certain how many of these books were actually written by him. He lived in a time of great intellectual activity and his powerful mind brought the same approach to medicine as was applied to other sciences at this time. He was born on the island of Kos about 460 BC, the son of a physician; he led a wandering life, teaching and healing as he went.

The Greeks held the dead body in such reverence that he could learn little anatomy by dissection, but by the careful recording of knowledge and cautious inference from it he became the outstanding physician of his time. He was gentle and humane, wise yet eager to learn. He preached no narrow specialization, but that the physician should understand the 'whole man'. He understood the limitations of man and respected the 'healing power of nature'. His humanity and high ethical standards mark him out as the ideal physician for all time. The Hippocratic writings are remarkable for the detail and accuracy of their observations and it is worth remembering that, after the thousand years of anarchy that followed the break-up of the Roman Empire, it was the careful reconstruction of the works of Hippocrates that helped in the renaissance of medicine.

The name of *Aristotle* must have special mention in the history of medical records. He also was the son of a physician, and although not a doctor himself his thought moulded the development of all the sciences, including medicine. He lived about a hundred years after Hippocrates and became the tutor of Alexander the Great. A philosopher and a biologist, he laid the foundations for the theory of evolution, for embryology and comparative anatomy, but above all he was the first classifier of ancient science, and his writings have an encyclopaedic greatness. They have moulded scientific thought for two thousand years and when the Greeks were finally overcome by the Romans his ideas were absorbed and replaced the primitive magic of native Roman medicine.

It was, in fact, a Greek who became the greatest Roman physician. *Galen* was born in Pergamum about AD 130 and became famous by treating and curing the emperor. His importance to this study is that he wrote with great industry and applied himself vigorously to accounts of anatomy and physiology. He has been drawn taking a history at the bedside in AD 170. His writings have been better preserved than those of any other non-Christian writer. He was a dull, contentious fellow compared with the lofty Hippocrates, but he founded his teachings on case reports and records. These he interspersed with long philosophical dissertations in which he expressed his belief in the fact that man's perfection was controlled by an all-seeing God: a development of the philosophy of the Stoics which influenced the world of his day.

Christendom and Islam

This belief led to his work being treasured by both the Christian Church and Islam equally. When Galen died in about AD 200 medical advance ceased. It has been said that with his death the light of learning in the Western world went out for twelve hundred years. Christianity had no place for the clay that was mortal man. The monasteries were set on higher aspirations than science and although conscientious monks preserved the writings of Hippocrates and the other ancient masters, they were not inclined to experiment or to spread their learning beyond the cloisters. In this way they were 'antiscientific' and the advance of medicine had to wait, as all science and art had to wait, until the early fifteenth century. It was not, however, only Christendom that preserved the writings of antiquity. The world of Islam lay along the eastern boundaries of the Roman empire and the language and culture of its people were influenced by these contacts. In the seventh century large areas of those lands which had formed the eastern empire of Rome were invaded and occupied by the Moslems. It was at this time that preservation of the ancient Greek medical writings by the people of this eastern empire became of such importance, for the ideas that they expressed were not alien to Islamic thinking. Translated into Arabic they soon became more widely known and understood than at any time since Galen.

The Middle Ages

The Goths, who occupied much of Europe during the Dark Ages, had no use for Greek or Roman learning and it was the invasion of Spain by the Moors in the eighth and ninth centuries which brought back to the Western world much of the stored up knowledge of the Greeks. This knowledge, although altered and confused in the process of translation from Greek to Arabic and then back into the Latin of the Middle Ages, provided some of the stimulus required for the renaissance of medicine.

Dissection of the human body was part of the formal instruction of students, but it was a distant and third-hand method in pre-renaissance universities. The professor mounted his lofty chair from whence he would lecture and describe, whilst far beneath him a servant would perform the actual dissection along the lines pointed out by one of the professor's assistants. *Mondino di Luzzi* (1270–1326) was one of the few who actually performed the dissection himself and thus contributed to the rebirth of anatomy.

During this period of medieval history medicine continued to develop, but it was so deeply rooted in the teachings of Galen and the ancient Greeks that real progress was hardly possible until a break with these traditions had been made.

THE RENAISSANCE OF MEDICINE

The reasons for the great awakening of intellectual activity that began in the fifteenth century were many and complex. Religious differences stimulated enquiry, exploration enlarged the boundaries of knowledge, and printing carried ideas to all parts of the civilized world. The translation of Greek and Latin, and especially the works of Hippocrates and Galen, provided a basis for advance, and schools of art, led by *Leonardo da Vinci*, *Michelangelo* and *Raphael*, created a demand for detailed knowledge of the structure of the human body.

Leonardo da Vinci became interested in the study of internal anatomy and was one of the first to question the writings of Galen. He kept beautiful notes and drawings and although these were not published in his lifetime they were not without effect upon his pupils.

The intellectual activity in anatomy that these drawings stimulated in Italy soon had its effect in wider spheres. *Andreas Vesalius* was born in Brussels in 1514 and went to the University of Paris. Teaching of anatomy here was based entirely on the works of Galen, and Vesalius soon tired of the dull readings and went to Padua where new methods were taught. Here he applied himself to dissecting and to lecturing and over the course of four years prepared his great work *On the Fabric of the Human Body*. This beautifully illustrated textbook stimulated a period of anatomical activity and it has remained the basis of modern anatomy to this day.

SCIENTIFIC SURGERY

This work had an effect not only on anatomical thinking but made possible the start of scientific surgery. During this period of the sixteenth and seventeenth century Europe was torn by great religious wars and the surgery of the day was largely the surgery of wounds. Military surgeons marched behind the armies and military surgery was rough and ready. *Ambroise Paré* was a French military surgeon, born in 1517, and was equipped with Vesalius's anatomical knowledge, an enquiring mind and a sense of compassion for the sick. 'I dressed him and God cured him' is one of his famous adages which typifies his humane approach. He was a careful writer whose books were translated into many languages. Wherever they spread they took with them the concept that it was a surgeon's duty to relieve pain, and they influenced surgical practice in every country. These surgeons began to keep careful records and in Amsterdam in 1622 *Dr Nicholas Tulp* wrote a book containing records of hundreds of interesting cases. Thus starting the idea of collecting information for later reference.

THE DEVELOPMENT OF CLINICAL MEDICINE

Just as surgery is based on anatomical understanding, so is medicine based on physiological knowledge, and until the seventeenth century medicine had lagged far behind. It is true that doctors had acquired a knowledge of the use of drugs from the Egyptians, from the Greeks and from newly discovered lands, but this knowledge was largely empirical. It was based on trial and error and not on physiological principles. New drugs might be helpful; more often they were harmless and occasionally dangerous. *Thomas Sydenham (1624–1689)*, called 'the English Hippocrates', applied himself to the careful clinical recording of the natural history of disease and, as Paré was the founder of modern surgery, so Sydenham was the founder of clinical medicine.

The scientific facts upon which clinical medicine could build were provided by another Englishman, *William Harvey (1578–1657)*. He had studied at Padua under Fabricius, the successor to Vesalius, and from him had learnt that veins had valves, so placed that the flow through them must be towards the heart. With this seed of knowledge in his mind he experimented and dissected for thirteen years before he was able to publish in his book, *Anatomical Studies of the Motion of the Heart and Blood in Animals* (1628). Nearly every step forward in medicine for the next two hundred years was based on this single idea. Even so, there remained a missing link. Blood flows to the heart in the veins, and away from it in the arteries, but it remained for *Malpighi (1628–1694)* to supply the answer to the question of how it gets from the arteries back to the veins.

The first microscope was developed from the telescope of Galileo, but even with the use of a single lens it was possible to reveal details of the tissue, which added impetus to the study of the human body. Malpighi saw in the capillaries of the frog's lung the way by which the blood was enabled to pass from the arterial to the venous side. He also described the microscopic structure of the kidney, spleen and liver and it was the Royal Society in London which published all these observations.

During the sixteenth and seventeenth centuries great advances were made in the understanding of anatomy and physiology, and at the same time mechanics, astronomy, chemistry and physics were all developing. Clinical medicine had need of new methods of communicating knowledge to students and of relating the more abstract sciences to disease and health. At the University of Leyden, in the early eighteenth century, a system of medical teaching was introduced which had a profound effect upon medical progress. Until that time medicine had been taught in an abstract manner by lectures to students, and it was *Hermann Boerhaave (1668–1738)* who introduced the system of clinical teaching that is now followed. His students learnt from the teacher and the patient at the bedside, and understood the importance of careful clinical notes and records made at the time.

The advent of post-mortem records was largely due to the work of *Morgagni (1682–1771)*. He was professor of anatomy at Padua and he realized the importance of relating the clinical history and clinical findings to the post-mortem appearances when explaining the nature of a disease. During the next seventy years his work was followed by that of others culminating in the publications of Rokitansky, based on careful records made during 30 000 post-mortems.

THE IDENTIFICATION OF THE GERM

The theory that disease might be caused by the transmission of minute bodies from one person to another had been advanced as early as the sixteenth century by *Fracastoro (1483–1553)*. Many people had made significant contributions to understanding the cause of specific infections between that date and the work of *Louis Pasteur (1822–1895)*, but at a time when the search for the 'germ' was occupying the attention of many people Pasteur stood out among his contemporaries. He proved by experiments that minute organisms could enter bottles of broth and cause fermentation to take place. He showed that without organisms fermentation could not occur and, furthermore, that there was a specific organism for each type of fermentation. Originally, the work of Pasteur was concerned with brewers' yeast but after his election as a member of the French Academy of Medicine he began to turn his attention to the germs that cause disease in man. Anthrax is a disease that commonly affects cattle but can be contracted by people who work with the animals, such as farmers, butchers and leather-workers. It was known that the infecting agent could lie dormant in a field or a hide for many months, and it had already been shown by *Robert Koch* (1843–1910) that the organism could convert itself into temporary dormant bodies known as spores. Pasteur managed to grow the organism in cultures and show that the inoculation of other animals with this culture would kill the animal. He demonstrated that some animals possessed a resistance to this infection, and that oxygen, the body temperature, and blood corpuscles were all factors in the development of this resistance. With the aid of this knowledge he was able to build up a theory of immunity and the nature of infection. At the same time Koch continued his work on bacteria and his studies of tuberculosis, cholera and sleeping sickness and so laid the firm foundations of bacteriology.

The application of this knowledge to the practical side of clinical medicine was not long delayed. In Vienna the work of *Semmelweis* (1818–1865) showed that puerperal fever, the infection (usually fatal) of women in the lying-in period, was carried on the hands of students and doctors from the post-mortem room. Unfortunately this work was at first largely disregarded and it was not until *Lister* (1827–1912) recorded his observations in 1867 that 'antisepsis' was widely accepted. He demonstrated that the mortality from infection after operation could be dramatically lowered by cleanliness and the use of carbolic sprays to kill the germs carried in the air. His own records of patients who had had amputations show the dramatic change this brought about. Of 35 patients on whom he operated without antiseptics no fewer than 16 died. After the introduction of his methods only 6 died out of the next 40 cases. From this work has developed all our modern ideas of 'asepsis' and the sterilization of medical equipment.

The last quarter of the nineteenth century was marked by great advances in the study of immunity. Methods were devised of so weakening the virulence of the toxin produced by certain organisms that it was possible to protect patients by injections of the toxin in its attenuated form. Typhoid and cholera were among the first of the diseases to be tackled in this way, followed by diphtheria and tetanus. This work still proceeds, and poliomyelitis, measles and the common cold are the most recent diseases to be treated in this manner.

In many other regions of the world the battle against infection has raged. Not the least of the benefits which was brought by the expansion of the British Empire was the investigation of tropical diseases. The names of *Sir Ronald Ross* (1857–1932) and *Sir Patrick Manson* (1844–1922) in the conquest of malaria will never be forgotten. Yellow fever, the dreaded 'Yellow Jack', periodically decimated the garrisons in the West Indies. When work on the Panama Canal had been brought to a halt by this infection, *Walter Reed* (1851–1902) showed that it was spread by the mosquito. This American sanitary officer in Havana set out to destroy the mosquito and treat the victims under mosquito netting, and within three months the city was free from infection for the first time for one hundred and fifty years.

THE DEVELOPMENT OF ANAESTHESIA

It must be remembered that none of the great advances in surgery would have been possible without the development of the science of anaesthetics. This not only relieved the pain and consequently the shock from which many patients died but gave the surgeon time in which to develop his techniques. Drugs such as the opiates, alcohol or nicotine had been used for hundreds of years to ease this pain, but it was the use of ether that first gave real anaesthesia. There was a famous controversy in America between Long, Wells and Morton as to who should claim the prize offered by Congress for this, but there can be little doubt that it was to *Crawford Long* (1815–1878) that the first credit should go. Wells can claim the credit for introducing 'gas' for dental extractions; *Sir James Young Simpson* (1811–1870) pioneered the development of anaesthesia in this country. At first he gave ether to his obstetric patients and published a paper advocating its use, but his researches for a more efficient anaesthetic led him to the use of chloroform. A great controversy arose in Great Britain fanned by bitter denunciation on both practical and religious grounds. There were those who regarded pain as a trial sent by God and who looked upon interference with the pains of childbirth as a sacrilegious act. The controversy was silenced at last when *Dr John Snow* (1813–1858), the first British anaesthetist, was sent for to administer chloroform to Queen Victoria for the birth of Prince Leopold in 1853.

CHEMOTHERAPY

Chemotherapy was the word coined by *Ehrlich* (1854–1915) for the method of treating infectious conditions by the use of chemical substances. It was Ehrlich who made the first great contribution to the science he had named. He was working on the use of synthetic dyes when he found that methylene blue would kill the malarial parasite. For many years scientists had known that some dyes had an affinity for certain organisms and Ehrlich set out to find substances which would attack organisms in the human body without harming the patient. He approached this by what was at the time a novel method, that of relating the biological effect of a substance to its chemical formula. This led him to the discovery of the organic arsenical salvarsan, and the demonstration of its anti-syphilitic properties. This was the first chemotherapeutic agent and it led to the setting-up of the great German drug industry. In 1932 *Domagk*, who was the director of the research laboratories in one of these firms, noted that one of the new dyes contained a sulphonamide group which was effective on infections in mice. This dye, prontosil red, was the precursor of the great range of drugs which came to be known as the 'M & B' drugs in the early 1940s.

In 1928 *Sir Alexander Fleming* (1881–1955) noted that the presence of a mould on the culture plates in his laboratory stopped the growth of the bacterium around it. He further observed that it had this effect even when diluted 800 times. This was the development of the first antibiotic and led *Lord Florey* (1898–1968) and *Professor Chain* (1896–1979) in Oxford in 1940 to introduce penicillin. Since then the search for new antibiotics has been pursued all over the world. It has led to the discovery of new antibiotic-producing moulds and also to the artificial synthesis of antibiotics. These will destroy most of the bacteria to which man is susceptible. The vast range of modern drugs and the rapidity with which new ones are produced for the treatment of disease and the alleviation of symptoms present many problems to the physician.

X-RAYS

The publication of *Röntgen's* paper in Würzburg in 1895 introduced the science of diagnosis by X-ray, and it is difficult now to imagine medical diagnosis without it. New techniques for visualizing the structure and function of organs and systems inside the body have followed at increasingly short intervals. It was the first bismuth meal that gave gastroenterology its place in medicine. Now visualization of the kidney by pyelography, the gall-bladder by cholecystography, the bronchial tree by bronchography, and the heart and arteries by cardiography and angiography are routine techniques in most X-ray departments.

The use of X-rays in the treatment of disease, mainly in its malignant forms, is the result of the work of *Marie Curie* (1867–1934). Her early studies of radium were the precursor of modern techniques using much more intense and accurate sources of X-rays such as cobalt 'bomb' therapy for the destruction of malignant tumours, and close cooperation between surgeons and radiotherapists now produces encouraging results in the treatment of many forms of cancer. This is often aided by new chemotherapeutic drugs, which exert their suppressive influence upon the malignant cells.

New rays will come to take their place in the field of therapy, and already ultrasonic and laser beams have been developed.

SURGERY

The revolution that Lister started has continued at an increasing pace. In the early days, much of surgery was concerned with the management of wounds and the drainage of abscesses, but after Lister's discoveries the whole body became available for surgical treatment. The abdominal cavity was the first area to be explored and German surgeons such as *Billroth*, *Trendelenburg* and *von Mickulicz* were outstanding.

Since then the cranial cavity and the chest cavity have attracted surgeons to specialize in these fields of work. In 1923 *Cutler* and *Levine* in Boston were the first to operate on the diseased mitral valve. The development of surgery of the heart has been one of the most dramatic developments of this century. In the 1940s surgeons were operating on the great vessels entering and leaving the heart. Today the introduction of techniques for rapidly cooling the body, and the later development of machines outside the body for maintaining the circulation, have led to the repair of holes inside the heart, the replacement of valves, and finally to the transplantation of the whole heart.

At the same time, equally significant but less sensational advances have occurred in the surgery of vessels, genito-urinary surgery and orthopaedic surgery.

One thing is certain, and that is that medicine will continue to progress. But wherever new advances lead us they will be accompanied by the age-old practice of meticulous recording. The doctor of the future will depend, just as his predecessors two thousand years ago did, on the careful management of medical records in order to practise his science.

3

The Origins of the Welfare State

The development of the welfare state had its roots in events which occurred 400 years ago. For several centuries before this, charity, shelter and medical treatment had been largely the prerogative of the monasteries. The poor of the land who sought this aid were, by and large, people displaced by war or pestilence, and the landholder, grazier or small farmer had a stability conferred upon him by his property. At the beginning of the sixteenth century the rural economic stability of the whole of Western Europe became disturbed. This was not so much the result of any single great upheaval but rather that of a steady accumulation of pressures on the economic structure. In England it was the economic instability of the wool trade with the continent which aggravated the problem. Alternate cycles of boom and slump produced much unemployment and, for the first time, this began to affect a different class of person—the small farmer.

Just at the time when this was occurring the monasteries were under attack by Henry VIII and they were too impoverished to help with the numbers of vagrants and beggars appearing on the roads.

The state was only concerned with this increase in poverty because it was recognized as a source of recruits for rebel armies, and for this reason, and not for charitable purposes, it took action.

THE STATUTE OF 1536

This was designed expressly to deal with the unemployed, destitute and vagrant. It could not by any stretch of imagination be regarded as a piece of legislation intended to aid the sick and it relied entirely on voluntary funds. Nevertheless during the course of the next 65 years there was a progressive development of state help for the poor.

An event of great importance occurred in 1547 when the City of London, recognizing that the funds produced by voluntary levy were insufficient to meet its needs, introduced a compulsory levy. It was this event which introduced the concept of national responsibility for the individual: an idea which is basic to the welfare state. In the next 20 years local towns, boroughs and cities all over England introduced schemes for classifying the poor and providing help financed by a compulsory rate. This had the unfortunate result of drawing into the town the poor from the surrounding countryside, and thus the burden on the town became too great.

16

In 1572 the state itself followed the example set by local boroughs and a compulsory national rate was introduced. This money was not only to be used for the relief of old people, infants and the sick, but also for providing work for the able-bodied pauper. Thus the 'Old Poor Law' was developed.

THE 'OLD POOR LAW' (1601)

The parish had long been the unit of local administration but the series of acts introducing the Old Poor Law consolidated their responsibilities and power. They were based on a system of compulsory levy of a poor rate on all householders. This money was to be spent in three ways: poor children were to be apprenticed, the elderly were to have cottages built for them on waste land, and work was to be provided for the able poor. During the next 50 years the Privy Council continuously exerted pressures on the parishes. It did this by a series of orders sent out to the local justices and to high sheriffs, and by the collecting of regular reports every three months. There is no doubt that these measures met with very real success, but with the outbreak of the Civil War in 1642 the central control and organization was lost and once again it was left to individual parishes to do as they thought best.

The restoration of the monarchy in 1660 brought back again the attempt of central authority to apply direction to the system, but in spite of this there was a lack of control which coloured all the attempts at poor relief. In 1662 an Act, known as the Law of Settlement and Removal, was introduced which controlled the administration of the Poor Law. It was designed to remedy a defect which was stated as 'Poor people are not restrained from going from one parish to another, and do therefore endeavour to settle themselves in those parishes where there is the best stock, the largest commons or wastes to build cottages and the most wood for them to burn and destroy'. This it did by providing that, where a person moved into a parish and was likely to become a burden on the rates, he could be moved back to his original place of settlement. This simple act of legislation had deep social consequences. Initially this law helped in the administration of the poor, but each section was eventually subject to abuses which undermined its value. Apprenticeship, which had been designed as a method of securing work for poor children, came to be used as a method of changing a child's place of settlement. The children were often compulsorily 'bound out' and when they ran away they swelled the numbers of vagrants on the roads. The limitations applied to the building of cottages on waste land led to overcrowding. This in itself had social consequences. Marriages were delayed, illegitimacy was common and the unmarried mother was treated with great harshness and driven on to the roads to prevent her becoming a burden on the rates.

The level of expenditure on Poor Law relief had been steadily rising and many parishes were complaining of the burden when, in 1832, a Royal Commission was set up to investigate the problem. Their report and recommendation was the basis of the Poor Law Amendment Act of 1834, commonly known as the 'New Poor Law'.

THE 'NEW POOR LAW' (1834)

This act was inspired by a new economic principle and like the old Poor Law was not governed by charitable objects. The principle was that of 'less eligibility'. The Commissioners argued that 'every penny bestowed that tends to render the condition of the pauper more eligible than that of the independent labourer is a bounty on indolence and vice'. Poverty was thought to be a crime and the workhouse became virtually a prison. This was deliberately applied so that the conditions of the poor became worse than the meanest labourer and led to labourers being prepared to accept appallingly low wages rather than go into the workhouse. The whole idea behind this new law was to force workers into the labour market, but, to be fair to it, it was thought that jobs were available for those who would work.

There was an inevitable reaction to this harsh treatment and many local authorities began to vary the strict rules in an attempt to ease the lot of the inhabitants of workhouses. For this they were bitterly attacked by the supporters of the 1834 principle, but as had happened on every occasion in the past, where local authority had led, central authority soon followed. By 1891 toys and books were allowed to be given to children; in 1892 tobacco could be provided; in 1893 visiting committees of ladies were permitted, and a year later tea, milk and sugar, were supplied. Finally in 1897 trained nurses were allowed to look after the sick. Improvements were gradually made and in 1918 inhabitants of workhouses were no longer made to wear the pauper's uniform. The social stigma of the workhouse is still remembered by people today, and it is the 1834 Act that is partly responsible for the widespread dislike of so many old, sick or poor people to accept help of a charitable nature.

This then was the scene which the Royal Commission of 1905 surveyed. Although the members of the Commission were unanimous in their condemnation of the principles behind the 1834 Act, there was no general agreement about what should be done to replace them. The majority felt that voluntary charitable action was important, and that the state should content itself with providing the minimum basic requirements. The minority argued passionately for a system of the best possible social services to be provided by specialist bodies and this seems to be the first pointer towards the setting-up of the welfare state. The Commission's report was published in 1909 and fomented great indignation against the established methods of gaining relief. No action was taken, however, for two further years.

FRIENDLY SOCIETIES

What had been happening to the medical services during this period? The nineteenth century was, after all, a time of great advance in medical science, and it is true to say that such organized services as there were, devoted themselves to the care of the lower classes. But this medical care was austere in the extreme and was governed by the same principle as had been the 1834 Act—an inner disdain for poverty. The upper classes had always been able to fend for themselves at home, and hospital treatment was confined to the lower classes. These hospitals took on some of the character of the workhouses and were, in fact, often built alongside them.

Domiciliary medical treatment for the lower classes was developed from the fact that it was necessary to band together in order to be able to pay for it; strange as it may seem the earliest British insurance societies were founded by French workmen 180 years ago and subsequently by semireligious bodies such as the Ancient Order of Foresters and The Hearts of Oak. Many of these societies were small local ventures encouraged by the squire or other prominent citizens, and yet others were, and still are, founded on the 'pub'. The voluntary insurance associations became known as the 'Friendly' societies, a name which is still applied.

NATIONAL INSURANCE ACT (1911)

This was the most important piece of medical legislation introduced prior to the National Health Service Act of 1946. It was introduced by *Lloyd George* (1865–1945) who was Chancellor of the Exchequer at that time and who had had an opportunity of studying the working of this type of legislation in Germany in 1908. As a result of this he proposed a scheme which applied the contributory insurance principle to the sick. This was to be a compulsory scheme and it was unpopular with all social classes, producing a series of political crises. It was only with much difficulty that the Bill was finally passed. The Act had certain great faults, some of which were the result of the compromises which its supporters had to accept in order to secure its passage. Apart from the fact that it applied only to wage-earners (self-employed people, however poor, could not be included) it only provided certain basic medical requirements. Additional benefits, such as hospital, dental and ophthalmic services, were limited to specific conditions.

Opposition to the bill had been led by the 'Friendly' societies and their members, and by the trade unions who were already in the health insurance business. As a result of this opposition an incredibly complicated administrative machine was set up. The GP and pharmaceutical services were administered by local committees of doctors, chemists and representatives of local authorities, but the cash benefits were distributed by 'approved societies'. These societies consisted of almost anyone who wanted to be in them: large insurance companies, trade unions, small local groups and so on. It is worth asking why insurance companies and trade unions wanted to become involved in such a scheme. The insurance companies represented a vested interest, and the health insurance scheme gave them an entrance into thousands of homes where they could sell other insurance policies and burial benefits. The advantages for the trade unions were even more obvious. They no longer had to use their capital on payments of sickness benefits, but could divert the whole of their resources to other trade union activities such as strike benefits, and as a result of this they enrolled many new members. Furthermore these 'approved societies' secured for themselves the right to refuse admission to anyone they considered to be a bad medical risk and it was just such people who most needed the system. Indeed by the beginning of 1939, it was becoming obvious that both the health insurance scheme and the public assistance organization, which now administered the Poor Law, were incapable of providing security. It was this widespread recognition that led directly to the concept of the welfare state.

THE WELFARE STATE

During the Second World War there was a rapid expansion of many public services which had previously borne the stigma of the 'Poor Law'. School meals services and certain pension rights were applied to the whole community and this started the idea of a service to all as a right. In 1942 *Sir William Beveridge* (1879–1963) planned a scheme of comprehensive social insurance. This scheme assumed that it was the duty of the community to provide an income for all those whose earning capacity had been interrupted by social circumstances beyond their control. Thus the poor were no longer to be treated as a separate group of people, and in 1944 the Coalition Government published a White Paper supporting the main proposals.

Apart from these insurance proposals the years from 1920 to 1946 had been marked by a series of investigations designed to show how better use could be made of the medical resources available. At this time the hospitals were divided into two groups: the voluntary hospitals supported by charitable donations and the public hospitals administered by local authorities. Charges were graduated according to the patient's ability to pay and thus the voluntary hospitals tended to select patients who could afford fees, and medical treatment was largely concentrated in these institutions. The public hospital tended to fill its beds with the aged, infirm and chronically sick. Specialist practice in both these types of hospital was largely 'honorary', the income of the Consultant being derived principally from work done in his consulting rooms or in the home. As most of his work was done in hospital, working for nothing, the specialist charged inordinately high fees to upper- and middle-class patients, who were thus subsidizing lower-class treatment. This meant that these Consultant services were concentrated in the relatively small areas of the country where such fees could be obtained.

At the same time the GP services were coming under close scrutiny and it became obvious that not only was there a maldistribution of services but the incomes and the clinical isolation of general practitioners presented other problems.

It was in the light of these and many other considerations that the National Health Service Act was introduced by *Aneurin Bevan* (1897–1960) in 1946. It has in many ways achieved its aims and in many other ways it has left problems as they were. There was a major reorganization of the Health Service in 1974 which is discussed in Chapter 5. Further reorganization removed the middle tier—the Area Health Authority—in 1982. The health service is still subject to stresses and strains both from within and without. There can be little doubt that these will produce changes just as the pressures from the past have led to its creation.

4

Medical Education and the Role of the Hospitals

During the 400 years that social and economic pressures were moulding the development of the 'welfare state' the same forces were gradually changing the pattern of medical practice. It is true that there were hospitals in existence 800 years ago, but these were all founded by religious institutions and were concerned more with sheltering the poor and needy than with healing the sick. St Bartholomew's hospital was founded in 1123 and is still flourishing today, but many of the old hospitals and lazars, as the leper hospitals were known, were swept away with the dissolution of the monasteries. It is really only in the last hundred years that hospitals have come to play an important role in the treatment of the sick.

In early Tudor times England was a very backward country in medical matters compared with Italy, France and other continental countries. The first true medical schools were established in Greece in the time when Hippocrates was alive, but it was the spread of the Christian religion over western Europe that brought the teaching that it was a Christian duty to care for and comfort the sick. Priests carried on the tradition of healing and teaching, and by the beginning of the twelfth century these monastic and cathedral schools reached their highest point of influence. However, they taught only those things that it was thought necessary for a monk to know and this did not satisfy more enquiring minds. Thus it was that 'studia' arose to teach subjects that were beyond this range of knowledge; Salerno, in Italy, became the first school to specialize in the teaching of medicine as long ago as the ninth century. By the thirteenth and fourteenth centuries a number of these 'universities' had been established all over northern Italy. Soon after, Paris, Prague and Cracow followed suit.

THE ROYAL COLLEGE OF PHYSICIANS

In England, Oxford and Cambridge began to teach medicine and degrees were issued to those who could afford them. The few physicians were not bound together by any order, and practised only in the great houses and large towns; much of medical practice, in Britain, was carried out by unqualified people. There was a generous supply of these 'quacks', people who had taken no form of examination, and they far outnumbered the medically qualified. The emergency produced by this situation led to the passing of an Act in 1511 by which the bishops were enabled to grant licences in their dioceses (a privilege still held by the Archbishop of Canterbury) and unlicensed practitioners were to pay a heavy fine.

This situation was not very satisfactory and in 1518 a group of physicians, led by *Thomas Linacre*, a gifted and brilliant scholar, petitioned Henry VIII who granted a charter setting up a Royal College of Physicians which was to license those who were qualified to practise, punish pretenders to medicine and to punish malpractice. The fellows and licentiates were drawn exclusively from the graduates of Oxford and Cambridge and although the College never did take any direct part in the training of those who were to become physicians, it instituted postgraduate lectures and selected its members from the élite of the profession.

THE BEGINNING OF SURGERY

In the mediaeval monastery the barber shaved the monk's head and if minor surgery was required, who better than the barber with his sharp razor to do it? These 'barber–surgeons' had a grant of arms in 1452, and in 1461 the Company of Barber–Surgeons was formed. Henry VIII reincorporated them in 1540 and gave them certain rights and privileges, one of which was to be called 'Master' or, as it became colloquially, 'Mister'. For this reason, in Great Britain, surgeons are still addressed as 'Mister' instead of 'Doctor'.

In 1800 the College of Surgeons was formed but it did not insist on high professional standards and the social status of surgeons was much lower than that of physicians. They were allowed to operate externally but not to give medicine internally.

THE APOTHECARIES

Unqualified medical men often made a living from shops selling herbs and drugs and were known as 'Apothecaries'. They were attacked by the more legitimate doctors and James I decided to protect them by forming a Society of Apothecaries in 1617. They were (essentially) tradesmen who had learnt their job during a five-year apprenticeship and were drawn from lower middle-class families. In fact they were at one time part of the Worshipful Company of Grocers.

In 1815 the Apothecaries Act gave the Society of Apothecaries the power to license and examine in medicine and this act reformed the whole system of medical training. Up to this time it had been conducted by a system of theoretical lectures and casual apprenticeship but, because of the apothecaries' insistence that examination and not apprenticeship should be the gateway to the profession, private medical teaching establishments sprang up. Those in Birmingham, Liverpool and Manchester developed into medical schools and became the nucleus of new universities.

Furthermore, the Society insisted on six months' hospital practice for all would-be doctors and there was thus a rush of students to the hospitals which had established medical schools.

By the end of the eighteenth century there were, thus, three strata of medical men catering for the different social classes of the country. At the same time there were two types of institution concerned with treating the sick: the workhouse, established by the parishes and developing along the lines laid down by the Poor Laws (see Chapter 3), and the voluntary hospital.

THE VOLUNTARY HOSPITALS

The voluntary hospitals were largely established on the initiative of laymen, and were founded by people on the top rung of the ladder of social success, or by those who were anxious to reach it. They were financed by the willingness of the rich to help the poor and subscribers were often given the right to nominate beneficiaries of the charity.

The very earliest of these hospitals paid their physicians and surgeons for the work that they did, but it became a mark of confidence to be nominated by the powerful patrons of the hospital to be a member of the medical staff and these posts thus became honorary in status. In any case recipients could hope to become the professional attendants of the governors themselves. The paid staff of hospitals was very small, although some hospitals employed resident apothecaries.

The patients of the voluntary hospitals, although poor, were not the very poor, for the hospitals did not wish to incur the expense of funerals. The well-to-do continued to receive their treatment at home and the very poor were consigned to the workhouse.

THE TEACHING HOSPITALS

The teaching hospitals then became the more select of the voluntary hospitals and large sums of money were obtained by the members of the medical staff from fees paid for instruction by the students. Promotion to honorary physician and surgeon was very slow as the occupants were reluctant to share the glittering prizes they had obtained. This produced a large number of keen but frustrated young doctors who, as medical science advanced, turned their attentions to narrower and more specialized fields.

SPECIAL HOSPITALS

The study of special diseases and the use of specialized treatments demanded the setting-up of units concentrating on these conditions. The older generations of physicians and surgeons fought tenaciously against these developments and resisted at every step what, as they saw it, was a whittling down of their power and responsibility. But in spite of this opposition the mid-nineteenth century saw the growth of specialized hospitals. Specialization was not only seen as a means of acquiring knowledge but it was widely condemned as a form of self-advertisement and bitter attacks were launched upon the special hospitals by all the leading 'great men' and the influential medical journals.

There is no doubt, however, that there was a great need for these hospitals. For example, maternity work was regarded by the surgeons as being part of the province of physicians, and yet the President of the Royal College of Physicians held, in 1827, 'that midwifery was an act foreign to the habits of a gentleman'. In the practice of midwifery there was the great danger of puerperal sepsis—a disease from which sometimes as many as one-quarter of the patients died. Thus the reason for excluding midwifery from the general hospital was the same as for the exclusion of smallpox and other infectious diseases. During this period of the nineteenth century special hospitals dealing with maternity work, infectious diseases, nervous diseases, eye diseases and so forth were established; there were even hospitals set up to treat cancer, the stone, diseases of the skin, ears and rectum. Most of these hospitals were set up and controlled by doctors, unlike the general, voluntary hospital. At this time there were, therefore, two types of hospital: the voluntary hospital, with its subdivisions of teaching hospital and the special hospital, and the public hospital developed from the old paupers' hospitals or workhouses.

THE COTTAGE HOSPITAL

Soon the hospital movement began to spread to the rural areas, and local subscribers led by the parson and landlord and assisted by philanthropists built cottage hospitals. These were staffed differently from the general hospitals and they were open to all local GPs who began to treat even the more serious surgical cases.

The GP had his origin in the dually trained apothecary and had done his stint of six months' training in the hospital. He was accepted as the doctor of the middle classes and he went into single-handed practice in the provinces and in rural areas. He began to challenge the rights and privileges accorded to the Fellows of the Colleges and obtained access to the Poor Law hospitals in the area in which he practised.

It was not long before the medical press was full of the evidence of demarcation disputes between the various sections of the profession. Furthermore the charitable work of the public hospitals was often bestowed upon people who could well afford to pay for it and the profession saw itself robbed of its just fees. This often meant there was less money available for those who really needed it. A system was therefore developed whereby hospital treatment was paid for according to the patient's means and this soon spread to nearly every voluntary hospital in the country.

REFERRALS

Another source of dispute between the hospital doctor and the GP lay in the nature of the consultation. General practitioners complained that when they referred a patient to a hospital doctor they never saw him back again, but the hospital doctor continued to treat him for a wide range of conditions that should rightly have been within the general practitioner's field of work. This argument was bitter and protracted but eventually was ended during the last quarter of the nineteenth century by the development of a system of referrals which still appertains today.

Firstly, it became obvious that the hospital doctor must become a specialist and from then on was termed 'a Consultant'. Such was the rate of progress in every branch of medicine that no GP could stay up to date in every field. Consequently there was a need to consult when a special problem arose or when the benefit of a deeper experience in a more narrow speciality was required. Then it became apparent that as there was not enough Consultant practice to go round at the rate of fees that were being charged, these fees must be put up. This had the double effect of keeping up the Consultant's income and preventing the drift away of the GP's living. It followed, as a result of this decision, that unpaid hospital work had to go and that Consultants during the early part of their careers, and before they had built up a practice, must be paid for their work. Finally it was established that, broadly speaking, it was the practitioner who consulted the specialist for advice about the management of the case, and not the patient who asked for advice about his condition. This still forms the basis of the relationship between these two branches of the profession, but, as both are working for the good of the patient, a considerable degree of give and take exists.

The question of the qualifications required to enable a person to practise medicine was settled in 1858 by the Medical Act of that year which established the General Medical Council (GMC) (see Chapter 9) and drew the outlines of the structure of the profession that exists today.

Qualifications which enable a doctor to seek admission to the register of the GMC are given by some of the universities, the Society of Apothecaries, the Conjoint Board of the Royal Colleges of Physicians and Surgeons, and, in Scotland, by the Royal College of Physicians and Surgeons of Edinburgh and the Royal College of Physicians and Surgeons of Glasgow. A detailed list of these qualifications and higher degrees will be found in the Appendix.

PAYING PATIENTS

As we have seen in the previous chapter, from the mid-nineteenth century onwards there were gradual moves towards easing the lot of paupers in hospital. The change from pauper hospital to public hospital was accelerated by the great smallpox epidemics of 1871, 1877 and 1881. The Metropolitan Asylums Board had been set up to provide special accommodation for the poor suffering from smallpox but when the three great waves of infection struck London the Board began to admit many cases apart from paupers, and in fact some were actually paying patients. This action made a breach in the wall built around the Poor Law infirmaries and changed their whole character, for people from the middle-classes were now coming into hospital. Until this time the voluntary hospitals also had been almost exclusively working class and the middle and upper classes showed no desire for treatment away from home.

There now began the era of the paying patient and a different class of patient sought and found admission. This move provoked further dissension because GPs were not permitted to follow their patients into hospital.

Thus the dissension which again shook the profession had the same root cause as that which had troubled it for the previous 100 years (see page 23). As hospital treatment became cheaper for the patient, and more effective, the GP saw an increasing danger to his livelihood. As more sophisticated methods of treatment could not be carried out in the home even the upper classes eventually sought hospital treatment. Initially this was carried out in private hospitals and nursing homes but soon the voluntary hospitals were adding private wards and private wings.

At the same time the infirmaries, as the new hospitals built under the Poor Law hospital service were called, began to admit a higher and higher percentage of acute sick. They were under the charge of salaried doctors, known as medical superintendents. These doctors wanted the acute sick admitted as they increased clinical interest and this gave grounds for the hope that medical instruction would occur in the public hospitals, thus raising their status.

MEDICAL PRACTICE AFTER THE 1911 ACT

The National Insurance Act of 1911 (see Chapter 2) brought comparative stability to the GP because, for the first time, he was assured of a steady income from his 'panel'. This was most important in poorer areas of the country where private medical fees were a heavy burden and often could not be afforded at all.

The years between the two great wars were marked by two other important changes which helped to mould medical practice as we see it today. The voluntary hospitals had for many years found that their income from charitable sources was not enough to enable them to pay their way, and many of them were heavily in debt. As they increased the fees, payable by those who could afford them, the public sought some means of providing for the burden which might have to be borne. Consequently there was an enormous growth of voluntary insurance and this paved the way for the compulsory insurance which is the basis of our present conception of the welfare state. Secondly, the public hospitals began to employ Consultants from the voluntary hospitals on a part-time basis and this inevitably led to some Consultants being employed almost wholly by a number of public hospitals.

The income of GPs at this time was drawn from two main sources. In working-class areas a high proportion was from the 'panel' patient and a smaller proportion from private fees. The position was reversed where the practice was composed mainly of patients from the middle classes. Apart from these the doctor had a variable income from other sources. Many practitioners were employed in the public hospitals, part-time, in a variety of different positions, and there were posts available with factories, schools and local health authorities, and as police doctors.

The Consultant was, with the exception of the medical superintendents, employed on a part-time basis by both voluntary and public hospitals and usually had a sizeable income from private practice. Aspiring Consultants were paid by the hospitals while they were in training and waiting for a vacancy on the staff.

Such was the position then, when the various health service plans were produced by the Labour Party, by the doctors, by Sir William Beveridge and by the Coalition Government of 1944. These plans were produced partly as a result of social pressures and partly because of pressure from the medical profession, but there was no clear point at which a health service was invented. It was in reality, the logical progression of the events of the previous hundred years.

5

The National Health Service (NHS)

'Be it enacted by the King's most Excellent Majesty, by and with the advice and consent of the Lords Spiritual and Temporal, and Commons in this present Parliament assembled and by the authority of the same, as follows:'

With these words was introduced the National Health Service Act of 1946, which governs our health service today. Some of the Acts which were amended or repealed by it date back to 1838 and it is worth considering in broad terms what it is that the Act sets out to do. It simply laid upon the Minister of Health the duty to promote the establishment of a service to provide to all patients, free of charge, all the necessities for the prevention, diagnosis and treatment of illness. The great difference between this Act and all previous Acts is that treatment is available to all and not only to those who have paid contributions. For this reason it is a completely new concept. The organization upon which it was based was one of function. It was recognized that the existing medical services fell into three functional areas: those concerned with the sick person within the institution, those concerned with the sick person within the community and those concerned with preventive medical services. These were fairly clearly identified with the hospital services, the GP services and those services provided by the local authority but excluding the school health services.

The NHS did not bring those areas together but relied upon some broad direction from the top and rather ad hoc relations developing lower down the structure. Thus the hospital service was administered by Regional Hospital Boards, of which there were fifteen in England and Wales, five in Scotland and a single authority in Northern Ireland. Under these were absorbed all the voluntary and public hospitals in the country, some 3000 all told, and national planning of hospital requirements was established. The take-over came just in time, for all were chronically short of money and some were on the verge of financial insolvency. Unfortunately, development has continued to be hampered by shortage of money.

The position of the teaching hospitals in England and Wales was a curious one. They were related to the Regional Hospital Boards only in that there was one in each region. They retained relatively independent Boards of Governors who were responsible directly to the Secretary of State. These arrangements were designed to preserve their rather special nature while allowing the quality of their service to permeate the region. In Scotland, however, they were included in the regional administration.

The GP services were organized through Executive Councils of which there were 134 in England and Wales and 25 in Scotland. These administered the family doctors' contract, the dental services, pharmaceutical services and the services for testing eyesight and dispensing glasses (supplementary ophthalmic services).

The 174 local health authorities looked after the preventive services, ambulance services, etc.

Each of these elements of the health services had different boundaries as well as different functions and different chains of command. The task of producing a proper balance between hospital and community services and establishing proper priorities became increasingly important. Successive governments began to consider unification of the service and the first major reorganization of the NHS took place on 1 April 1974; however a further major reorganization of the NHS took place in 1982 and the middle tier of administration, the Area Health Authority, was abolished.

There were a number of factors which helped to prepare the way. Central government was reorganized into departments with a wider range of responsibilities. Local government areas were drastically reshaped so that the 148 major local authorities responsible for health programmes (county councils and county borough councils) in England and Wales were reduced in number to 72 local government counties and metropolitan districts outside London. The personal social services had been drawn together under the Local Authority Social Services Act of 1970 so that aspects previously under a health committee were included with children's and welfare topics under one committee. Thus it became possible to combine many of the functions within large areas that had the same boundaries as local government.

SERVICES WITHIN THE NHS

These are:
1 The hospital and specialist services:
   (a) in-patients
   (b) out-patients
   (c) accident and emergency
   (d) laboratory, radiology, and other diagnostic services
   (e) physiotherapy, etc.
2 The family practitioner service
3 The school health service and the following services previously controlled by the local authorities:
   (a) ambulance services
   (b) epidemiology in the community
   (c) family planning
   (d) health centres
   (e) health visiting
   (f) home nursing and midwifery
   (g) maternity and child health
   (h) preventive services including vaccination and immunization programmes
   (i) registration of nursing homes

The local authority remains responsible for the special education requirements of handicapped children, educational psychology, personal social services and all the measures needed to prevent the spread of infection, such as food safety and hygiene, port health and health aspects of workers' environments.

ORGANIZATION OF THE HEALTH SERVICE

The Department of Health and Social Security (DHSS) is headed by a Secretary of State, who is responsible to Parliament for the strategy of health care throughout the United Kingdom. The Department assists him by settling the balance and scale of services provided in the various regions and areas, by guiding and supporting the authorities within the regions and by providing certain specialized services. He is advised by the Central Health Services Council which is itself advised by a number of Standing Advisory Committees for medicine, dentistry, nursing, mental health and other services. Six of the members are ex officio Presidents of Royal Colleges; the remainder are appointed by the Secretary of State himself.

The structure below the central department differs in the four countries making up the United Kingdom (Fig. 5.1). In England there are 10 Regional Health Authorities (RHAs) outside Greater London and four within it. Each region consists of a number of complete health districts which are responsible for operating health services and collaborating with local government. They each serve a population of between 150 000 and 500 000. Wales is treated as a separate 'region' under the Welsh Office with nine districts each with a varying

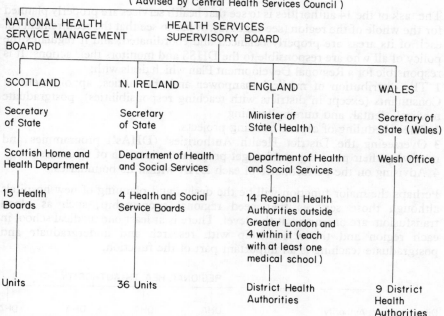

Fig. 5.1 The structure of the health service.

number of 'units'. Scotland is divided into 15 areas served by Health Boards and Northern Ireland has four Health and Social Service Boards with 36 'units' below them with delegated authority. The principle behind this organization is to attempt to provide authority and make decisions as close as possible to the point where patient services are supplied.

Management of the Health Service

The NHS is one of the largest undertakings in western Europe in terms of money and people. Management of such an organization is a complex task. The Secretary of State for Social Services is chairman of the Health Services Supervisory Board, whose other members consist of the Minister of State for Health, the Permanent Secretary (who is the 'top' civil servant in the DHSS), the Chief Medical Officer, the chairman of the National Health Services Management Board and two or three others. Their task is to decide on the objectives and the resources available to the health service. They are assisted by a National Health Services Management Board whose chairman is a member of the Supervisory Board and who is the national 'General Manager' of the health service. The Management Board is small, multidisciplinary and responsible for finance, personnel, property and planning, and is responsible for management all the way down to Regional and District Authorities, each of whom have their own General Managers.

REGIONAL HEALTH AUTHORITIES

The task of the 14 authorities is to see that health services are properly planned for the whole of the region (see Fig. 5.2). It has to see that the requirements of each of its areas are properly balanced and coordinated, and it regulates the policy of all who are responsible to the DHSS and monitors their actions. It is responsible for a Regional Development Plan which deals with:
1 The distribution of medical manpower and specialities, appointment of Consultants (except in districts with teaching responsibilities), postgraduate medical, dental, and nursing training.
2 The scheduling of capital building projects.
3 Overseeing the District Health Authorities' (DHAs') programmes and reviewing their planning and budget proposals, allocation of resources.
4 Advising on the performance of each DHA within its boundaries.

Perhaps the major function will be the design and planning of new hospitals although those services that need regional sponsorship, such as blood transfusion, are organized at this level. There is at least one medical school in each region and the relationship with research and undergraduate and postgraduate teaching is an important part of the function.

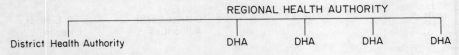

Fig. 5.2 The structure of Regional and District Health Authorities.

Members of the RHA are all appointed by the Secretary of State after consulting the main local authorities, the universities and the main health professions. There are usually about 15 members, and the chairman, also appointed by the Secretary of State, can be paid part-time. It is important to recognize the very substantial responsibilities of these bodies. They deal with a population of several million people, dispose of a budget of tens of millions of pounds each year and employ many thousands of people. It is obvious that to do their job they need a large staff and also a powerful advisory machinery of professional people. The principal regional officers are: the Regional Treasurer, Works Officer, Nursing Officer, Administrative Officer and Medical Officer and they form the team to carry out planning at this level.

THE DISTRICT

The point at which all the services begin to concentrate on the individual patient and his needs is the district. This is a locality within which it is possible to satisfy most of a patient's health needs and thus contains either a district general hospital or several hospitals, 50 to 100 GPs who mainly use that hospital, and a larger number of paramedical workers such as midwives, nurses and health visitors. The population served by such a district varies between 150 000 and more than 500 000. There may be as many as 15 districts in one region.

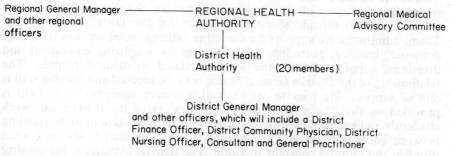

Fig. 5.3 The organization of the Regional and District Health Authorities.

District health authority (DHA)

The DHA's responsibilities include the following.
1 Hospitals, i.e. day-to-day running (the medical care of a patient attending hospital as an in-patient or an out-patient is the sole responsibility of the Consultant in charge of the case)
2 Maternity and child health services in hospitals and the community
3 Health visiting
4 Community nursing (district nursing and domiciliary midwifery)
5 Vaccination and immunization
6 Health education
7 School health (in cooperation with the local authority)

8 Ambulance transport (in the smaller areas where the RHA is not responsible)
9 Community health clinics, such as chiropody, occupational therapy, dental services, contraceptive clinics, etc.
10 Health centres

The DHA is not, however, responsible for the contracts of GPs, ophthalmic medical practitioners, dentists, opticians, and pharmacists, who are independent contractors, not employees of the NHS. These contracts are administered by Family Practitioner Committees (FPCs) (see Chapter 6).

The DHA consists of a chairman appointed by the Secretary of State and 20 other members, 16 appointed by the RHA and 4 by the local authority. They consist of one local hospital Consultant, one local GP, one nurse, midwife or health visitor, one university representative, a member recommended by the trade union, four members appointed by local authorities and eleven other members appointed for their individual contribution by the RHA.

The health authority is served by a number of full-time officers, of whom the General Manager is directly responsible to the authority for the achievement of objectives set by the authority.

District General Manager

This is the senior officer of the health authority. Amongst other tasks he is responsible for most of the support services for the district hospital and therefore has to provide secretarial support for the District Management Team, administrative support for the other officers, hotel services (catering, domestic, laundry, portering, etc.), services for sterilizing equipment and dressings, supplies and all the services related to medical records. The relationship of the District General Manager to the medical and nursing staff is one of support. He tries to see that all necessary equipment and help is provided so that the nursing and other services of the district can work efficiently and enable doctors to do their job. The promotion of understanding between administration and the medical side of the staff is always a great problem and requires constant attention. The General Manager is keenly alive to this and will constantly remind all members of his staff that the only function of a hospital is to treat patients. This may seem such an obvious point that it is hardly worth stressing, but it is only too easy for administration to become an end in itself and for the welfare of the patient to be forgotten in the interests of efficiency.

The other main officers are the District Community Physician, District Nursing Officer and District Finance Officer.

District Community Physician

The District Community Physician has two main tasks: to help plan the development of services in the district and to coordinate the preventive services, e.g. immunization and screening for disease.

District Nursing Officer

This officer is responsible for all the nursing services, hospital and community, within the district. This involves general nursing, nurse training, midwifery, psychiatric nursing and community nursing.

District Finance Officer

The budgeting of all services within the guidelines laid down by the authority is the responsibility of this officer.

Medical Representatives

Prior to the most recent reorganization the officers listed above formed a management team together with a Consultant and a GP elected by the District Medical Committee (which represents all doctors in the community). The chairman of a DHA now has the task of involving doctors more closely with the management process but the exact structure by which this will be done is not agreed and may vary from district to district. Fig. 5.4 illustrates the structure of the team prior to 1985 and this structure may still operate in some districts.

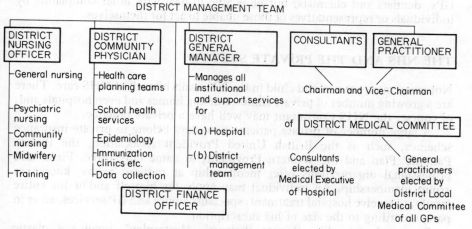

Fig. 5.4 The district management team.

COMMUNITY HEALTH COUNCILS (CHCs)

These were established in 1974 to increase participation of 'consumers' in health service matters. There is one council in every health district in England and Wales, 201 in all. One-third of membership is drawn from voluntary organizations, one-half appointed by local authorities and one-sixth by the RHA. They comment upon local services and are consulted by authorities on future plans. They have a right to visit health centres, to veto hospital closures, which then have to be referred to the Secretary of State, and to attend DHA meetings. While CHC members may visit hospitals to observe and obtain the views of staff, they are not entitled to confidential information about patients and cannot actually investigate any specific case. The CHCs have a duty to provide information to the public and can advise and help in the presentation of complaints about the NHS, directing them to the correct department and so ensuring follow-up; similarly, they can channel queries and suggestions. They may have working groups relating, among other things, to services for the elderly and handicapped, the mentally ill, child health and maternity care, and to hospital services.

HEALTH SERVICES COMMISSIONER

Complaints of a general nature can be dealt with through CHCs or the appropriate authority, but there has been an important extension of the ombudsman principle with the appointment of a Health Service Commissioner. An individual with a complaint against the NHS may remain dissatisfied even after it has been dealt with by the health authority. The Commissioner is an independent third party to whom such an individual can have direct access. It is not intended that he should deal with matters of clinical judgement or those which should go to a court or to the Service Committee in the case of GPs, dentists and chemists, but he is able to deal with other complaints by individuals or representatives of those unable to act for themselves.

THE NHS AND THE PRIVATE SECTOR

Not every man, woman and child in the UK avails himself of NHS care. There are a growing number of private clinics, nursing homes and even hospitals and, of course, the NHS Consultant may well have a private practice.

A large number of private patients nowadays belong to private insurance schemes, such as the British United Provident Association, the Private Patients' Plan and the Western Provident, to name only three. Firms and professional organizations offer membership at reduced terms, known as group membership. An individual may apply for himself and/or his entire family, to receive hospital treatment, specialist advice and GP services, all or in part, according to the size of his subscription.

Some schemes, like Private Patients' 'Masterplan', involve a plastic membership card which is taken as a request to the hospital to send accounts for private beds direct to the insurance company. Under other schemes the patient settles the fees himself and claims them afterwards from the insurance company.

6

The Family Doctor Service

The position of the GP underwent a profound change with the 1946 Act. Until that time he was a free agent and could move from one area of the country to another at will. He bought his practice and with it the goodwill (existing list of patients) when he entered practice. This was not the burden that it sounds, as it was related to the income and was paid for over several years. With the advent of the NHS the sale of goodwill was abolished and a sum of money set aside to compensate those who had bought their practices prior to 1946. The GP lost most of his private practice overnight but gained a regular income from capitation fees. Freedom of movement was lost in England and Wales because the country was divided into areas and Executive Councils would not accept doctors on their list if the area already had sufficient doctors, but this had the effect of making the distribution of GPs more even throughout the country. In Scotland certain areas are designated as 'open' if there is a scarcity of doctors in them.

In 1974 the Executive Council was replaced by a Family Practitioner Committee; its area of responsibility coincides with the local authority area. However, there are no FPCs in Scotland or Northern Ireland. GPs are able to receive earnings from other sources, but their main income is received from their contract of service with the FPC.

Since the advent of the NHS there has been a steady growth of partnerships. In these the doctors share premises, staff and equipment. Often they share responsibility for the patients of the practice, but in other practices each partner may look after his own 'list' of patients. In 1951 43% of doctors were single handed, today less than 13% are, and more than half the total number of GPs work in groups of four or more doctors. The government has set up schemes to enable groups of doctors to build and alter premises and employ staff.

More than one-quarter of all GPs work in health centres owned by health authorities and more than one-quarter of all patients use them. In Northern Ireland, where a particular policy of developing these health centres exists, more than 60% of all GPs work within them. There are now more than 30 000 GPs in Britain of whom about 20% are women. In addition there are 2000 GPs in training.

THE FAMILY PRACTITIONER COMMITTEE

FPCs are autonomous bodies responsible to the DHSS and are entirely independent of the administrative structure of the DHA. The Committee consists of 30 members. There are 15 professional members—eight doctors,

35

three dentists, two pharmacists, one ophthalmic optician and one dispensing optician. These are appointed by the health authority and four by the local authority. The chairman is appointed by the Secretary of State. The staff of the FPC are appointed by the health authority and include an administrator who acts as secretary. Through these FPCs are administered the contracts of doctors, dentists, chemists and opticians, arrangements are made for paying them, and certain disciplinary procedures are arranged.

THE GENERAL PRACTITIONER

The doctor enters into a contract with the FPC in whose area his patients reside. He may, therefore, be under contract with one or more such Committees but his form of contract does not vary. It is the responsibility of the Committee to pay the doctors on its list and this it does by maintaining a record of the number of patients on the doctor's list on the first day of each quarter and paying a fee for each patient.

The doctor is thus paid for his responsibility and not for the amount of treatment given. He is notified of the number of patients on his list each quarter and is given an opportunity of disputing it—an event which must be very rare! The doctor is also paid certain other fees and allowances for the care he gives to the patients on his list, and these have to be claimed from the Committee.

The doctor is paid on the last day of each quarter for the number of patients on his list on the first day of that quarter. Consequently if a patient enters and

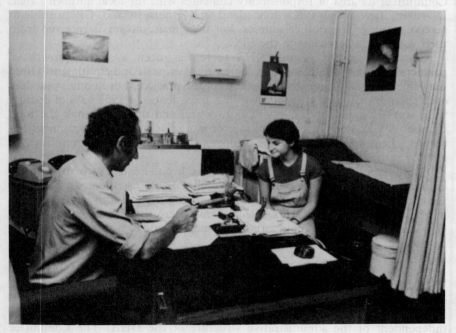

Fig. 6.1 A general practitioner consulting.

leaves his list during the same quarter he is not paid for that patient. But similarly if the patient enters his list during the last week of one quarter and leaves his practice in the first week of the next, then he is paid for a full quarter's responsibility. In practice this arrangement works in a reasonably fair manner.

As well as this list the Committee records the names and addresses of all patients who are registered with doctors under contract with it. By this means the Committee can ensure that a patient's medical record envelope is in the possession of his doctor.

It might be thought that this is a foolproof method of ensuring that each patient is recorded only once on a doctor's list, but inflation of lists does occur. People often use different names, reverse the order of hyphened names or Christian names. Occasionally 'nicknames' are used. When a patient dies the registrar should collect his medical record card, or if he emigrates the embarkation authorities should collect it. This does not always happen and in order to prevent this inflation a central National Health Services register is maintained at Southport, Lancashire. The FPC notifies the central register of each patient registered on a doctor's list in their area. All registrations are recorded in the central register in NHS number order, but in case there is doubt a supplementary register in alphabetical order is also kept.

To sum up, the FPC keeps two registers: one in a long alphabetical run to show the patients registered in the area and the other to show the patients on each doctor's list. The Committee also runs an 'account' ledger which shows the total number of patients on each doctor's list so that his quarterly cheque can be calculated.

THE CHEMIST

It is the FPC's duty to arrange for the provision of drugs, dressings and appliances, and to do this the Committee enters into contract with chemists who wish to provide these pharmaceutical services. The chemists will dispense all prescriptions handed to them on the NHS prescription form (FP 10). They are normally open from 9.00 a.m. to 6.00 p.m.. If asked to do so by the council they will provide a 'rota' service, usually staying open an hour later in the evening in order to dispense prescriptions from patients who have attended an evening surgery. (A copy of this rota is often available from FPC's offices and can be displayed at the doctor's surgery.) The chemist on rota duty also opens for an hour on early closing day and for an hour on Sundays and Bank Holidays. For these rota duties they are paid a fee above that which they get for the dispensing of medicine.

If a prescription is marked 'urgent' and the chemist dispenses it outside normal hours he is paid an extra fee.

There is a special list kept by the doctor of dressings and appliances which he may prescribe on form FP 10 and the chemist is paid only if he dispenses from this list.

In 1983 well over 300-million prescriptions were dispensed in England and Wales. These are checked at a number of pricing bureaux in various parts of the country and the chemist is then paid for each prescription he dispenses.

The total paid is equal to the cost of the drugs and the cost of dispensing, plus a standard profit allowance.

THE GENERAL PRACTICE TEAM

Care of a patient within the community often calls for the application of skills possessed by a number of specialist workers apart from the doctor. It is important that, although several people are involved, care should not become fragmented. If this happens the patient becomes bewildered by conflicting advice and there may be overlaps or gaps in the care. It requires considerable skill to weld such a group into a cohesive team and this is only possible if each member understands the role of other members and the lines of communication are clearly defined. The medical secretary will play a key role in ensuring that there is efficient and coordinated interaction between the members of teams.

Members of the practice team may either be employed by an outside authority (usually part of the health authority) or directly and privately employed by the doctor. Staff employed by the health authority are nurses, health visitors and midwives. They may either be 'attached' to the practice in which they are responsible for all the patients in the practice or, less frequently, responsible only for those patients who live in a particular geographical area. Directly employed staff usually consist of receptionists, medical secretaries, practice managers and practice nurses, but some larger practices may subdivide administrative responsibilities and employ specialist telephonists, bookkeepers, filing clerks, dieticians, physiotherapists and clinical psychologists. Whoever employs the staff, and whether they are 'attached' or not, they can only work as a team if they meet frequently, keep good records and develop a corporate responsibility towards 'the practice' (see Table 6.1).

Sometimes case discussions have to be arranged at which everyone involved takes part. Sometimes practice meetings are needed to discuss general policy

Table 6.1 A typical primary health care team of more than 20 people looking after 9000 patients.

Team members	Numbers
Secretary/receptionists (part-time)	6
Practice manager	1
Practice employed nurses	2
Attached nurses	3
Health visitors	1 or 2
Community midwives	1
General practitioners	4
Trainee doctors	1
Part-time clinical psychologist and dietician	1

decisions. Much of the exchange takes place during coffee breaks or tea-time in the practice office or common-room. It may also be necessary to develop systems in which messages are written and their receipt acknowledged.

HEALTH AUTHORITY EMPLOYED STAFF

Community nursing Sisters (district nurses)

As well as nurses working within the hospital service there are a large number of nurses whose sphere of activity is confined to the community outside the hospital. They are employed by the health authority, and come under the management of the District Nursing Officer who is a member of the District Management Team (see Chapter 5). These district nurses are registered general nurses who have taken a special course in community care. They originally worked independently of general practitioners, but in recent years they have been to a large extent (over 80%) attached to practices, so that they work with the doctors and are identified with their patients. This has led to a much greater understanding between the two professions and to a much wider use of nursing skills. They have access to the medical notes, frequent meetings with the doctors, and carry out home treatment, routine follow-up, visiting, and a variety of other tasks as mutually agreed between the GP and the District Nursing Officer. Many of them also have treatment sessions within the doctor's surgery. A lot of their work is concerned with the seriously handicapped patient and the dying patient. It can involve heavy lifting and nurses may have to work in pairs. Visits may need to be made twice daily.

Largely due to the increasing age of the population their numbers have been greatly expanded and there are now 20 000 full-time district nurses, about two for every three GPs in England. District nurses are often aided by nursing auxiliaries who are state enrolled nurses and carry out less highly skilled tasks.

The Social Services Department may supply nursing equipment such as beds, bedding, air-rings, plastic sheeting, bedpans, backrests, and walking frames.

Health visitors

These are registered general nurses who have either a midwifery qualification or completed a twelve-week obstetric course as part of general training and who are specially trained in health visiting. Their role is in the field of preventive medicine, health education and counselling. They are employed by health authorities, most frequently attached to practice in a similar manner to the district nurse, give advice to expectant mothers, mothers with young children and the elderly. They have an important role in the early detection of disease in the young and the old, so that they may be screening infants for congenital dislocation of the hip, young children for hearing defects, and old people for difficulties in looking after themselves. Frequently they will take part in well-baby sessions within the practice. Like the district nurse they are important members of the team and have easy access to the doctors and to the case notes. There are in Britain more than 9000 whole-time equivalent health visitors.

Midwives

Midwives are generally fully trained nurses who have passed the midwifery examinations of the National Boards. They are provided, free of charge, to attend mothers confined at home. In most areas they conduct their own antenatal examinations at a local clinic or in the patient's home. They attend during the delivery and in the lying-in period (10 days). They are encouraged to cooperate closely with the GP who is looking after the mother, and in many areas antenatal examinations are carried out jointly, either at the clinic or the doctor's surgery. Where a mother is discharged from hospital, within the first 10 days after a confinement, they will continue the nursing care at home. Midwives often run their own 'parent-craft' and relaxation classes at the clinic and distribute welfare foods. In rural areas the duties of midwife, district nurse and health visitor are often combined. In most areas midwives are attached to a practice. There are now very few babies born at home and in most cases the midwife follows her own patients into the hospital to deliver them either in special GP obstetric units or within the obstetric department. They are concerned with 'normal' cases.

Where medical abnormality is likely, or has been discovered, before, during or after labour, the patient is usually put under the care of the hospital doctors. Close liaison is established with the health visitor as she will take over supervision of the baby after the first 10 days. Antenatal care is shared with the family doctor, the patient perhaps being seen alternately by one or the other. This close liaison between all those caring for an expectant mother is an important element in the development of personal care given by a team of involved people. There are 3500 whole-time equivalent community midwives in Britain.

DIRECTLY EMPLOYED STAFF

Practice nurses

These are trained (RGN or SEN) nurses working generally within the practice premises on an extended range of services under the supervision of the doctor. Amongst their tasks will be dressings, assisting at minor operations, injections, ear syringing, taking electrocardiographs (ECGs), blood pressures, cervical smears, audiometric tests and so on. They complement the important work of the community health workers and work mainly in the treatment room, but may occasionally visit patients in their homes. There are now more than 4000 whole-time equivalent practice nurses at work in Britain.

Practice managers

These are the senior administrative staff in the practice. Their job is to secure the smooth running of administration so that clinical staff can get on with their jobs. More detail is included in Chapter 28 but they supervise the employment, training and method of working of staff, 'housekeep' in the premises and bookkeep for the accountant.

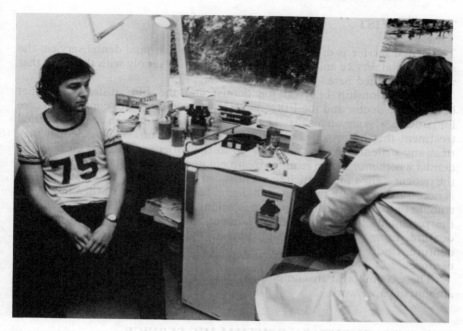

Fig. 6.2 Nurse and patient in a treatment room.

Medical secretaries, receptionists, etc.

There is not a sharp division between the tasks done by administrative staff and many of the duties such as reception of patients and telephoning will be shared. Correspondence is the particular responsibility of medical secretaries and 'receiving' in person or on the telephone that of receptionists. The latest figures are that there are more than 45 000 whole-time equivalent secretaries and receptionists working in general practice in Britain.

FAMILY PLANNING

Contraceptive advice is free under the NHS and the supply of contraceptive pills and some devices is free on prescription. There are two sources of advice: the main one is the family doctor and the Family Planning Clinic is the other. Most doctors regard family planning advice as an integral part of the family medical care to which the doctor, health visitor, nurse and reception staff will all contribute. Some patients, particularly the young who are anxious about information reaching their parents, prefer to seek advice from a clinic outside the practice but the clinic will always notify the practice about advice they have given. Confidentiality is, as always, a very important principle.

Contraceptive advice and sexual counselling is an important part of 'well-woman' care—preventive medicine—and will usually include advice on other topics such as self-examination of breasts to aid in the early discovery of lumps, advice about cervical smears, blood pressure, smoking and diet.

THE DENTIST

The dental service is divided into three parts: the hospital dental service, the school dental service and the FPC dental service. It is only with the latter that we are concerned here.

The relationship between the dentist and the FPC differs from that between the doctor and the FPC. As we have seen the doctor contracts to care for patients who are on his list. The dentist has no list and each course of dental treatment that he provides constitutes a separate contract. The dentist may treat any patient privately and it is up to the patient to make it clear to the dentist whether or not he requires treatment under the NHS. On each occasion the patient signs a form which the dentist completes to show the treatment that is necessary to restore the patient to dental health. The dentist then fills in the amount of treatment that the patient is willing to have. This is done because, if the patient declines part of the treatment and is then fitted with a partial denture, he may at a later date complete the treatment and require a full denture. Under these circumstances the NHS may refuse to supply the partial denture.

These claim forms are complicated and involve the dentist in a considerable amount of paper work.

THE SUPPLEMENTARY OPHTHALMIC SERVICE

(See page 264.)

7

Local Authority Services

THE LOCAL HEALTH AUTHORITY

The local health authorities were in many respects the senior branch of the NHS. For, as we have seen, the hospital service and organized general practice had developed along local lines until 50 years ago, whereas public health had the framework of a national service for over 100 years.

The early eighteenth century was the time when the conception of protecting the health of the community was stimulating men to act. The health of the army and navy came under scrutiny at this time and manuals were published outlining steps which needed to be taken. At the same time the congestion and squalor caused by the industrial revolution were producing grave disquiet and in 1795 the first Board of Health was set up in Manchester by *Thomas Percival* (1740–1804), a local doctor. The repressive measures of the 1834 Poor Law had been introduced by *Edwin Chadwick* (1800–1840), who became one of the Poor Law Commissioners and it was not long before he saw that the burden of helping the poor was only one aspect of the expense of prevention of disease. At first he concentrated on the engineering problem of providing new towns with water supplies and drainage, and he soon came to realize that some central control of this activity was necessary. This resulted in the remarkable series of Public Health and Sanitary Acts which were produced between 1848 and 1875. It seems odd that the man who inspired the ruthless approach of the Poor Law was able to construct such a humane series of legislative acts. The answer to the paradox lies in the fact that disease and fever, which started in the slums, soon spread to the homes of the rich. The Poor Law Commissioners themselves were stirred into action by the great cholera epidemics of the early nineteenth century and during the next 50 years the Commissioners helped to smooth the way for acts dealing with water supplies, sewerage, the health of dwellings, inspection of food, burials, and the control of the spread of infectious diseases.

The Public Health Act of 1848 set up a General Board of Health to act as a controlling body, but, after only 10 years, it was dissolved and the powers transferred to the privy council acting through the independent local authorities. This very independence enabled some local authorities to carry out far-sighted plans.

Liverpool led the way by appointing the first Medical Officer of Health in 1847 and London soon followed. It was recognized later that special training was necessary, and in 1888 an Act of Parliament laid down that every Medical Officer of Health who had to look after a population of more than 50 000 must hold a special diploma, thus ensuring the quality of the men who had to administer the public health laws. Birmingham, at this time (1873–1876), had a Lord Mayor *Joseph Chamberlain* (1836–1914). He summoned a conference of local sanitary authorities in 1875 and thus began the movement for the healthier organization of town life, characterized by slum clearance, new streets and parks, gas and water supplies and open spaces in the city.

In 1919 the Ministry of Health was formed and it at once became a centre for all the local health authorities, advising, helping and coordinating them. It introduced a proper scientific attitude of public health problems and led to the introduction of a series of measures dealing with slum clearance and housing, tuberculosis, factory conditions and mental treatment. In the succeeding years nearly every aspect of public health was reorganized upon a national scale culminating in Part III of the NHS Act of 1946 which was designed to draw all these activities into one medical service. During these 200 years the health picture of the British Isles had changed out of all recognition. The expectation of life had increased from around 35 years to more than 65 years; infant mortality had declined from 20% to less than 2%. In 1836 of all the children born, half died before the age of five. These changes have had profound effects on the field of work of public health authorities and the tendency is for them to be less involved with diseases and more with welfare work.

Local government was reshaped in 1972 by a series of measures which brought together the government counties and metropolitan districts in England, eight local government regions in Scotland, eight county councils in Wales and four in Northern Ireland.

The local authorities have responsibilities for all social services and public health services, and it is these two roles that are considered in this chapter.

SOCIAL SERVICES

These services, whilst not strictly part of the health services, play an important role in the management of health needs of major groups of the community. Responsibility for the overall provision of services devolves upon the Secretary of State for Social Services, advised by a Personal Social Services Council. The local authority areas each have a single social services committee with organizing and coordination functions. The principal officer within the local authority is the Director of Social Services.

Prior to 1970 local authorities had fairly considerable responsibilities for personal health services, but those have now been removed. There is, of course, a problem in this area because the needs of an individual or a family in trouble in the community are often a blend of health and social matters. For example, a deprived family may have housing problems and educational problems as well as containing individuals who are physically ill or psychologically disturbed. Chronic ill-health may be the result of social circumstances and at other times the cause. Wherever a division of responsibility exists there will be problems caused by that division, and the separation of health and social services has created some problems as well as helping others. It requires considerable effort in the communication and coordination of services to avoid making matters worse and the medical secretary may exercise an important role in this area.

Broadly speaking the functions of the local authorities' social services departments can be grouped under three headings: services for children,

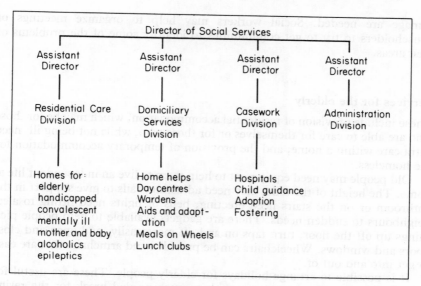

Fig. 7.1 The structure of the social services.

services for families and services for the elderly. When a medical secretary rings the social services department she will speak first to a telephonist who will probably refer her to the duty social worker. It is his or her job to decide whether it can be dealt with now or needs to be referred to one of the specialist divisions.

Services for children

Social workers scrutinize fostering and adoption applications, write social inquiry reports for courts when young people present before them, and receive and supervise children and young persons taken into care under a court order if provisions for home care are not possible. This is usually a last resort measure. They also arrange and supervise 'intermediate treatment' schemes for young people who have got into trouble and scrutinize applications for day nurseries, hostels and group homes.

Services for families

The care of pre-school children by child minders or by the establishment of day nurseries meets an important need in some areas.

The unsupported mother can be helped by the provision of assistance in the house or by the establishment of mother and baby homes.

Other groups of people with special needs within the family are the deaf, the blind, the educationally subnormal, the chronically disabled and so on. All have special needs and requirements of the social services, often requiring residential accommodation.

Sometimes the family or part of the community can be threatened by local disaster and plans for dealing with emergencies caused by flooding or fire damage are needed. Social workers may help to organize meetings of householders to try to get communities to identify some of the problems of their areas.

Services for the elderly

These include provision of residential accommodation, which may be for those who are able to care for themselves or for those who, while not being ill, need extra care within a home; and the provision of temporary accommodation for the homeless.

Old people may need equipment to help them to live an independent life at home. The height of the toilet may need adjusting, rails to give support in the bathroom or on the stairs need erecting, bells or lights need fitting to alert neighbours to sudden needs. There are gadgets available to help people pick things up off the floor, turn taps on and off more easily, and open and close doors and windows. Wheelchairs can be provided and armchairs that are easy to get into and out of.

It is possible to arrange holidays for elderly people. These are useful for those living alone but can also provide a much needed break for the caring relatives of those going on holiday.

Chiropody services for the elderly or handicapped are very useful and a laundering service for incontinent patients will help families with problems in this line, for the ordinary laundry will often not accept badly soiled sheets. A wide range of medical equipment such as commodes, bedpans, incontinence pads, walking frames and sticks, and adaptations to homes to accommodate dialysing equipment, etc., may be provided.

It can be seen that the knowledge of how to arrange those supporting services is of great value.

Other services

Home helps

These important members of the caring team deserve a heading to themselves. Very often they are the major factor in preventing the complete breakdown in the social competence of a person within the community. They are provided by the local authority and provide domestic help in such cases as ill-health, old age or maternity. They will clean and tidy, do fires and washing up. Often they will help with shopping and collecting prescriptions. Perhaps their most important contribution is in making contact with people who would otherwise be isolated.

Some repayment may be requested from households which can afford it. Home helps are in great demand and as much notice as possible should be given when sending in a request; in maternity cases for example it may be possible to estimate weeks ahead and this will enable the home help to visit the mother before the baby is born. Most authorities employ an organizer who will visit the home and assess the amount of help needed and the repayment to be made.

Social workers

These are the most skilled workers in the social services team. Traditional training is changing rapidly, but usually she will either have a good university degree followed by one year of training, or will be a more mature person with two years of special training. Previously social workers were often trained for special aspects of work. Thus we had medical social workers, psychiatric social workers, child health officers and so on. Today, the training is more general and designed to fit a person to work in any area of the profession.

Her task falls into two main areas: effective provision of resources, and casework.

She has a very detailed knowledge of the social services and can assess the patients' problems. This enables her to identify the needs and then recruit the appropriate official or voluntary help to meet the needs. Often this is a very specialized need which can only be provided by identifying the particular society or charitable trust.

Casework is a very particular skill which not only requires long training but is also very time-consuming. It has a considerable element of psychology in it and is designed to enable the client with relationship and personality difficulties to understand their problems and work out their own solutions. This often involves working with the whole family.

Probation officers

Many of the organizations mentioned in this chapter will receive help and advice from the probation officer. He is appointed by the probation committee composed of local magistrates, has special training and usually a university diploma in social studies.

Voluntary services

Meals-on-wheels

Some authorities provide this service or organize it through a voluntary body. A hot lunch may be provided on certain days of the week, usually for the elderly. A nominal charge is often made.

Unmarried mothers

Most local health authorities use the voluntary welfare association to help unmarried mothers. These are mainly run by the religious denominations and the moral welfare workers are provided by the largest of these—the Church of England. Jewish, Catholic and other organizations may also provide workers. They assist with the making of arrangements for the care of the baby and also with admission of the mother to one of the association's Mother and Baby Homes for a period from six weeks before to six weeks after the birth.

Citizens' Advice Bureaux

These organizations have, since 1948, been largely financed and supported by the local authority but maintain their independence of the public authority.

They are helped and advised by a national council and staffed by specially trained voluntary or paid workers. They will give expert advice on a wide variety of problems, especially preliminary advice on legal problems.

Old people's welfare councils

Quite independent of the local authority, these are often supported by financial and other help. They are advised by a national council and help to integrate and encourage local schemes for old people.

Marriage guidance councils

These are supported by grants from the Home Office and together with the Catholic Marriage Advisory Council give advice on a wide range of matrimonial problems.

Adoption

Over 20 000 adoption orders are made annually by the courts of Great Britain and Northern Ireland. Adoption is now regulated by acts passed in 1950, 1958 and 1976, and the Registrars-General keep registers of all adopted children.

The local authorities (in Northern Ireland, the Ministry of Home Affairs) keep registers of all the adoption societies—there are over 80—and through their children committees may act as adoption agencies.

Family casework

Mention must be made of the development in London of family casework services. There are three voluntary organizations doing this type of work: Family Service Units, The Invalid Children's Aid Association and the Family Welfare Association and these all accept students for training. The principal feature about the work they do is that they offer a complete social service to families that are in distress and they are, therefore, able to provide a coordinated service which is sometimes lacking with other bodies.

Many other voluntary services are available including the National Society for the Prevention of Cruelty to Children, organizations helping special groups such as cancer sufferers, the deaf, blind, patients who have strokes and people suffering from multiple sclerosis. The secretary should know such groups are available and know where the register of these organizations is kept with their addresses and telephone numbers.

PUBLIC HEALTH SERVICES

Environmental health

Public health inspectors are appointed by the local authority to carry out such duties as the inspection of shops and slaughter-houses, the regulation of markets and the inspection of food and deal with the problem of housing, where it constitutes a danger to health, as in infestation and with smoke and noise nuisances.

These may all be areas where medical services are required. The control of infectious disease, imported through air and sea ports, is the responsibility of the local authority's environmental health officers.

Education of handicapped children

It is the responsibility of the local authority to provide services for children who need special education due to mental or physical handicaps or to emotional or social deprivation. The health authorities have to provide the medical services required for identification and treatment but over a thousand special schools are maintained for the blind, partially sighted, deaf, educationally subnormal, severely epileptic, maladjusted, delicate and physically handicapped children. All services are provided free of charge.

Mental health (see also p. 193)

The law relating to mentally ill patients is set out in the 1983 Mental Health Act. An application for compulsory admission to hospital for assessment may be made on the recommendation of two doctors for a period of up to 28 days, or for treatment if this is necessary for up to six months, or as an emergency for up to 72 hours in the first place.
1 One of the doctors involved must have been specially approved for this purpose by the Secretary of State and both must have examined the patient.
2 Approved social workers may also make application for admission to hospital and this may be upon the request of the nearest relative of the patient.
3 The Act also governs the setting up of Mental Health Review Tribunals and the management of property and affairs of patients.

Social workers will also be involved in the care of the mentally ill in the community in a variety of ways.

8

Occupational Health Services

The father of occupational medicine is Bernardino Ramazzini (1633–1714). It was in 1700 that the first edition of the work to which he owes his immortality, *De Morbis Artificum Diatriba*, was published. He inquired into the conditions of work and the occupational diseases of many different types of worker, and advocated rest intervals in heavy work, better ventilation, and more suitable conditions generally in many trades. He said that when a doctor visited a working-class type of home he should always ask the patient, 'What is your occupation?'.

But industrial medicine was born with the Industrial Revolution in England. Charles Turner Thackrah (1796–1833) of Leeds investigated the health hazards of workers in Yorkshire and Lancashire, and wrote of tuberculosis in tailors, lung disease in miners and metal grinders, and lead poisoning in glaze dippers. He wrote of children in the flax mills: 'Many from six to seven years of age, roused from their bed at an early hour, hurried to the mills and kept there, with an interval of only forty minutes, till a late hour at night, kept moreover in an atmosphere impure. . . .'

Thackrah's book on *The Effects of the Principal Arts, Trades and Professions* was published in 1831. Also in 1831 a Royal Commission on the Employment of Children in Factories was established, which resulted in the Factories Act of 1833. This act forbade night work for persons under 18 and limited their working hours to 12 a day and 69 a week. It also established factory schools for children under 13 and stipulated the production of doctors' certificates to affirm that children were of normal strength and appearance for their years, nine years being the minimum age of employment.

Much of the evidence for this act had been collated by Sir Robert Peel the elder, who was Home Secretary and himself a mill-owner and had secured the passing of earlier acts in 1802 and 1819.

The most important provision of the 1833 act was the establishment of a Factory Inspectorate, with four inspectors to cover the whole country. These inspectors tried to arrange for special medical men to perform certifying duties in each area, but it was not until the Factories Act of 1844 that power was given to them to appoint doctors for the purpose of examining young persons brought before them.

HEALTH AND SAFETY AT WORK ACT

The Health and Safety at Work Act came into action in 1975. It gives power to the Secretary of State for Employment to draw up regulations and codes of practice on health and safety measures. It puts duties on employers, creates a

Health and Safety Commission which is responsible for control, gathers all the various government inspectors into a new body called the Health and Safety Executive and tidies up all the previous legislation.

The Act itself, whilst being described as 'brief', still runs to over 40 000 words and puts a general responsibility on all employers to ensure the safety, health and welfare at work of all employees. There is special safety legislation covering most groups of workers including those employed in the medical and dental services and applies to the safety of machinery, hazards from chemicals and the general conditions of work including lighting, overcrowding, temperature, cleanliness, sanitary arrangements and so on.

EMPLOYMENT MEDICAL ADVISORY SERVICE (EMAS)

This service consists of about 100 full-time doctors and nurses who are employed under the umbrella of the Health and Safety Commission.

They are located in all the major industrial areas and have clear responsibilities:

1 To give advice to young people about medical aspects of employment (this particularly concerns those people identified as handicapped at school).
2 To examine people employed in certain hazardous industries such as mines, quarries, chemical works.
3 To maintain contacts with hospitals, family doctors and others concerned in personal health services.
4 To advise on training and resettlement services, the employment of people on the disabled persons register, etc.
5 To study health hazards in industry.

There are EMAS area officers in most regions who will help with problems that arise. Leaflets and advice are issued by the service, covering a wide range of occupations.

MEDICAL SERVICES BY INDUSTRY ITSELF

At the same time as public legislation was making its contribution to improvements in working conditions, private concern was active. In 1830 an employer in worsted spinning appointed a Medical Officer to visit the factory daily. In 1855 a Dr Lewis was appointed as a full-time Medical Officer to establish the Post Office Medical Service, but progress was slow and up to 1939 only 50 such people had been appointed.

In 1940 Ernest Bevin, then Minister of Labour, realized that if war production was to be kept going every available pair of hands was needed and no time could be lost through avoidable sickness or injury. He therefore issued an order requiring all factories engaged in war production to organize medical and nursing services, and he put the responsibility for this upon industry itself. When the NHS was introduced these services were not included and they remain entirely voluntary. But today some 650 factories employ full-time, and some 4500 factories part-time, doctors and the ordinary membership of the Society of Occupational Health is about 900.

Where a firm is too small to establish its own medical services it may combine with a group to provide joint services. Such groups operate in Dundee, Harlow, from the Central Middlesex Hospital, and in Rochdale, Slough and West Bromwich.

There is therefore much scope for medical secretarial work inside industry. Apart from this, contact between the general medical service, the hospital service and the occupational health service becomes increasingly important.

THE MEDICAL SECRETARY IN INDUSTRY

Much of what is said in this book about the type of work done by the GP's secretary and the Consultant's secretary is applicable to work in industry. Sometimes she will be one of a team of secretaries working under a supervisor, and there will usually be nursing staff, perhaps a Chief Nursing Officer, for her to turn to for advice on clinical problems. Conditions will vary considerably from one industry to another, and as well as her medical vocabulary the secretary may need some command of a technical vocabulary.

The main functions of a medical department are:
1 Certain statutory obligations under the various factory acts.
2 General advisory services concerning such matters as occupational hazards and health education, canteen, sanitary and washing arrangements, sickness absence statistics, etc.
3 Routine examinations:
(a) pre-employment (this includes examination on return to work after an illness)—to ensure fitness to perform the work
(b) periodical—when there is some special hazard involved in the work and particular tests are necessary
4 Personal services to individuals including:
(a) first-aid treatment and reference to hospital or family doctor when necessary
(b) advice and reference to family doctor for treatment when necessary
(c) continuing treatment after liaison with the family doctor, including rehabilitation after prolonged illness
(d) advice to management regarding an individual's capacity to do a particular job

In all these functions the medical secretary may play a part, particularly in the keeping of records.

Statutory records

These include:
1 A register of accidents.
2 A notification to the factory inspector of accidents causing:
(a) loss of life
(b) loss of full earnings for more than three days
3 A record of periodical examinations in industries where special regulations apply.

Records for routine examinations

1 *Pre-employment.* The type of record used will vary from one factory to another. The secretary may be required to obtain basic information for this: name, address, sex, date of birth, marital state, family accommodation, details of previous employment, check number, department, etc. (Figs 8.1a,b,c).

2 *Periodical examination.* Again the type of record will vary from industry to industry. A review index card will need to be made out and filed under the appropriate date so that the patient can be recalled at the correct time. Certain very important ethical considerations apply to these individual clinical records, and they must be known and observed by the medical secretary. Unlike the records of NHS patients, these are the personal property of the doctor who recorded the facts. They are not the property of the firm or of any director or

---

MEDICAL RECORD — FITNESS FOR EMPLOYMENT

Date

CONFIDENTIAL

F.1032

Crane Driver	Solder Planisher
Lorry/Artic. Vehicle Driver	Foundry Worker
Test Driver Mechanic	Work's Policeman
Locomotive Driver	Fireman
Shunter	Plastics Worker
Disabled Person	Canteen Employee

Name
Address

Check No.

Department

Present or Last Job

Panel Doctor
Address

Service Medical Category   Year

Date of Birth   M. S. W.

Registered Disabled Person   Yes/No

HISTORY

Occupational

Dust and Toxic Exposure

Job changes on health grounds

Accident involvement

Present Health

Cough, breathlessness, wheezing, chest pain or indigestion

Last Chest X-Ray   Result

Last saw Doctor   Reason

Fig. 8.1a Pre-employment medical record.

EXAMINATION

Ht.		Wt.	Urine	Albumin	Sugar
Vision—Far	Right	Left	Vision—Near	Right	Left
Unaided			Unaided		
Aided			Aided		
Eyes	Right	Left	Ears	Right	Left
Fundi			Drums		
Visual Fields					
Colour Vision			Hearing. F.W.		
Physique			Hernia		
General Mobility			Varicose Veins		
Hygiene					
Cardiovascular System			Skin		
P.R.	B.P.	Atherosclerosis	Skeleto Muscular		
Heart					
Cyanosis			X-Ray		
Respiratory System			E.C.G.		
Dyspnoea					
Oral Cavity			Others		
Abdomen					
Nervous System					
Mental			Haemoglobin	Punctates	

OPINION

Signature...

Fig. 8.1b Pre-employment medical record.

employee. Furthermore the facts cannot be divulged to anyone else without the patient's consent (unless the doctor is ordered to produce them in court). This consent should always be obtained in writing. The records should, therefore, be kept in locked drawers and suitable arrangements made for the custody of the keys. If the doctor leaves his employment with the firm, he will hand the records over personally to his successor. If, for any reason, this is impossible, he will destroy them. These notes are commonly typewritten and the rules will be known to the secretary.

Requests for disclosure frequently come from solicitors or the DHSS. It is important to determine in the case of solicitors whether disclosure to the solicitors acting for both sides is required and, if so, to obtain the appropriate consent.

X-rays and ECG recordings may need separate filing.

Medical History

Bronchitis___	Nervous Disease___
Pleurisy___	Mental Disorder___
Pneumonia___	Epilepsy, Fits, Faints, Blackouts___
Asthma___	Giddiness or Headaches___
Tuberculosis___	Ear Disease___
Heart Disease___	Defect of Sight or Hearing___
Hypertension___	Recurrent Nose or Throat Infection___
Rheumatic Fever___	Skin Disease, Dermatitis___
Rheumatism, Fibrositis, Sciatica___	Blood Disorder___
Gastric or Duodenal Ulcer___	Hernia, Varicose Veins, Piles___
Kidney or Bladder Disease___	Bone and Joint Disease or Injury___
Alimentary Infection___	Other illness, injury or operation___
Other Abdominal Disorder___	
Diabetes___	

Difficulty in standing, stooping, kneeling, lifting, pushing, pulling or gripping___

Night or Shift Work. Yes/No___ Dates___ Difficulties___

Difficulty in driving at night or in distinguishing colours___

Family___

Fig. 8.1c Pre-employment medical record.

Records for personal services

Apart from the entries that have to be made on the clinical records, the medical secretary will have important liaison duties to perform.
1 When emergency or first-aid treatment is required, the patient's own doctor must be informed. This will usually be done in writing on a standard form, but in some cases a telephone call to the doctor's secretary may be an additional help.
2 If further treatment is required and could helpfully be given at the factory, this may be done with the consent of the patient's own doctor. In this case a form will be sent to the doctor requesting his consent.

The same is true of both rehabilitation and physiotherapy treatment, but the former, generally of a lighter nature while complete recovery is taking place, may be ordered by the factory doctor.

It must not be thought from this that the liaison is a one-way service from factory to surgery. Most GPs are frequently consulted by patients about their fitness to do certain work, and they may write to the industrial Medical Officer requesting changes in occupation. However, in many cases the GP does not really know what the conditions of work are, nor does he know the standard of physical fitness required, and he will therefore write to the factory doctor asking for his help with the problem. The importance of this type of cooperation can be readily understood when one considers the large proportion of life that is spent at work.

At times the patient may not know the name, address or telephone number of his GP, and the details on his clinical record card may be out of date. Then the FPC willingly supplies the details by telephone.

The medical secretary will be well advised to make a list of local doctors and include in it their surgery hours and telephone numbers.

When patients leave their employment or die, their clinical records should be kept for five years in case they are required for legal purposes.

Records for management

In many large industries, detailed accident statistics are kept in addition to those that are statutorily required. From the daily list of works accidents the secretary may be required to make a monthly return; this is often analysed in terms of parts of the body involved—hands, feet, eyes, etc.—and departments of the factory where the accidents occurred. In some very large factories, computers are used to relate these data to types of machines, foremen's reports on how injuries occurred, and periods of time spent off work. This information can then be used to advise on safer methods of working.

Further duties in industrial medicine

1 *Arrangements for travel abroad.* Many companies send representatives abroad, and often at short notice. The World Health Organization publishes a book on the vaccinations required for each country, but this does not take into account the fact that the plane or ship may stop at other countries en route to the particular destination. For this reason the travel agency or airline will have to be consulted. Further details are given in Chapter 33.

2 *Specialist appointments.* Some firms pay for employees to have private consultations under benevolent schemes, and the secretary may have to make the arrangements.

3 There are many other tasks that may be undertaken by the good medical secretary, such as: making preparations for visiting groups of doctors; arranging for industrial Medical Officers to attend conferences and seminars; claiming travel allowances; and collecting references for lectures and articles. Remarks on these activities will be found elsewhere in this book.

II

General Secretarial Duties

9

Ethics and Etiquette

The relationships between one doctor and another and between a doctor and his patients are governed by the professional ethics and etiquette of medicine which have developed over many centuries. These have been designed to protect the high reputation and standing of the profession, to protect the patient from the unscrupulous and to develop mutual trust and confidence between doctors. As such they are the basis of all the work done by the doctor and the secretary must clearly understand and respect them.

The ethics of medicine are the professional standards of what is morally right and wrong. The earliest declaration of ethics was made in the *Hippocratic oath* in about the fifth century BC. In its present form the oath is of a very much later date than Hippocrates himself, but some of it may be even earlier, and certainly reflects the spirit of the Hippocratic physicians. Undoubtedly it represents a standard of ethics that has never been surpassed. It is in the form of an indenture between a physician and his apprentice and whilst the modern doctor may not affirm it formally he accepts its spirit as the ideal standard of professional behaviour.

> I swear by Apollo the physician, and Aesculapius and Health, and All-Heal, and all the gods and goddesses, that, according to my ability and judgement, I shall keep this Oath and this stipulation—to reckon him who taught me this Art equally dear to me as my parents, to share my substance with him, and relieve his necessities if required; to look upon his offspring as my own brother, and to teach them this art, if they shall wish to learn it, without fee or stipulation; and that by precept, lecture, and every other mode of instruction I shall impart a knowledge of the Art to my own sons, and those of my teachers, and to disciplines bound by a stipulation and oath according to the law of medicine, but to none others. I will follow that system which, according to my judgement, I consider for the benefit of my patients, and abstain from whatever is harmful to them. I shall give no deadly medicine to anyone if asked, nor suggest any such counsel: and in like manner I shall not advise a woman to procure abortion. With purity and holiness I shall pass my life and practise my Art. Into whatever houses I enter, I shall go into them for the benefit of the sick. Whatever I see or hear, in the life of men, which ought not to be spoken of abroad, I shall not divulge, as reckoning that all such should be kept secret.

The terrible lapses from this idea which occurred in certain countries during the Second World War led doctors to feel that this oath needed restating in modern times. On the initiative of the British Medical Association the *Declaration of Geneva* was made by the World Medical Association in 1947, and this now sets down the guiding principles of all professional behaviour.

> I solemnly pledge myself to consecrate my life to the service of humanity. I will give to my teachers the respect and gratitude which is their due.

59

I shall practice my profession with conscience and dignity; the health of my patient will be my first consideration: I shall respect the secrets that are confided in me; my colleagues will be my brothers; I shall maintain by all the means in my power the honour and noble tradition of the medical profession: I shall not permit considerations of religion, nationality, race, party politics or social standing to intervene between my duty and my patient; I shall maintain the utmost respect for human life from the time of conception; even under threat, I shall not use my medical knowledge contrary to the laws of humanity.

The *Declaration of Geneva* is based upon an International Code of Medical Ethics which applies both in times of peace and war. The English translation is as follows:

A doctor must always maintain the highest standards of professional conduct.
A doctor must practise his profession uninfluenced by motives of profit.

The following practices are deemed unethical:
(a) Any self-advertisement except such as is expressly authorized by the national code of medical ethics.
(b) Collaboration in any form of medical service in which the doctor does not have professional independence.
(c) Receiving any money in connection with services rendered to a patient other than a proper professional fee, even with the knowledge of the patient.

Any act or advice which could weaken physical or mental resistance of a human being may be used only in his interest.
A doctor is advised to use great caution in divulging discoveries or new techniques of treatment.
A doctor should certify or testify only to that which he has personally verified.
A doctor must always bear in mind the obligation of preserving human life.
A doctor owes to his patient complete loyalty and all the resources of his science. Whenever an examination or treatment is beyond his capacity he should summon another doctor who has the necessary ability.
A doctor shall preserve absolute secrecy on all he knows about his patient because of the confidence entrusted in him.
A doctor must give emergency care as a humanitarian duty unless he is assured that others are willing and able to give such care.
A doctor ought to behave to colleagues as he would have them behave to him.
A doctor must not entice patients from his colleagues.

Some of the principles in this code need further definition.

PUBLICITY

Broadly speaking self-advertisement is unethical. If it is necessary for a doctor to notify his patients of a change in address or telephone number he may put a notice in his waiting room, but any notice sent by post must be in a closed envelope and only sent to patients known to be on the doctor's list. Difficulties these days arise more often in press publicity, television or broadcasting. The secretary must never make or give any statement to the press without consulting the doctor. He will wish to preserve his anonymity at all costs if the principle of no self-advertisement is to be maintained. Only if it is of public importance to provide authoritative information will he depart from this principle.

CERTIFICATION

All doctors are liable to issue certificates and reports from time to time and many of these, such as death certificates, National Insurance certificates, etc., are duties that are statutorily imposed upon him. The secretary should be careful to observe that the doctor is not placed in a position where he is asked to certify improperly. This applies in particular to declarations of a patient's illness that have not been verified personally by the doctor, or to statements that an examination has been made on that day when, in fact, a relative attended for the certificate. This means that the exact wording of any certificate that is issued must be complied with.

THE CONSULTATION

The doctor cannot and does not practise in isolation. He relies for advice and support on his professional colleagues and will turn, from time to time, to a colleague who by reason of his special skills in one branch of medicine will be able to advise him. There are occasions when a patient will need to be examined by a doctor acting on behalf of a third party such as an insurance company, a factory doctor, or the Regional Medical Officer. The method of consultation between two doctors has been developed over many years and is carefully observed.

Consultation with another doctor on behalf of the patient

As we have seen in Chapter 4 it is the Consultant who is applied to for advice by the practitioner and not by the patient. This advice is given for the instruction of the practitioner in the management of the case and not for the instruction of the patient. Properly speaking it is then up to the practitioner to pass the Consultant's advice on to his patient if he considers it appropriate to do so.

In practice these somewhat rigid rules are modified because the specialist will have the confidence of the practitioner and the consultation is a cooperation between the doctors in formulating the diagnosis, prognosis and treatment. It is in these circumstances that etiquette as well as ethics applies.

Etiquette is the established custom and is followed meticulously. We have seen that it is the duty of the practitioner to summon another doctor when circumstances dictate and he will agree to a consultation if the patient's or relative's request for one seems reasonable. It is the practitioner's duty to find out what fees will have to be paid and to notify the patient in advance. When both doctors are attending the consultation punctuality is important and the secretary should ensure that the doctor is notified correctly of any arrangements made by her and that these arrangements fit in with other appointments that he may have.

In private practice, and under the NHS, consultations may take place at the patient's home. When these are arranged for a NHS patient they are known as 'domiciliary visits'. The service is available to those patients who, for medical reasons, are unable to attend an out-patient department at hospital.

A list of Consultants who are prepared to make domiciliary visits is published by the RHA and a fee is paid to the Consultant for each visit up to a certain number each quarter. (There are minor differences in the scheme between full-time and part-time Consultants.) The claim form for the fee has to be signed by the practitioner as well.

Consultations under the NHS for patients who are well enough to travel will be carried out at the hospital out-patient department and for private patients either at the hospital or at the Consultant's rooms. Although these consultations may take place when both doctors are present, more often the patient is seen by the Consultant alone, the attending practitioner having sent a brief history of the case to the Consultant.

After examining the patient the Consultant forwards his opinion and advice in a sealed envelope to the practitioner. During the course of the consultation the patient will expect to have his questions answered and possibly his fears allayed, but the Consultant will exercise great discretion about the information he gives to the patient and his relatives.

The secretaries of both doctors must ensure that the letters between the doctors are sent off as soon as possible to ensure that the Consultant is never asked to see a patient without a letter and that the reply is received by the practitioner without undue delay so that he has it before the patient consults him again. Any arrangements for further consultation or additional investigation should be effected only with the foreknowledge and cooperation of the patient's doctor and copies of any correspondence between one Consultant and another about the patient should be sent to the patient's doctor.

Consultation with another doctor on behalf of a third party

Under these circumstances the first point to be observed is that the patient consents to this examination and to the disclosure to the third party of any information obtained. The second point is that nothing must be done to disturb the confidence that the patient has in his own doctor or to interfere with any treatment.

PROFESSIONAL CONFIDENCE AND SECRECY

Every patient expects his doctor not only to use his skill but also to observe absolute secrecy about any information that he receives as a result of his examination and treatment, and on this understanding of professional confidence rests the relationship between the doctor and his patient. He should never break this confidence unless statutorily obliged to do so. This occurs in circumstances such as the notification of infectious diseases and in death certificates. The doctor may also be ordered by a court of law to disclose matters that he would not otherwise wish to disclose and may wish to register his protest before complying with the order.

ACCEPTANCE OF PATIENTS

Here there are two simple rules.

1 No doctor will accept for treatment a patient who is already receiving active treatment for the same condition by another doctor, unless he is satisfied that

the patient has notified the first doctor that his services are no longer required. 2 In the event of the patient's own doctor being temporarily unavailable, another doctor may give what treatment is necessary but will afterwards notify the patient's regular medical attendant. This happens as a result of emergency or when the patient is taken ill away from his home district. Doctors who work in the NHS find that the regulations about acceptance of patients allow them to conform to this proper ethical standard in just the same way as do doctors who are in private practice.

THE DENTIST AND THE DOCTOR

When the doctor considers that his patient needs dental treatment he will refer the patient to his usual dentist. If the patient has no dentist of his own, there is no objection to the doctor recommending one. There are occasions when a patient may, in the doctor's opinion, require major dental treatment necessitating specialist advice. In such cases the doctor will consult with the patient's usual dentist before arranging the consultation.

CHAPERONING

The doctor and the dentist are particularly at risk from accusations by female patients that they have been indecently assaulted. The presence of a third person, usually a female, is an insurance that the doctor or dentist will always wish to have. Many women are emotionally or mentally disturbed when they are consulting a doctor, and dentists are often exposed to such charges by patients who have become hallucinated under anaesthesia. Furthermore the presence of a chaperone may relieve the patient of some embarrassment. When the secretary has to act in this capacity she should try to be completely unobtrusive. She can do this best by occupying herself with some quiet task in the examination room and should so arrange matters that there is a small job that can be done. She will then be in a position to help the doctor if he needs an extra pair of hands, and the patient if she needs help in getting on or off the couch or in dressing herself. If the patient has a friend or relative in attendance he or she can be asked to help the patient dress. Most doctors will establish a custom about chaperoning procedures with their secretary and it will then be a routine procedure but the secretary should ensure that she does not leave the doctor without a chaperone at any time. It may not be necessary for her to be in the examination room to exercise this function; it will often, indeed usually, be considered a sufficient insurance for her to be within ear-shot.

SUMMARY

From this description of the ethics and etiquette of medical practice the secretary will be able to appreciate those items which particularly apply to her work.
1 She must always remember that her work is strictly confidential. Nothing that she learns from a patient, from the doctor, from the medical records or from the correspondence must ever be disclosed to anyone else.

2 She must never discuss the details of her work or the personal affairs of the doctor with anyone else.

3 The treatment or behaviour of another doctor must never be criticized in the hearing of a patient.

4 She must be circumspect when talking about the doctor to any other person. She would be wise never to praise his accomplishments unduly.

5 It will be her duty to help foster the good relationship between doctor and patient and to do everything in her power to enable the doctor to treat his patients.

THE GENERAL MEDICAL COUNCIL (GMC)

This body is now the only one with the powers to license practitioners, that previously vested in the Royal College of Physicians being abolished with the passing of the Medical Act (see page 25). The GMC has several functions. Firstly, it has to keep a register of those who have obtained qualifying degrees entitling them to practice at large; it has also, by a subsequent amendment of the Act, to keep a separate register of those who have obtained higher degrees. Secondly, the GMC has to prescribe standards of medical education, to supervise this in approved teaching centres, and to visit such centres. Thirdly, the publication of the *British Pharmacopoiea* is the responsibility of the GMC. This is a book 'containing a list of medicines and compounds and the manner of preparing them, together with the true weights and measures by which they can be prepared and mixed . . .' Finally it has the duty to administer discipline. It is to the GMC that members of the medical profession or members of the public may make complaints if a doctor has behaved disgracefully or has been convicted by the courts. The council can then, if the charge is proved, direct that his name be erased from the register ('struck off').

OTHER PROFESSIONAL BODIES

There is a very wide range of professional societies and associations to which the doctor may belong. These organizations may be concerned with clinical, benevolent or medico-political matters, or with a combination of these, and there can be very few doctors who are not members of some of them. A list consisting of the names, addresses and secretaries of the more important is to be found in *The Medical Directory* and details of the work and scope of some of these is covered here.

The British Medical Association (BMA)

This association was founded in 1832 by Charles Hastings of Worcester. It now has nearly 65 000 members and is the largest medical association in Britain. It is concerned with nearly every aspect of medicine and medical affairs and is recognized as one of the principal bodies representing British doctors. Thus it is represented on the Central Health Services Council (see page 29). Through the General Medical Services Committee it is the principal negotiating body for GPs, and the Central Consultants' and Specialists' Committee acts on behalf of consultants. These latter two committees have autonomous powers in respect of matters relating to the NHS even though they are a part of the machinery of the association, and they have their local constituent bodies in the Local Medical Committees and the Regional Consultants' Committees.

The BMA itself is governed by the representative body which comprises elected members of all the regional divisions of the BMA and a number of ex-officio members and representatives. The Council of the BMA consists of some seventy doctors elected annually with a few ex-officio members, and is the executive of the association. The divisions are the units of the association and may be grouped together into branches, and each of these has its executive committee.

The other work of the association may be divided into four groups:
1 *Publishing.* Eighteen journals are published regularly of which the *British Medical Journal* has the widest circulation. This is sent out weekly and contains original papers, book reviews and articles, a correspondence section and classified advertisements about practices, hospital appointments and locum tenens. *Abstracts of World Medicine* covers the whole field of clinical medicine and there are sixteen specialist journals.

A number of books and pamphlets are published by the BMA Family Doctor Publications for health education purposes. There are at present about 70 titles in the series covering many aspects of health. Titles include *Having a Baby*, *Slim Safely*, *Facts of Life for Children* and *The Change of Life*. Although some doctors have supplies of them, they are most readily obtained from chemists or directly from Family Doctor Publications, 47/51 Chalton Street, London, NW1 1HT.
2 *Clinical.* The association organizes an annual clinical meeting and an annual scientific meeting which are held in different parts of the country from year to year. Branches and divisions will often arrange a programme of clinical meetings throughout the year and there are regional offices of the BMA in fourteen cities in the British Isles.
3 *Benevolent.* A number of medical charities are organized by the BMA and supported by functions arranged by divisions.
4 *Insurance.* The Medical Insurance Agency (MIA) was started in 1907 to obtain the best possible insurance terms for individual doctors.

The medical practitioner's union

This has about 5000 members drawn mainly from general practice. Although a much smaller organization than the BMA it covers the same varied fields of work, and has representation on various bodies that negotiate for the whole profession.

The 'Royal' colleges

The Royal College of Physicians of London
The Royal College of Surgeons of England
The Royal College of Physicians, Edinburgh
The Royal College of Surgeons of Edinburgh
The Royal College of Physicians and Surgeons of Glasgow

The Royal College of Physicians in Ireland
The Royal College of Surgeons in Ireland
The Royal College of Obstetricians and Gynaecologists
The Royal College of General Practitioners
The Royal College of Pathologists
The Royal College of Psychiatrists

These are examining bodies. They represent their membership on official committees and publish journals. They are also concerned with postgraduate education and research.

The Royal Society of Medicine

The Royal Society of Medicine is a clinical society with headquarters in London. It is divided into a number of sections, each of which covers a particular aspect of medicine. Proceedings are published every month.

10

Typescripts

Communication of medical facts between one doctor and another is normally carried out by means of a letter. This provides a permanent record and, as we shall see in later chapters, becomes an integral part of the medical record. The medical secretary, whether she is working in a hospital or for a doctor outside, will find that a great deal of importance is attached to the quality and accuracy of her work in this field. This applies not only to the letters that she types, for a personal secretary should also be able to compose a letter from brief notes. She may also be asked to type reports, minutes of meetings, manuscripts and scientific papers. The important points to be observed in all this work will be considered in this chapter.

THE MEDICAL LETTER

The medical letter is written from one doctor to another and is the confidential communication of medical facts between them. As in all her work the extreme importance of the confidential nature of these letters cannot be too highly stressed. Letters are sometimes dictated to the secretary and taken down in shorthand, but they may be typed at the time of dictation or typed from a recording machine.

Letters are an ambassador and an advertisement for the person sending them so it is essential that they are well displayed. Each doctor may prefer a particular method of display, but the following illustrate the principal letter styles: fully blocked (see Fig. 10.1) or semi-blocked (see Fig. 10.2). Many organizations are now using open punctuation in business letters. This means that no punctuation is inserted in the reference, date, name and address of addressee, salutation, complimentary close and any wording below.

1 *Reference.* A form of reference may be used to enable identification of the letter or typist. This usually consists of the initials of the dictator followed by the initials of the typist, e.g. REG/PET would mean that REG had dictated the letter and PET had typed it. When the patient is identified by a number, as in hospital, this number may follow, e.g. REG/PET 39600. This may be typed at the left-hand side of the page underneath the heading of the paper or in the bottom left-hand corner. When it is in reply to a letter already bearing a reference number this is typed as

> Your Ref.: PGB/BNS
> Our Ref.: REG/PET

A letter written by the typist will only bear the reference PET/–. The reference is typed two spaces below the heading and begins at the left-hand margin.

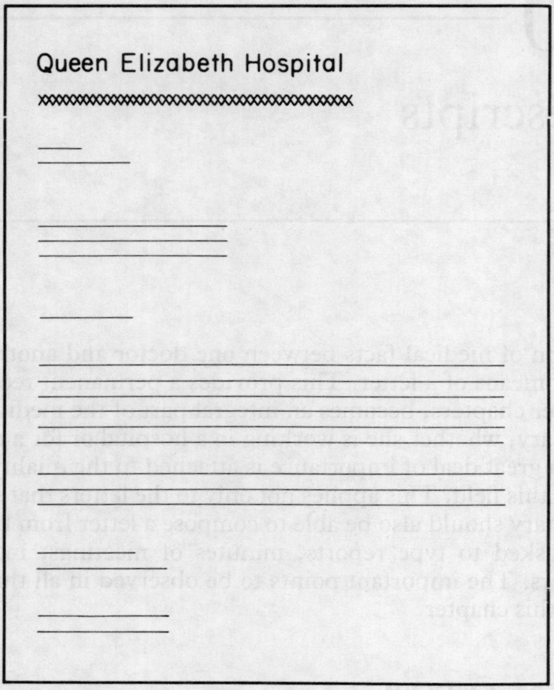

Queen Elizabeth Hospital

Fig. 10.1 An example of a fully blocked letter, each line begins at the left-hand margin.

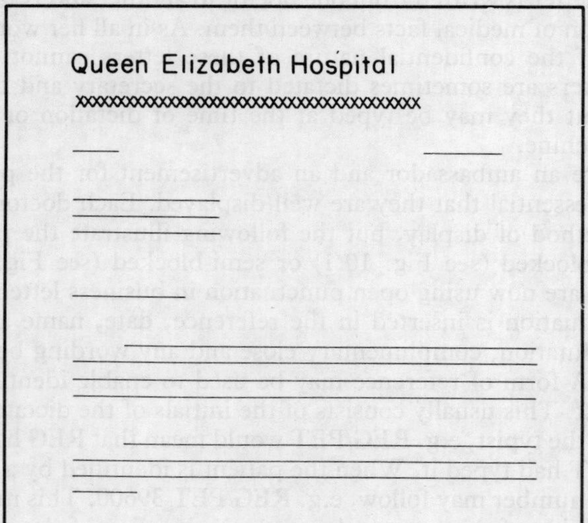

Queen Elizabeth Hospital

Fig. 10.2 An example of a semi-blocked letter with the date and complementary closing phrase as shown and the first line of each paragraph indented.

2 *The date.* This is typed in the order of the day, month and year:

22nd January, 1986

It is often typed two spaces below the heading on the paper, opposite or slightly lower than the reference and should end at the right-hand margin. Where the heading or printed address is in the centre of the notepaper the date is also centred.

3 *Inside address.* The inside address is typed on to the letter so that the retained carbon copy will show to whom the letter was sent. It is normally written two line spaces below the date and each line starts at the left-hand margin. In private correspondence this address is sometimes typed at the end of the letter, and when the letter is of a very personal nature may be omitted. In this case the secretary should remember to type it on to the retained carbon copy.

4 *Line spacing.* This will usually depend on the length of the letter and the size of the paper, but a turn over should be avoided if possible. Letters are normally centred with equal margins on both sides and at the bottom.

5 *The salutation.* This is usually typed two spaces below the reference and beginning at the left-hand margin. It is normally typed as:

Dear Dr Brown, (the full-stop after Dr or Mr is often avoided nowadays).

When the letter is of a personal nature the salutation may be hand-written by the dictator.

6 *The subject heading.* In medical letters this is normally the name, age and address of the patient referred to in the letter. It is centred over the writing line, two lines below the salutation, is underlined and there is no full-stop at the end:

Dear Dr Brown,

Mr Charles Harris, aged 50
120 Laburnum Grove, Fordhill, Lanchester

7 *Paragraphing.* A new paragraph is used every time the subject changes. If the paragraph is an exceptionally long one it may be broken at a convenient point as it is preferable to avoid one paragraph only. It is convenient to break most medical letters into three parts.

    (a) An acknowledgement:

        'Thank you for seeing this lady for me.' or 'Thank you for your letter about Mrs Jones who attended my clinic today.'

    (b) The body of the letter containing factual information such as the history and medical findings.

    (c) The final paragraph which contains an account of the action that is to be taken.

Each paragraph is normally indented five or more spaces, depending on the size of the type. When using blocked style leave two lines between paragraphs and start at the left-hand margin.

8 *The subscription.* When the letter has opened with the salutation 'Dear Mr Jones,' the subscription will be 'Yours sincerely'. If a greater degree of familiarity is shown by an opening of 'Dear Ted', the close will be:

With kind regards,
Yours sincerely,

or more familiarly, 'Yours' or 'Yours ever'.

The subscription will start five spaces to the left of the centre of the writing line and it is usual to type the name and sometimes the description of the signatory five lines below the subscription and ending at the right-hand margin, thus leaving room for the signature:

Yours sincerely,

R. E. GREEN, FRCS
Consultant Surgeon.

9 *Enclosures.* If reports or separate papers are enclosed with the letter the word 'Enc.' or 'Encs.' is typed at the bottom left-hand corner so that the recipient will not leave anything undiscovered in the envelope.

10 *Envelopes.* These should be of an appropriate size and should match the paper when possible.

11 *Continuation sheets.* The top of a continuation sheet should be typed with the headings:

Name of addressee   – 2 –   Date

In official documents a catchword is used at the bottom of each page and repeated at the top of the next page, e.g.

referred to me by his dental surgeon and I shall be
/admitting

'admitting' is then the first word of the first line upon the next page.

ADDRESSING DOCTORS

The mode of addressing a doctor is always a problem to the layperson and it is one that the secretary in her written communications will have to face daily.

In America and in all other European countries every medical person is addressed as 'Doctor', but there are historical reasons why surgeons, in Great Britain, are addressed as 'Mister' (see page 22). This applies to anyone who is a Fellow of the Royal College of Surgeons, but also includes the more specialized branches of surgery such as obstetrics and gynaecology, ophthalmological surgery, ear, nose and throat surgery, dental surgery, etc. (Lists of the various qualifying degrees and further qualifications are to be found in the Appendix.)

In personal communications diplomas and degrees are normally omitted, thus one doctor writing to another will address him as Dr J. Brown, Mr M. Jones, Professor B. Black, etc. In formal and business communications when diplomas and degrees are included the following rules are adopted:

1 Honours and decorations come before university degrees or diplomas, e.g. Sir John Dunn, KBE, CB, FRCS. (For the order in which decorations should be put the secretary must refer to *Whitaker's Almanack* or other reference books.)

2 Medical degrees take preference over surgical degrees, e.g. Mr J. Dunn, MD, FRCS.

3 Surgical degrees come before obstetrical qualifications, e.g. Mr J. Dunn, MD, FRCS, FRCOG.

When postgraduate degrees are held qualifying degrees may be omitted, e.g. Mr J. Dunn, FRCS (omitting his qualifying degree of MD, ChB).
4 University degrees take precedence over the qualifications of the Royal Colleges, which precede diplomas, e.g. Mr J. Dunn, MB, ChB, MSc, FRCS, DMR.
5 A useful device when writing to the medical profession is to drop the courtesy title and address the letter to J. Dunn, Esq., FRCS, not Mr J. Dunn, FRCS. Although 'Esquire' has, more or less, been dropped in the commercial world, it is useful inasmuch as some secretaries have difficulty during their early days divining which title to attach to which degrees; thus 'Esq.' eliminates the risk of inadvertently causing offence.

When the name and degrees appear as the author of a medical publication they will be written as J. Dunn, MD, FRCS (a surgeon's MD should always feature in his degrees). The secretary will see from this that there may be a number of different ways of addressing an individual doctor depending on the circumstances.

THE WRITTEN NUMERAL

A problem which sometimes confuses a secretary when typing medical manuscripts is when to use numbers in figures and when in words. The usage varies from journal to journal but these rules are safe to follow.
1 *Figures should be used for:*
   (a) dates—the day and year of the date, e.g. 1st June, 1986
   (b) quantities and measurements
   (c) the time when it comes before 'a.m.' or 'p.m.'
   (d) ages
   (e) statistics, and accounts of case series
   (f) references
   (g) addresses
2 *Words should be used for:*
   (a) the number ONE on its own and to start a sentence, e.g. 'Fourteen hundred and sixty-two white blood cells in each . . .'
   (b) round numbers over one hundred, e.g. six thousand
   (c) the time, when it comes before 'o' clock'
   (d) vague amounts, e.g. six or seven times
   (e) figures in legal documents
   (f) numbers up to 'ten'. However, if numbers both under and over 'ten' appear in the same piece of work words should be used for all numbers.

The most important rule is to be consistent.

SCIENTIFIC PAPERS

Much research work and investigation is undertaken by doctors and whilst it will not all be submitted for publication a great many doctors will publish papers recording their investigations in scientific journals. All medical and scientific writing should conform to a conventional pattern and this will usually fall under ten headings:

1 *Introduction*. This should state clearly and concisely what the paper is about and what points it hopes to establish. It is not a summary of conclusions but a statement of intention.

2 *Objects*. This will give an account of why investigation is being carried out and will often give a summary of the state of knowledge on the subject being investigated. It will usually contain a brief review of the relevant literature.

3 *Material*. This section will describe the material being investigated. This may consist of an account of the ages, social status or other facts about the group of patients investigated, details about the disease treated, the drug being tested, etc.

4 *Method*. The way in which the investigation is carried out is set out in this section. There will often be a detailed account of technical procedures, operations and accounts of the way in which measurements have been obtained.

5 *Results*. These will be set out as simply as possible. They may consist of descriptions of individual cases or they may be a statistical analysis of many results. Graphs, tables or histograms (numbers shown as different-sized blocks on graph paper) are used if this makes the results more easily understood.

6 *Discussion*. This is a comparison of the results obtained with the results of investigators in the same field. It will draw attention to points of similarity and points of difference.

7 *Conclusion*. The discussion of the results will lead the writer to certain conclusions and these will be set out clearly and unequivocally in this section.

8 *Summary*. This is always an important section. Most doctors or scientists are very busy people and there are a very large number of scientific publications appearing each week. The summary is added to the paper to enable people to see rapidly whether the paper is concerned with a subject or draws a conclusion that interests the reader. If it does the paper can be studied in detail at a more convenient time.

9 *Acknowledgements*. These are the acknowledgements to those who have helped or advised on the preparation of the paper.

10 *References*. The reason for listing references in a paper is to provide the reader with the source of evidence for statements made by the author. They have to be accurate, consistent in style and contain sufficient detail to allow them to be easily found by the reader.

In one system they are numbered sequentially in the text and then listed at the end of the paper in the same order. In an article a statement 'it has been shown[4]' would be the fourth to be mentioned and would be in fourth place in the list of references at the end.

Discussions are taking place to produce an international standard of references. Most medical journals use the 'Vancouver Agreement' and list them in this order: author(s), title of article, journal title, publication date, volume number and inclusive page numbers, e.g.

4 Jones, XY. Haemoglobin levels in Scottish schoolchildren. *Br med J* 1986; **12**: 361–365.

References to books indicate: author(s), or editor(s), the title, edition (if not the first), place of publication, publisher and date:

Smith, AB. *Medical memories*, 2nd ed., London, Baillière Tindall, 1986.

Other publications use a name/date system (e.g. Harvard system) in the form 'it has been shown by Smith (1986)'. The *Instructions to Authors* of the publication should always be consulted.

Manuscripts

These should be typed on A4 size paper, with double spacing, leaving a one-inch margin to each side and to top and bottom. Only one side of the paper is used. Two copies of the typescript should be sent to the publisher, including the top copy. One copy should always be retained. The pages of the typescript should be numbered consecutively starting with page one on the first page of the first chapter and going straight through to the last page of the last chapter. The title-page, preface, list of contents, etc., should be numbered separately in large or small roman numerals. Page numbers should be in the top right-hand corner and if there is any mistake in page numbering, or if extra pages have to be added, either renumber throughout or, more simply, call the new pages 125A, 125B, etc. In this case add at the foot of page 125 'pages 125A and B follow' and 'pages 125A and B precede' at top of page 126.

Headings, sub-headings, etc., should be standardized throughout the text. Headings and words calling for special typographical treatment are marked lightly in the text and a number pencilled in the margin which refers to a list, e.g.

1 chapter headings
2 chapter sub-headings
3 chapter sub-headings
4 side sub-headings
5 words requiring prominence in text
6 words requiring sub-prominence in text

Corrections to the text are made in ink, above the line to be altered or where the insertion is to be made and not in the margin. If a large section is to be altered or inserted, it should be typed out on a separate sheet, which should state its position in the text, while the text itself should be marked to show that an insertion is to be made.

It may sometimes be necessary for the secretary to send work directly to the typesetter. In this case she must state her employer's requirements as to the type-sizes and style to be used, the quality of the paper on to which the work is to be printed, quantity of copies wanted, etc.

Whether she is dealing with the typesetter or the publisher she will receive two sets of proofs. One should be checked carefully against the manuscript, but before demanding alterations she must consider what they will cost. (The cost of the typesetter's own typographical errors are usually borne by him; the cost of any other alterations is very high.)

The proof is then marked in both the text and margin by the correction signs shown in *Copy Preparation and Proof Correction*. Should the corrections be so many that a further proof is required from the printer mark it 'Revise'; otherwise, they should be marked 'Press after Corrections'. The second set of proofs is given identical marks and kept for reference.

INFORMATION RETRIEVAL

Advances in medicine are generally first reported in scientific journals but the information explosion that has occurred in the last 20 years has meant that the number of journals published has risen so dramatically that no doctor doing research work can keep abreast of developments by reading the journals. To help him find the information sophisticated methods of indexing this mass of material have been developed. These consist of either the printed book or computer systems.

Index Medicus is the most widely used book-based system but even this is produced by a computer-aided method to increase speed. The first step in retrieving information is to consult the list of medical subject headings (known as MeSH). This is updated every year and contains the most commonly used medical terms, but as these are added to every year it is possible that the 'MeSH' heading you are looking for was not used in earlier years.

To begin with you can establish that a heading exists in MeSH for the subject you are looking for. If you look up the term 'hemicrania' you will find—HEMICRANIA *see* MIGRAINE. This shows that all papers on 'hemicrania' are listed as 'Migraine'. It may also list with it related terms under which you will find articles of interest, e.g. with Mental Health Services

see related   Halfway Houses,
Hospitals, psychiatric departments,
Hospitals, psychiatric.

Next, by a numerical code you are guided from Section 1 to Section 2 in which the subjects are listed in a progressively more specific manner,

e.g.   gastrointestinal diseases   C6.405
intestinal diseases   C6.405.469
colonic diseases   C6.405.469.158
colitis   C6.405.469.158.188
ulcerative colitis   C6.405.469.158.188.231

The final article is always listed under the most specific heading available, so ulcerative colitis will only be found under that heading and not any of the previous ones and this saves looking through a long list of irrelevant articles.

Index Medicus is published each month and provides references from more than 3000 journals. In the first half, references are listed under these subject headings. If, for example, 'Ulcerative Colitis' is looked up, all articles on ulcerative colitis that have appeared in the year of this volume are listed with the English language references first, followed by those in foreign languages. The second half of *Index Medicus* consists of an author index which enables you to search for papers written by a particular individual.

Searches through *Index Medicus*, although very much more speedy than searches through the indexes of many journals, are always somewhat time consuming and it is now possible to question a central store of records kept in a computer and obtain a list of all the references printed out at a terminal in about seven minutes. There are now a number of commercial firms that provide the supply service to libraries, information centres and individuals although they do not themselves set up the central data base. Major data base suppliers include British Library (BLAISE), Lockheed Information Systems (DIALOG) and System Development Corporation (ORBIT).

The search is carried out at a computer terminal using a form of typewriter linked to the computer by a telephone line. The researcher asks for references on a subject such as 'asthma'. It is possible to refine this by combining it with a set of references on 'hypnosis' so that the final list, shown either on a visual display unit (VDU) or printed out, refers only to articles in which hypnosis has been used to treat asthma.

The researcher can, through this system, have a regular 'tailormade', up-to-date list of references sent to him on the subject of his particular interest, although he does, of course, still have to find the original articles and read them.

COMMITTEE WORK

Many doctors serve on committees. They may be staff committees, local medical committees, or committees concerned with outside interests and the secretary may be asked to type the agenda or the minutes.

The agenda

This is a programme of the work to be done at the meeting. It is usually prepared by the chairman and there is a standard order of procedure. Sufficient copies of the agenda should be prepared so that each member of the committee can have one. These are the standard headings that commonly appear on the agenda:
1 the place, date and time of the meeting
2 apologies for absence
3 minutes of last meeting (these will be read, confirmed as correct and signed by the chairman)
4 business arising out of the minutes
5 correspondence

After this is taken the main business of the meeting in order (5 to 7). This may include reports by members of the committee. Finally
8 any other business
9 date of next meeting

The minutes

These will normally be kept by one of the committee members who has been nominated as the secretary of that committee. The minutes record the name of the committee, the place, date and time of meeting. The members present are listed, followed by those who send apologies for absence. The minutes then follow the items on the agenda noting, in particular, any decisions that have been made. In typing the minutes the secretary may come across certain unfamiliar words which are peculiar to committee work or to the procedure at meetings.

- Ad hoc—means 'arranged for this purpose'. An ad hoc committee is one arranged to deal with a specific problem
- Addendum—means 'an addition to'
- Amendment—a proposal to alter a motion by adding or leaving out words. It is voted on before the motion
- Casting vote—second vote used by the chairman when an equal number of votes are cast for and against a motion
- Cooption—the power a committee has to elect additional members to the committee
- Ex-officio—meaning 'by virtue of office'
- Motion—the words framing the proposal under discussion. When put to the meeting it becomes 'the question' and when passed 'the resolution'
- Nem Con—means 'no one contradicting', or no one voting against (some may abstain)
- Unanimous—when everyone present votes the same way

11

The Secretary and Finance

In general practice and Consultant private practice it will be the responsibility of the secretary to manage the normal day-to-day financial affairs of the practice. This will usually consist of three duties:
1 paying bills
2 sending accounts to patients and receipting where necessary
3 keeping the books for the accountant

In order to understand the processes involved in this work it is essential to have knowledge of the mechanics of the banking system.

THE CHEQUE

When a cheque is written it is an order for a bank to pay to the account of another person a certain sum of money. In fact there is no passing of cash between the banks. They make use of the Clearing House at the Bank of England. A bill is paid by issuing a creditor with a cheque. This cheque is paid by the creditor straight into his account. The creditor's bank does not demand a cash payment from the debtor's bank but uses the cheque as part of the balancing settlement in the Clearing House. An example of the way this works can be set out as follows.

As a secretary to a doctor you send, on his behalf, a cheque to John Harris Ltd, from whom he has bought some books. This cheque for £6.00 is paid by John Harris Ltd into their bank (Lloyds, High Street) who credit the account of John Harris Ltd with this amount. The cheque was drawn on your bank (Midland, East Gate Street) and at the end of the day that £6.00 will form part of a balancing settlement between Lloyds Bank and the Midland Bank and will either increase or decrease the accounts of Lloyds and Midland at the Bank of England. The cheque will then be returned to the Midland Bank, East Gate Street, who will debit the doctor's account with £6.00. Thus the debt has been settled without any cash being transferred.

Opening an account

This can normally be done by anyone who pays a sum of money into the bank. As a means of securing themselves against fraud and default the bank will make certain other demands. They will want a personal recommendation from someone who is already known to the bank and they will also require two references from people who are acceptable to them.

Before they issue a cheque book they will require a specimen signature and each cheque must be signed in exactly the same way. Cheques are normally issued in books containing from 10 to 500 blank cheque forms. Accounts are handled by computers and each cheque will have printed on it the cheque number, the customer's account number, the bank branch number and the name of the customer.

It is possible for accounts to be opened in the names of two or more people. Commonly this is done with husband and wife but joint accounts, as they are known, are opened by partnerships and thus cheques can be signed by any one of the partners.

There are two types of account: (1) current account, and (2) deposit account.

The *current account* is the one on which cheques are normally drawn and into which sums of money are paid. Transactions can take place immediately and the bank may make a charge for keeping the accounts.

If the account becomes overdrawn the bank will charge a fixed rate of interest on this sum; this is usually about 2% above the Minimum Lending Rate, which is the rate of interest that the Bank of England is prepared to lend money at. If the account remains above a specified credit balance it is common for the bank to make no charge for keeping the accounts.

Deposit accounts are really reserve accounts in which a sum of money is put aside. The depositor agrees not to withdraw the money without giving notice, and thus the bank is able to use this money. The bank will pay a rate of interest of about 2% below the Minimum Lending Rate for this use. The current account cheque book cannot be used to withdraw money from the deposit account.

Drawing a cheque

The cheque is usually made out by the secretary but can only be signed by the person in whose name the account stands, or in the case of a joint account by

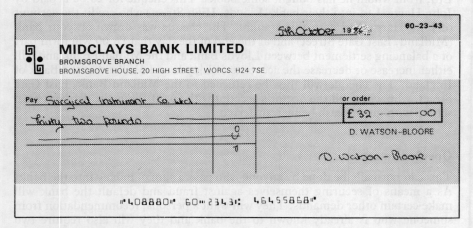

Fig. 11.1 A specimen cheque.

one of the holders. There are certain details which must be correctly inserted on every cheque (Fig. 11.1). These are:

1 the date, month and year
2 the name of the person to whom the cheque is to be paid. This should be the same wording as that on the account
3 the sum of money to be paid, written first in words and then in figures
4 the signature, which must be the same as the specimen signature that the bank holds

Certain important points must be made here. The entries on any cheque must start as near as possible to the left-hand side of the appropriate space on the cheque and any gap in this space which is left after the words have been inserted should be filled with a dash or the word 'only', so that no other words or figures can be added. Any alteration which is made to a cheque must be either signed or initialled by the person who has signed the cheque. The importance of these points lies in the fact that whereas the bank is liable to pay any loss incurred when a cheque has been altered and not signed, it is not liable to pay if the cheque has been drawn so badly that an alteration has been made possible because of this fact.

Cheques may be made out 'To order' or 'To bearer'. This enables cash to be drawn by the person presenting the cheque, but he must write his name on the back of the cheque. This is known as 'endorsing' the cheque. It used to be common to make cheques out 'To bearer', but this is now rarely done because these cheques may be cashed without endorsement and are therefore liable to abuse. Prior to 1957 it was necessary for the payee to endorse every cheque, but the Cheques Act of 1957 lays down that it is no longer necessary to endorse cheques which are paid directly into a payee's account. When a cheque is drawn it is very important to fill in the counterfoil or 'stub' accurately as this will be used to check the bank statement.

Crossing a cheque

A cheque may be presented at the bank on which it was drawn in exchange for cash, but, as mentioned before, it must then be endorsed on the back by the payee. It will be seen that it is possible for someone else to present a cheque which they have found or stolen in exchange for cash. In order to prevent this occurring a system of 'crossing' a cheque has been developed. This consists of drawing two lines across the front of the cheque. It is usual to write the words 'and Co.' between these lines, although in point of fact this is not necessary. The effect of crossing a cheque in this manner is to ensure that it can only be paid into a bank account and cannot be exchanged for cash unless the cheque is specifically made out 'Please pay cash', or to 'cash'. Some cheques are printed 'crossed'. If cash is required the payer must write 'pay cash' over the 'cross' and sign it.

Paying-in

When cheques and cash are paid into the bank one of the paying-in forms issued by the bank should be used (Fig. 11.2). These are issed in books. Each one consists of two portions, one of which is retained by the bank and the other

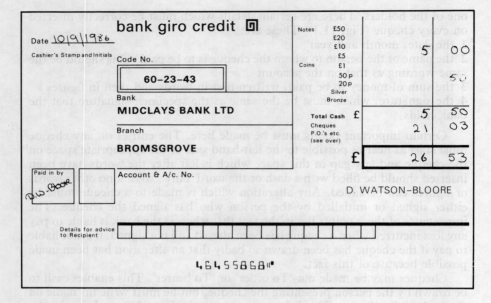

Fig. 11.2 A specimen paying-in cheque.

retained by the person paying in. It is important to see that both portions are correctly filled in and that the portion retained by the secretary is both initialled and stamped by the bank. This official receipt is an important protection. It is wise for the secretary to pay cheques and cash into the bank as soon as possible. Money should always be kept under lock and key, and large sums should never be kept in the surgery as there is a limit to the protection given by ordinary insurance coverage.

Stopping a cheque

This process is used when a cheque has been lost or when it is necessary to cancel a cheque that has been sent out. The cheque is 'stopped' by asking the bank to stop payment if the cheque is presented. The bank will need to know the name of the payee, the date and the number of the cheque.

Bank statements

Every bank keeps a list of the credit and debits passed through a customer's account. At intervals agreed with the customer, they send out a loose-leaf sheet called a statement (Fig. 11.3). They may include with this all the paid cheques that are dealt with in the statement. These statements are numbered so that they can be placed in the holder kept by the customer in the correct order. Cheques used to be identified on the statement by the name of the payee, but it is customary now to identify them by the last three figures of the serial number on the cheque. Debits and credits are listed and the balance is brought down at each entry.

Date	Detail	Debits	Credits	Balance

D. WATSON–BLOORE
46455369

In account with
MIDCLAYS BANK LTD

1986

BROMSGROVE   60 2343

Date	Detail		Debits	Credits	Balance
18JUL	Balance forward	406315	58.55		691.84
		406316	93.63		539.66
19JUL	DD STANDARD LIFE		3.49		
	DEPOSIT ACCOUNT	TR	15.00		
	CASH/CHEQUES			13.75	
	TR FROM D/A			500.00	1,034.92
22JUL		405197	79.20		955.72
23JUL		406317	20.00		935.72
24JUL		405199	160.18		775.54
25JUL		406321	15.00		760.54
26JUL		406319	17.77		
		406323	38.27		
	DEPOSIT ACCOUNT	TR	15.00		689.50
30JUL		406320	4.50		
		406324	10.00		
	CASH/CHEQUES			67.21	
	CASH/CHEQUES			84.42	826.63
1AUG		406325	10.00		816.63

Abbreviations:	CD Cash Dispenser	DV Dividend	TR Transfer	O/D indicates an
	DD Direct Debit	SO Standing Order		Overdrawn Balance

Fig. 11.3 A bank statement.

It is the responsibility of the secretary to check this statement against the counterfoils of cheques which have been retained. It should be noted that the statement will also include details of bank-charges, standing orders and credit transfers. The *standing* or *banker's order* to pay a regular sum to the same payee on a given date each week, month, quarter, etc., is an instruction given to the bank. A *credit transfer* is a means of paying an account by a direct transfer of money from one bank to another. Until this system was introduced it was necessary to write a separate cheque and use envelopes and postage in each case. With credit transfer one fills in a form for each of the bills to be paid and sends or takes the forms, with a list and one cheque covering the total amount, to the bank. The bank will then pay to the accounts of the various payees the appropriate amounts. Thus, however many bills are paid only one cheque and one envelope are needed. These slips are then distributed to the branch bank and then to the payee as an advice.

DIRECT DEBIT (VARIABLE DIRECT DEBIT)

A direct debit payment differs from a standing order in that it is the payee who initiates payment by sending an order, previously signed by the payee, to the bank, and not the bank that starts it off. It is possible to arrange a variable direct debit so that subscriptions, say, can be increased periodically to take account of inflation, without having to go back to the subscriber each time.

CREDIT CARDS

By the use of credit cards it is possible to make a purchase of goods or services and to pay at a later date. This avoids the necessity of carrying large quantities of cash. Cards are issued by some large stores for use by customers in any of their branches, by banks whose cards may be recognized in shops, hotels, railway booking offices and so on, and by companies such as American Express that are recognized internationally. They certainly are convenient, but, owing to the rates of interest charged, are a relatively expensive way of obtaining credit. Many businesses will only accept a cheque in payment for goods and services if the person paying produces a bank card at the same time.

AUTOMATIC CASH DISPENSER

Many banks have installed machines whereby customers can draw a limited amount of cash, say £100.00, by tapping out a personal code number and inserting a special voucher. These machines can be used at times when the bank is closed.

BANK CHARGES

Banks may make charges for the services they provide such as the transactions of paying in money, drawing out cash and so on. These charges can be minimized by observing the various tariffs adopted by the particular bank. For instance if the amount left in an account never falls below £50.00, or if the average amount kept on account for a half-yearly period is not less than £100.00, services may be free. A good secretary will make it her responsibility to advise her employers how these arrangements can be best used for their particular circumstances.

PAYING ACCOUNTS

Accounts may be paid by cheque or by cash. It is customary to pay sums of £1 and over by cheque and lesser amounts in cash. Before paying any account the secretary should satisfy herself that the account is correct and has not previously been paid. It is often wise to get the doctor to initial an account as an approval of payment. It is a normal custom to collect amounts together for payment so that this can be done at the end of each month.

If a receipt is needed then the account should be returned with the cheque and a formal receipt requested.

Filing receipts

When these receipts mentioned above are returned, the secretary will file them in a simple sprung box file. She will file with these the unreceipted accounts to which have been attached the appropriate cheque returned by the bank with the statement. This serves as a receipt in this case. Included in the receipt file are the remaining returned cheques settling debts for which no account was rendered, e.g. wages and salaries. When these are filed in the correct order, a true record of all accounts paid, apart from standing orders, is achieved.

SENDING OUT ACCOUNTS

Accounts will be sent out by the secretary only to patients treated privately. Here it should be noted that a doctor may be called upon to attend another doctor. In these circumstances he will abide by the traditional practice of not making any direct charge for treating him or his dependants. It is not customary to specify the services rendered but the account is couched in general terms 'To Professional Services rendered'. It is usual to send these accounts out monthly or quarterly but a certain amount of flexibility is required here. It is not tactful to send out an account to a patient who has been seen on the last day of a month so that he receives it the next day. On the other hand, the executors of a patient who has died will not thank the doctor who delays matters by waiting three months before sending in his account.

These accounts are kept either in a ledger form or card-index form, so that a note can be made of the fee chargeable and the date on which the attention was given.

Specially printed ledgers and account cards for doctors can be obtained.

BOOKKEEPING

Bookkeeping systems have been in use since ancient times. Records of commercial contracts have been found in the ruins of ancient Babylon. Very excellent systems of double-entry accounting were those of the Massari of Genoa in 1340, so the system must have been in use long before then.

As far as the medical secretary is concerned, the simplest method of bookkeeping is the best. There are a number of different methods of recording the accounts but all are intended to record, classify and summarize the financial transactions.

A doctor's bookkeeping system is usually based on an *Analysis Cash Book* (Fig. 11.4). In this book all receipts and expenditure are listed in columns under the appropriate headings. It is possible to buy analysis cash books specially designed for doctors or, depending on the type of work done, the headings can be written in by the secretary.

It is customary to enter all receipts on the left-hand side and all expenditure on the right-hand side where a single analysis book is used. It is possible to run two books, one for receipts and one for expenditure, but items have a habit of getting put down in the wrong book. It must be stressed here that the job of the secretary is not one of accountancy. It is only necessary to record

RECEIPTS				PAYMENTS			
DATE	DETAILS	FOLIO	AMOUNT	DATE	DETAILS	FOLIO	AMOUNT

PAYMENTS ANALYSIS

SUNDRIES

RENT RATES AND INSURANCE	REPAIRS RENEWALS AND MAINTENANCE	SALARIES AND WAGES	PETTY CASH	BANK LEGAL AND ACCOUNTANTS CHARGES	DRESSINGS DRUGS AND INSTRUMENTS	TRANSPORT EXPENSES

Fig. 11.4 An analysis book.

expenditure and receipts in a simple logical way. By this means it is possible for the accountant to do his work at the end of the financial year without having to ask numerous questions and without missing items of expenditure that have not been recorded.

In the analysis book the top and bottom lines on each page are left blank in order that the accountant can add each column of figures. Each item is recorded twice: once in a column which will give the sum total of all expenditure and receipts and then separately, analysed under the appropriate heading. By this means it is possible to find out not only what the total expenditure is but also what fraction has been spent on, say, drugs and dressings. It is important to be very neat and very accurate at this work.

Petty cash

There are always a number of small transactions in the running of a business. There are postage-stamps and milk to be paid for and cleaners who want to be paid in cash. It is to deal with all these that the petty cash box is kept. This is started with an 'imprest' of a sum sufficient to cover cash expenses for a week. This imprest, a sum of say £5.00–£20.00, is drawn from the general account by a cheque through the main cash book. A separate petty cash book is maintained analysing all expenditure and at the end of each week a sum of money is drawn by cheque to restore the figure of the float to the original sum. There are certain accounts which are normally paid by cheque, such as car expenses, which occasionally it may be more convenient to settle in cash when the sum is small. In these circumstances a petty cash slip (see example, Fig. 11.5) is filled up recording the date, details of the expenditure and the amount paid. The sum should then be entered in the 'sundries' column of the petty cash book and identified so that the accountant, when analysing total expenditure, can identify it as belonging to a column of the analysis cash book.

1 See that the cash box is kept under lock and key at all times.
2 Never remove money from, or add it to, the cash box without completing a petty cash slip and entering the amount in the petty cash book.
3 Never keep a large sum of money in the cash box.

INCOME TAX

In the normal course of events the medical secretary will have little to do with the preparation of figures for Schedule D Income Tax. It is, however, necessary to explain the nature of this tax so that she can understand the importance of accurate bookkeeping. Schedule D Tax deals, amongst other items, with incomes derived from professions and vocations not included under other schedules. These last words are important because a doctor who receives a salary from an employer will find that that part of his income is taxed under Schedule E. The distinction between the two lies in the special allowances which may be claimed. These allowances are based on the expenses that are incurred in the pursuit of the profession. In Schedule D it is expenses incurred wholly and exclusively in earning the income, and in Schedule E it is expenses incurred wholly exclusively and *necessarily* in earning the income. Thus it is important to see that all expenses incurred are properly recorded.

PAYE

Pay-as-you-earn is the name applied to the method of deducting tax related to the weekly, monthly or annual salary or wage. It is part of the Schedule E section and under it the employers are responsible for making the correct deduction before paying the salary. In practice the doctor will probably expect his secretary to do this for him. Full details will be found in *Employers' Guide to 'Pay as you earn'* issued by the Board of Inland Revenue, but the basic facts are given below.

1 the amount of tax deducted depends on:
  (*a*) the employee's total gross pay since the beginning of the income tax year
  (*b*) his income tax allowance for the same period (determined by his 'code number')
  (*c*) the total tax deducted on previous pay days.

2 Every pay day the employer adds the pay due to the total already paid to the employee from 6th April to that date. He then finds in the free pay table (Table A) for the employee's code number the employee's allowances up to that date and subtracts this from the previous figure. Then he looks up this resulting figure in the taxable pay table (Table B) and this shows the total tax due to date. From this he deducts the tax already deducted and this gives him the amount of tax due on the pay day in question.

This procedure is simplified by keeping a *Wages Book* (Fig. 11.6) which shows not only wages and PAYE but National Insurance contributions as well.

Deduction cards, known as form P11, are provided by the Inland Revenue for each employee. Column one shows the amount of Graduated Pension deducted (shown in the tables provided by the DHSS), column two shows the weekly or monthly gross earnings, column three the total gross pay to date. The total free pay is found in Table A as above and entered in column four. This amount subtracted from the gross pay gives the figure for column five. Reference to Table B gives the figures for the last two columns, six and seven.

Any new employee who has been working before will bring with them Parts 2 and 3 of form P45. This will have details of previous earnings and tax deductions in the current year and these are entered on the new PAYE deduction card. Part 3 will then be sent to the local tax office.

When an employee leaves form P45 is completed, part 1 sent to the tax office and parts 2 and 3 are given to the employee.

NATIONAL INSURANCE SCHEME

In April 1975 radical changes took place in the method of contributing to the National Insurance scheme. Contributions are now based on earnings and deducted in a similar way to PAYE. The National Insurance cards and stamps have been abolished. The medical secretary should acquaint herself with the regulations. Information leaflets may be obtained from local offices of the DHSS and these include leaflets NP15, NP7 and NP18. Forms with which the secretary will be involved are detailed in Chapter 29.

CASH RECEIVED			DATE	CASH PAID	VOUCHER NO.	PETTY CASH
DATE	FOLIO	AMOUNT		DETAILS		AMOUNT

Fig. 11.5 A petty cash book.

NO.	NAME	TAX CODE	HRS.	RATE	OVER-TIME	GROSS PAY	GROSS PAY TO DATE	FREE PAY TO DATE	TAXABLE PAY TO DATE	TAX DUE TO DATE	TAX REFUNDS

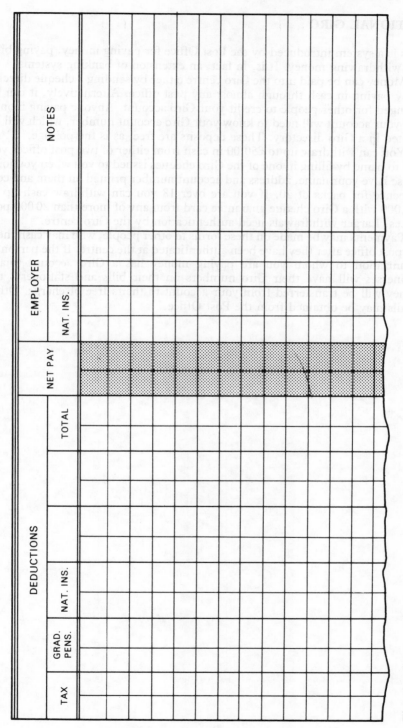

Fig. 11.6 A wages book.

NATIONAL GIRO

This is a system introduced by the Post Office for paying money, paying bills and withdrawing money. It is, in fact, an extension of banking systems.

Money can be paid into the Giro centre either by sending a cheque directly or by paying in cash through almost any post office. Alternatively, it can be arranged for other people to credit your Giro account. Anyone paying money into your account will need to know your Giro account number, which will be printed in a Giro directory. These deposits are free, as is the postage.

You can withdraw up to £50.00 in cash from either of two post offices you care to name by filling in one of the Giro cheques issued to you when you join. These have your name, address and account number printed on them and cost 10 pence for packs of 20. If you are over 18 you can withdraw cash up to £50.000 with a Giro cheque guarantee card from any of more than 20 000 post offices. Larger withdrawals need authentication by the Giro centre.

Payments may be made on these forms to other people, who may cash them at a post office after they have been authenticated at the centre. If the person or organization to whom you are paying money has a Giro account (many businesses will have their Giro numbers on their bills and stationery) the money will be transferred from your account to theirs free of charge. Other details may be obtained from the Post Office.

12

The Telephone and the Post Office

In Great Britain there is one telephone for every six persons in the country, more than in any other European country. The telephone has thus become of increasing importance in everyone's life and the medical secretary is not excluded. Thirty years ago her work consisted almost entirely of written correspondence; today an equally important part is taken by the telephone.

The advantage of the telephone is that it is often cheaper and quicker than writing a letter. An answer to a problem may be obtained at once and it has been calculated that, when dictator's and typist's time have been taken into consideration, as well as stationery and stamps, it may cost more than 40 pence to send a single letter. The disadvantage of the telephone is that no permanent record of decisions and opinions is kept and when medical details have to be communicated this is a very important factor. It is, therefore, necessary for the medical secretary to develop a good technique for using the telephone and to have a clear understanding of different telephone systems and methods.

RECEIVING A TELEPHONE CALL

The medical secretary is regarded by the person who is making the call as the representative of the doctor, and she should develop a clear and courteous manner of speaking.

When answering an incoming call:

1 Speak clearly and slowly and never say 'Hallo'. The correct form is to tell the caller to whom he is speaking by saying 'Dr Jones' secretary' or 'Dr Jones' consulting rooms', or 'Dr Jones' surgery'.

2 Pitch the voice at a low level (higher notes are more difficult to hear), do not speak too loudly and enunciate consonants very clearly.

3 If the caller is cut off before completing the message, the secretary should replace her receiver. It is the responsibility of the person who is making the call to re-establish the connection. Similarly it is the custom for the person originating the call to end it by saying 'Good-bye' when the conversation is finished.

4 A notebook and pen must always be kept by the telephone; messages written down on loose scraps of paper will be lost.

Recording a message

As mentioned before, all messages should be written in a book provided for this purpose. The telephone receiver should be in a position on the desk so that it can be picked up with the left hand; this leaves the right hand free to write. Every message should be preceded with the date and time of receipt and should have the name, address, and, where necessary, the telephone number of the caller. The message should be written down and important details, such as names, addresses, doses of drugs or descriptions of illnesses repeated to the caller so that they can be checked.

If arrangements have to be made on the telephone by the secretary they should depend on positive action; for example, never say 'If you don't hear from me you will know that I have heard from him'. The correct action would be 'I will ring you to confirm that I have heard from him'. This way there is no room for doubt.

If a message is received by the secretary which calls for action that she cannot take herself, she should make a note of the caller's name, address and telephone number and then take one of four steps:
1 Transfer the call to someone that she knows is able to take positive action.
2 Arrange for the caller to be rung back.
3 Ask the caller to ring back at a time when she knows action can be taken.
4 Take a clear message and undertake to see that action is taken.

At no stage should the caller be left for any long period in silence on the telephone. There should be a periodic reassurance that the matter is in hand and an apology for delay.

The secretary will normally find herself acting as the intermediary between the doctor and the caller and she should remember that this is an important part of the job that she has been trained for. On no occasion should a telephone call be put through to the doctor without informing him first and making sure that he wishes to take the call. The telephone in the doctor's consulting room may be on the same line as the telephone in the secretary's office, but a special device will prevent the doctor's telephone bell from ringing and all outside calls will be taken by the secretary. Here is an example of the procedure that should be followed:

Secretary: Mr Edwards' consulting rooms. Good morning.
Caller: May I speak to Mr Edwards, please?
Secretary: Who is calling, please?
Caller: Mrs Mary Jones.
Secretary: Would you hold the line, please, Mrs Jones. I will see if Mr Edwards is available.

The secretary can then speak to Mr Edwards on an internal communication system and if Mr Edwards does not wish to, or is unable to take the call, she can say: 'I am afraid that Mr Edwards is engaged at the moment. May I take a message, Mrs Jones?'

In most cases the secretary will be able to judge from experience whether the caller needs to speak to the doctor. If it is another doctor on the telephone that will almost invariably be the case but at most other times the secretary will endeavour to discover the gist of the matter herself. She may then find that she can deal with some of the problems herself, or arrange for them to be dealt with by someone else later, or she may have to seek advice on the right course of action to be followed from the doctor.

There is a great variety of types of equipment available today and if more than one or two internal telephones are in use, say in a group practice or when several Consultants share rooms for private consulting, there will be a small switchboard enabling outside calls to be held or a variety of internal connections to be made.

MAKING A TELEPHONE CALL

Before making any out-going calls the secretary should be quite clear to whom she wishes to speak and what she wishes to say. These may seem rather elementary points but a great deal of time and energy can be wasted if the secretary has not considered them. It is no good pouring out a long story to a junior clerk, who is not capable of answering a question or making a decision, only to find that it all has to be repeated to the superior. Similarly it is a waste of everyone's time to embark on a telephone conversation and then find that the facts required are not to hand.

The out-going call may be made from a direct outside line, in which case the number can be dialled as soon as the dialling tone is heard. If it is an extension line in a hospital, then it is necessary to say to the switchboard operator, 'Would you get me . . . please?' or if you have a receiver with a dial 'Would you give me a line, please?' When the dialling tone is heard the number can be dialled. Dialling should be done slowly and deliberately and when long combinations of letters and numbers are to be dialled, they should be written down first.

There are certain rules to be observed when asking an operator for a number.

1 Give the numbers in pairs; e.g. 4131 would be said, four one—pause—three one.

2 A pair of numbers is referred to as a double; e.g. 4431 is double four—pause—three one.

3 The figure 0 is referred to as a nought, two noughts become a hundred, and three noughts become a thousand; e.g. 4000 is four thousand.

It may be necessary to spell words on the telephone, and the standard GPO alphabetical code should be used for this purpose:

A for Andrew	J for Jack	S for Sugar
B for Benjamin	K for King	T for Tommy
C for Charlie	L for Lucy	U for Uncle
D for David	M for Mary	V for Victory
E for England	N for Nellie	W for William
F for Frederick	O for Oliver	X for Xmas
G for George	P for Peter	Y for York
H for Harry	Q for Queenie	Z for Zebra
I for Isaac	R for Robert	

If a caller is connected to a wrong number the caller should apologize for any inconvenience caused even though the fault may not be hers. The secretary should also avoid sending or receiving personal telephone calls unless they are urgent. She should maintain a complete and up-to-date list of any telephone numbers likely to be used frequently. This may be kept in a book but a strip index board provides a quick and convenient method.

TELEPHONE SERVICES

There are a wide range of telephone services with which the secretary should be familiar

Local calls

These are made to another line on any exchange in the area shown on the map in the front of the telephone directory. The current scale of charges is shown in every telephone directory.

Trunk calls

These are calls to areas outside the local area which are charged according to length of call and distance. There are three rates: peak rate from 9.00 a.m. to 1.00 p.m., Monday to Friday; standard rate from 8.00 a.m. to 9.00 a.m. and from 1.00 p.m. to 6.00 p.m. Monday to Friday; and cheap rate at all other times.

Subscriber trunk dialling (STD)

Most subscribers are now on exchanges that are reached by direct dialling using the code number. These codes now also apply to many other countries in the world and details of these can be found within the telephone directory.

Telephone calls from coin boxes are made after inserting coins and the call proceeds for the length of time 'bought'. It is also possible to use a special 'credit card' in certain coinless boxes.

Personal calls

The charge for a timed call begins when the number is answered. If a 'personal call' is made charging does not start until the caller speaks to the person required, or a substitute who is acceptable. If he cannot be traced only the personal call fee is payable. With STD it may be cheaper to dial a call and ask for a message to be given to the person required asking him to ring back.

Transferred calls

If the person being called is willing to pay the charge this can be arranged by asking the operator for a 'transferred call' to be made.

Credit card (See also Subscriber trunk dialling)

Calls can be made from any telephone and charged to your own account by the use of a credit card. The caller must quote the number on his card to the operator.

Other services which are available include emergency calls (999), telemessage, weather forecasts, time, a recorded recipe, test match scores, and alarm calls (calls from the General Post Office [GPO] made at specified times, usually to waken people in the morning). Details of these are given in the telephone directories.

Telephone transfer arrangements

Certain arrangements may have to be made in private consultant practice or general practice to have calls attended to when the telephone is unmanned. There are three available methods.

Internal switchboard. Incoming calls can be diverted from one number to another by the use of a small internal switchboard installed by the GPO (Fig. 12.1).

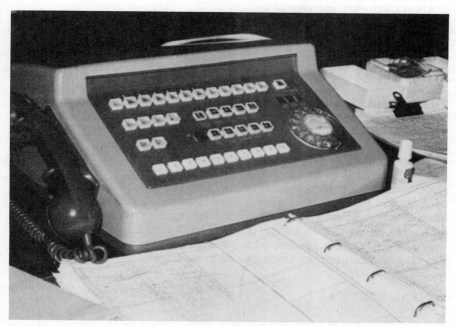

Fig. 12.1 A switchboard at the appointment desk.

Interrupted call. Arrangements can be made for calls to be intercepted by the GPO and redirected to another number on request.

'Ansafone'. This piece of equipment is a tape-recorder which can be connected to the telephone and which will deliver a recorded message, or record an incoming call. When a call is made to a number connected to such an instrument a voice may be heard saying 'Dr Jones is not on duty, please call Bloxwich 7477', or 'This is an "Ansafone". Please give your name and address and record the message you want to now ———'. Phrases like this will be heard

by any caller and the tape bearing the answer can be played back at a later date. The GPO will install a tape-recorder connected to the telephone which, whilst not recording an incoming message, will deliver a message. These should be clear and precise, such as 'This is Bloxwich 7477, doctor's surgery. The surgery is now closed until 8.30 in the morning. In case of emergency please ring Dr Jones at Bloxwich 4269, Bloxwich 4269'.

Radiotransmitters. Whilst not strictly a telephone transfer system, secretaries should be aware that some practices, especially in rural areas, are equipping themselves with radio transmitters and receivers to enable urgent or time-saving contact to be made with the doctor who is out visiting. Radio-pagers or 'bleeps' may be used in most areas of the country.

To summarize the important points in telephone technique:

1 Identify yourself correctly and promptly.
2 Always obtain the name and address of the caller.
3 Always write the message down.
4 Speak clearly and politely.
5 Do not make private calls unless they are urgent.

INTERNAL COMMUNICATION SYSTEMS

All hospitals and most surgeries have some form of internal communication between departments or between doctor and secretary. Hospital communication systems are examined in Chapter 23. In the surgery there may be simply a light or buzzer for summoning the next patient, or there may be an internal telephone system, or even a small loudspeaker in the waiting room, allowing the doctor to speak to his partners and his secretary. Occasionally the internal and external system is combined: a figure being dialled for internal calls and a code number followed by figures for an external call. Where there is a separate internal and external system, it enables the secretary to intercept incoming calls and consult the doctor on the internal system before putting the call through. This can also be done on an external line with extensions, but only if there is a manually operated switchboard in the surgery.

POSTAL SERVICES

The secretary should be conversant with some of the more important services that are provided by the Post Office. The charges for these services will vary from time to time and are listed in the *Post Office Guide*, which can be obtained from any post office. Different postage rates apply to:

1 inland postage and Eire
2 HM Forces overseas
3 Europe
4 outside Europe (airmail)
5 surface mail to all countries

For inland postage and Eire there is a 1st class service for letters, cards and packets which will normally be delivered the day after posting, and a 2nd class one which will follow at least 24 hours later.

Packets weighing more than 750 g cannot be sent by 2nd class service.

All envelopes should be sealed, but the sender's name and address on the back will help in the return of undelivered mail. 'Non-returnable' should be written on mail that is not to be sent back.

Apart from these there are certain other ways in which material can be sent by post.

Business reply service. This is commonly used by hospitals as a licensed business reply folder, addressed to the medical records department. It contains a request for an appointment and a clinical letter from the doctor and does not require a stamp.

Freepost. A reply paid service where pre-printed cards or envelopes are not available.

Datapost. This service provides same-day collection and delivery in many areas, either locally or intercity. Individual items are accepted up to 27.5 kg in weight.

Intelpost. This provides high speed, facsimile transmission for sending copies of documents between more than 100 towns in the UK and many overseas.

Royal Mail special delivery. This guarantees delivery in the next working day after posting.

Advice on delivery. This can be obtained by completing a form at the time of posting or subsequently.

Recorded delivery. This is used where it is necessary to be able to prove that a letter or package has been posted or delivered. It provides limited compensation in case of loss or damage and there is an additional fee. Compensation is, however, limited and is not paid for cash or jewellery. The receiver must sign a receipt, and if a further additional fee has been paid the sender will be notified of receipt.

Registered letter service. (Those containing money or jewellery must be registered.) The minimum fee will provide limited compensation, but higher compensation can be obtained by paying higher fees. The letter or parcel should be crossed with blue lines and marked 'Registered'. Special envelopes can be obtained from the GPO on which this is already done. Knots in string must be sealed with wax and a certificate of posting obtained. The receiver must sign a receipt.

Express post. Priority delivery of a letter by a special messenger may be secured by paying an additional fee, marking boldly the words 'Special Delivery', and crossing the packet with a broad blue or black line.

Data post, Data post same day, and data post overnight provide courier delivery services.

Cash on delivery (COD). When parcels that have not been paid for are sent COD the amount specified will be collected by the post office if a special form has been completed by the sender.

Poste restante. Letters and packets can be sent to any post office to await collection by an addressee who will be asked to prove his identity if the address of the post office is headed 'Poste Restante'.

Pathological specimens. These must be sent by 1st class letter post and never by parcel post. They must be well wrapped and conspicuously marked 'Fragile With Care' and bear the words 'Pathological Specimen'.

Postal codes. This is a group of letters and figures issued to all addresses as an aid to automatic sorting. All addressed correspondence should bear a postal code.

Post office preferred envelopes. These must be within the size range from 8.5 × 13.5 cm to 11.5 × 23 cm and meet certain other requirements of shape and quality of paper. This is an international arrangement to facilitate electronic sorting. Envelopes not conforming to this size will be charged at the next highest rate if the mail weighs less than 60 g.

Postcards must be within the size range from 8.5 × 13.5 cm to 10 × 14.5 cm.

13

Medical Statistics and Data Handling

The word *statistics* was first used in the eighteenth century to describe a series of facts and figures collected together, which related to the state, such as figures about trade, the number of the population and the mortality from diseases. It is believed to derive from the Italian word 'statistica', meaning statesman. It is used now in two different senses. Firstly, it means a collection of numerical facts, rather in the same way as it was originally applied. These facts do not now relate only to the organization of the state but to any subject in which quantity can be expressed numerically. Secondly, the word statistics is used to refer to a method of analysing collected numerical facts and drawing deductions and conclusions from them.

THE STATISTICAL METHOD

It is a curious thing that the word statistics engenders more heat and passion in the non-mathematical mind than almost any other. Scorn and abuse are poured on any idea which is expressed statistically and it has often been said that statistics can be made to prove anything that is wanted of them. These views are evidence that the person holding them fails to understand that facts are not altered by statistical methods, but only handled so that the most accurate conclusions can be drawn from them.

In medicine we are concerned with statistics in both senses of the word. Bed states, out-patient attendances and the incidence of disease are all presented numerically. The statistics may be set out simply and clearly in a number of ways:

1 *Typed tabulations.* These are columns of figures with a 'details' or explanatory column (Table 13.1).

2 *Graphs, single and multi-line (Fig. 13.1).* Upward and downward lines demonstrate increases and decreases in, say, the incidence of disease: comparisons are indicated by a second or third line, which are perhaps drawn in different colours, e.g. between adults and children, or between males and females.

3 *Bar charts—vertical and horizontal.* Sometimes called 'pillar graphs', these are most useful for purposes of comparison. *Histograms* (Fig. 13.2) are similar to bar charts: these have the blocks or pillars joined so that a continuous line is created. Both groups are most often used to show a time factor or frequency distribution, such as the total number of admissions during a certain period.

101

Table 13.1 Attendances at an out-patient department

Month	New patients	Old patients
January	22	111
February	27	119
March	23	142
April	28	173
May	27	161
June	30	154
July	19	101
August	12	81
September	17	119
October	21	165
November	30	154
December	24	121

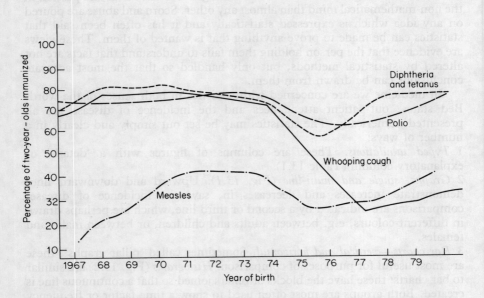

Fig. 13.1 The immunization status of two-year-olds between 1967 and 1979.

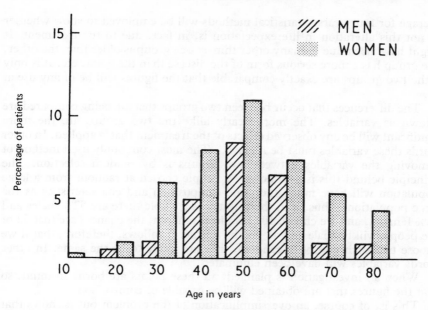

Fig. 13.2 A histogram showing the age distribution of people with varicose ulcers.

4 *Pie charts.* A pie chart is a circle representing a total (100%), with wedges marked off to illustrate the component parts; for example, the whole might represent one clinic session, and the segments the percentage of time given to specific treatment, follow-up cases, chronic patients seen at regular intervals and so on.

5 *Display and control boards.* These are boards with movable parts, magnetic studs, pegs, discs, etc. They demonstrate a changing position so that figures can be 'lifted' at any time. One of these is often used to indicate how many beds are occupied in a hospital ward at any particular time. Known as the bed board, this has sections representing all the wards in the hospital. Each section is headed by the name or number of the ward and shows how many beds exist therein. A stud or peg is attached to the occupied beds. The board is checked periodically against the bed-states forms, filled in by the Sisters, and against the waiting list.

Whichever of these methods is chosen the facts remain unaltered but will be shown more clearly.

The same methods may be used to demonstrate numerical facts obtained by doctors in the course of research. For example they may be used to demonstrate ages of groups of patients, duration of symptoms, time taken for treatments under investigation to be effective, etc. These statistics will consist of different units according to the figures they relate to: that is, they may be given in years, hours, kilograms, etc. As well as this the figures will probably need to be analysed by statistical methods in order to demonstrate their significance mathematically. For example, it is found that a group of patients suffering from a certain condition will live, on average, for five years if untreated. It is found that another group treated by method A will live on average for four years. Statistical methods will be employed to show whether or not this alteration in life expectation is, in fact, due to the treatment. It might have been due to many other things: one group is older than the other, one group has a more serious form of the disease than the other, etc. It is only if the two groups are exactly comparable that the figures will be of any use at all.

The differences that occur between two groups that are being compared are known as variables. The more nearly alike the two groups are the more significant will be any observed effects of the treatment that is applied. In other words these variables must be removed. The most commonly used method of removing the variables between two groups is by random selection. The principle behind this is as follows. A sample chosen at random from a large population will have much the same composition and characteristics as the large population. Thus, if in the country as a whole there are 52% males and 48% females, and we choose 100 people at random, the chances are that 52 of the people will be male and 48 will be female. It follows, therefore, that if we choose two such groups at random, they are likely to be the same. In other words variables will have been eliminated.

When an investigation is planned, all these points are borne in mind, so that the figures that are obtained will be capable of comparison.

This is, of course, an oversimplification of the problem but it shows that data so obtained are important. The role of the secretary in this may be in the collection of figures, or in the lay-out and typing of results and it is obvious that accuracy in this type of work is of great importance. This is nowhere more important than in the collection of figures, for here she must be scrupulously honest with herself in making sure that no prejudice or bias in favour of an answer is present. There is often a temptation, when a certain result is desired, to interpret figures in such a way as to make them support one's views. This has to be eliminated if the two basic problems that statistics sets out to deal with can be answered. These are:

1 The significance of results, by which we mean the reliability of the difference between two sets of figures.
2 The conclusions that can be drawn from differences which can be shown to be significant.

Punched card systems

There are many different ways in which collected material can be stored for later statistical analysis. When the investigation is on a small scale, involving few patients or only a few details about a larger number of patients, it is often possible to record them simply in notebooks or on cards which are appropriately indexed. If there is a lot of material and a large number of index cards it is often necessary to use a punched card system so that information can be recorded and extracted rapidly.

These punched cards are capable of storing a very large number of facts in a very small space and systems have been devised to extract information manually or automatically. The basic principle of the punched card is that a hole or slot is cut in a previously programmed card recording a certain fact. When it is necessary to pick out all those cards that record the same fact a bar or needle can be slid through the punched holes. If it is desired to pick out of a

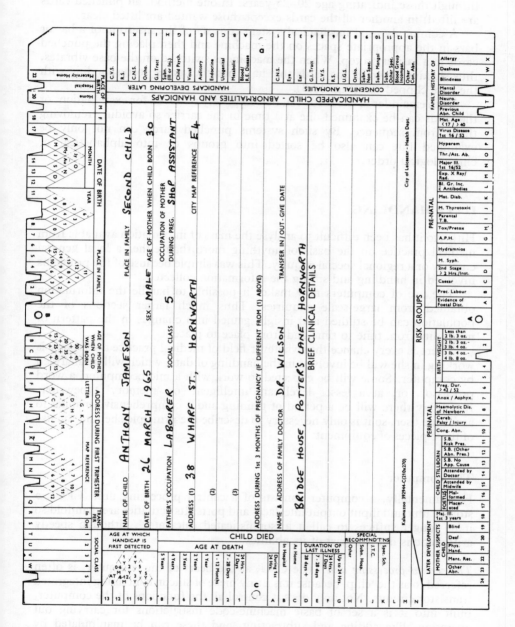

Fig. 13.3 An 'edge' punched card, which is used with the 'fact-finder' for extracting statistical information.

series of index cards all those females in the age group 20–25 years, a needle will be slid through all the holes corresponding with female and another through those indicating age 20–25 years. In one method, all punched cards are lifted: in another all the cards except those wanted are lifted clear.

A commonly used mechanical system consists of the insertion of a bar or bars in the appropriate spaces on the machine and then placing the punched cards in a carrier on top. When the machine is switched on the base vibrates, thus shaking down all the cards that have had the spaces corresponding with the bars clipped out (Fig. 13.3).

The remainder of the cards can be completely removed for examination, or the cards can be examined one at a time in the carrier so avoiding removing them from sequence. By such systems punched cards can not only be examined but can also be sorted into groups or into alphabetical or chronological order.

DATA HANDLING

Hitherto it has been difficult to analyse the mass of information available from medical practice on the basis of anything more than either a local general enquiry or a regional special enquiry. This was simple because of the problems involved in handling and sifting the information collected.

The use of computers now makes it possible to handle the information obtained from large-scale enquiries. Thus much larger sections of the population can be studied and insight gained into changes in the pattern of morbidity from time to time and from place to place.

There is every chance that whatever field of medical practice a secretary is working in she will be involved in the handling of data, which will be analysed by computer. Some will be expected to work with a microcomputer, a word processor, or, at a lesser level, an 'intelligent' or 'memory' typewriter. Invariably there will be a period of training and a comprehensive manual to assist the user, so it is only necessary to describe the principles behind the use of these pieces of equipment.

The computer

Fundamentally, a computer consists of a central processing unit (CPU), a storage unit and input/output interfaces and ports. Its activities are manifold so it no longer suffices to call it a 'sophisticated calculator', although speedy arithmetic is not the least of its abilities.

The central processing unit. The CPU, at the heart of the computer, is often referred to as the 'chip' because it is a tiny piece of silicon containing integrated transistor circuits. Not only does it control all the functions of the computer, built into it is a set of basic machine-code instructions for carrying out operations like adding and subtracting, and these can be manipulated by programs to do accounting, word processing or game-playing. The CPU also stores information in its circuits; this is called the 'primary' (or 'internal') memory.

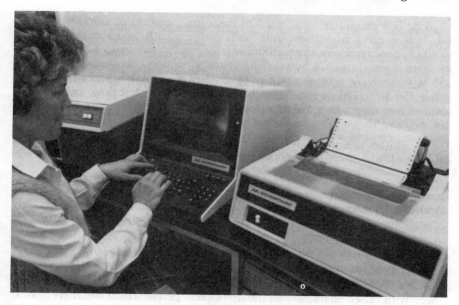

Fig. 13.4 A microcomputer at work in the surgery.

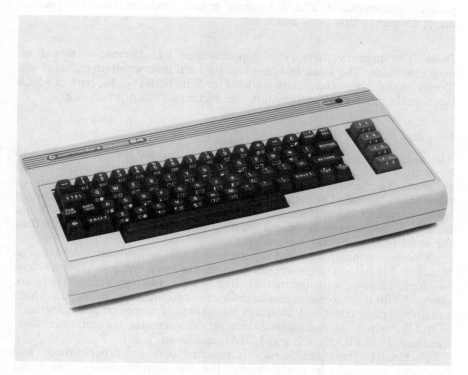

Fig. 13.5 The Commodore 64 computer (shown without VDU).

Byte is a computer term, used to measure 'memory' or storage capacity. But byte is not a convenient unit when working with 'small' computers and word processors, where the memory is large, and so kilobyte (K) is used (one kilobyte is equal to 1024 bytes). The primary memory runs between 8 K and 256 K—the average typewritten page contains about 1.5 K and a floppy disc about 150 K or 150 pages. A small Winchester disk (see below) may contain about 5 megabytes or more than 3500 pages.

Storage. Often described as the 'memory', it might equally well be regarded as a filing unit since it stores data that can be worked upon, changed or retrieved.

Interfaces. These are attachments where peripherals, such as keyboards (input) or VDUs, disk drives or printers (output), can be linked, commonly through the input and output ports at the back or side. It is essential that interfaces match the particular peripheral.

Printers. Printers may be fast or they may be slow and produce attractive work, rarely both. Letter-quality (slow) printers use a metal or plastic 'daisy wheel' with raised characters on the tip of each 'petal', which hammers against the inked ribbon. The noisy printers are best accommodated away from the input unit and VDU, so proofreading on the VDU before printing is of paramount importance. The 'dot-matrix' printer produces characters consisting of a series of tiny dots, and is fast.

Disks. The primary memory is supplemented by information stored on magnetic disks. The small business and personal microcomputer usually use 'floppy' disks. Large computers use hard (or Winchester) disks, both of which can contain much more information (see section on word processing).

Language

The instruction lists which enable computers to execute specific tasks have to be written in binary numbers—noughts and ones—and there are several versions. The instructions can be processed at the rate of hundreds or thousands a second. The language met by the medical secretary will depend on which computer she encounters. (She needs to be flexible because it will not necessarily be the same as the one she used at school or college, any more than the word processor will be the same.)

The most popular language at present is BASIC—Beginners' All Purpose Symbolic Instruction Code—because, instead of using symbols, it comes close to simple English, with instructions like 'Read', 'List' or 'Print'. There are others: COBOL—Common Business Orientated Language; PASCAL, which usually operates faster and facilitates the writing of more complex programs; FORTH, which is complicated but provides greater control over data-handling; FORTRAN; 'C'; and LOGO, and so on.

Fortunately, language fluency is essential only for programmers, and programs are available commercially, but the secretary must master the commands explained in the instruction manual accompanying her computer.

Programs

Information (data) that is to be put into a computer is usually introduced in a coded form. That is a small group of numbers is used to indicate the subject. For example, a classification of diseases might code 'bronchitis' as '115'. These coding systems are very carefully constructed and are often agreed nationally or internationally so that data from different sources can be combined or compared.

The portable computer (Fig. 13.6)

There is no such thing as the definitive portable computer but, as there are almost a hundred systems available, one may well have a purpose in a hospital somewhere.

Usually it is a single unit with a carrying handle and a fold-down keyboard, powered by mains electricity, designed for moving from office to office or from office to home. Portable computers are designed for specific operations, i.e.

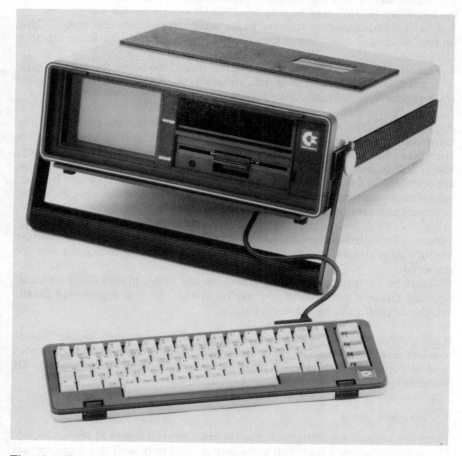

Fig. 13.6 The SX-64 portable computer.

data collection, and can be an electronic alternative to a notebook and shorthand.

The pocket computer comes next!

Use of computers in hospital

This varies from hospital to hospital. The computerization of patient administration is a complex subject and, depending on the skill brought to it, has no boundaries. Some of the subjects involved are: the master index; registration (e.g. labels); bed states; waiting lists; admissions and discharges, TCI (to come in) letters; hospital activity analysis and statistics; operation schedules; departmental administration, e.g. X-ray and casualty; investigation results; prescriptions; drug reactions; appointments systems; management information; and there may be links with nursing and community systems, e.g. FPCs. (For use of computers in general practice see pages 234–236.)

The master index. When a computer print-out is not wanted, computer output on microfilm (COM) may be employed. COM occurs in two ways:
1 The COM equipment is attached to the computer to create film images. This on-line method is quick but it uses time that may be required more urgently elsewhere.
2 The off-line method makes the computer record the index on magnetic tape which is then used as a form of data entry into the COM system so that once the tapes have been created, the computer is free.

Appointments. Not only can all out-patient appointments be listed, the computer can sort out relevant details from its base and incorporate them elsewhere, for example into letters concerning appointments. In this way, letters will go automatically to guardians in the case of children, and when an appointment has to be cancelled the computer will issue an apology. Because subsystems can interface with each other a notification of death will automatically cancel an entry in the appointments system.

Clinics. Clinic lists are produced, often with semi-adhesive labels containing identification details, which are stuck onto tracers when the case notes are retrieved.

Lists are in appointment time order, usually with a master check-list, and pointing out new patients, in one way or another, so that registration details can be checked prior to the consultation.

Waiting lists. Names, conditions and degrees of urgency, etc., enable doctors to select cases for admission. They also make it easier for clerks and secretaries to deal promptly with queries from general practitioners and patients. Of course it is important that details are kept up-to-date.

The computer system

There are various configurations; the system may well evolve at regional level. The majority of users may well come into contact only with the departmental VDU and printer. Each would probably be allocated her own password in order to gain access; then of course, unit numbers would be used to call up a great deal of the information required. Confidentiality prevails. The short-term memory is erased when the machine is turned off, but some screen displays are deleted automatically after a certain period of time so that sensitive data cannot be exposed indefinitely.

The use of computer systems in hospitals

1 A data bank for reference and from which subsystems can be implemented, when all identification details of patients are stored, and a computerized appointments system is easier to institute.
2 Computer systems provide a quick certain way of retrieving patients' identification details.
3 Broader access to information; it is no longer centralized in its own department.
4 Swift retrieval of data.
5 Speed in collecting and presenting statistics.
6 Label printing, even with adhesive backing.
7 Dependable information as a result of the many checks and the discipline imposed by the computer system.

Filing

It is the paper print-out that has given rise to complaints about the computer's paper mountain and print-out plague. The continuous stationery on which output is printed is not only expensive, it is heavy. It also needs to be sorted and secured. Usually there is a button available for a print-out of only what is on the screen (e.g. a page), so the user needs to ask herself if she really needs it and, if so, how much.

The print-out paper is filed in special binders; these may be loose-leafed and suitable for sprocket-punched continuous stationery. Machines called 'bursters' will separate the sheets and decollaters will remove carbon paper. Filing may take place in drums when using very big machines. Floppy disks can go into special binders; whatever method is used, careful protection is necessary. There are storage units for rigid disks in which they are placed flat on withdrawable shelves; ideally, disk packs and magnetic tape reels need fireproof safes. There is a vast variety of equipment available so the choice depends upon available space and frequency of retrieval.

All the usual rules about indexing apply to computer material, *and* a control procedure for retrieval and return.

This is a problem that information technology can solve—with the paperless office.

Information technology

This could be described as the transmission of knowledge between computers or other equipment, or the handling of vocal, pictorial, numerical and textual information by means of an electronically based combination of computing and telecommunications. Advances in this field have produced electronic mail, word processing, viewdata, teletext and data bases.

So important does the Government consider information technology it has appointed a Minister for Information Technology within the Department of Trade and Industry to coordinate activities in this field.

As students of general office administration will have seen, there is scarcely an area of our lives that information technology cannot influence. Not only can it create the paperless office, it has led to, among other things, medical-interviewing machines.

In one program a questionnaire is presented to the patient on a terminal in order to reduce the doctor's routine note-taking and to establish basic facts or symptoms. The patient presses a button to indicate 'Yes', 'No', or 'Don't understand'. Then on the basis of this response, the computer poses the next question. At the end of the session a summary is printed.

The medical secretary can help by explaining the procedure to patients and by pointing out that not only do the strict rules about confidentiality still apply but that there is often a control incorporated into the unit so that only one doctor has access to important information, particularly legal information. It has been claimed that, far from objecting to these 'mechanical' interviews, some patients answer the computer more candidly, or at least with less embarrassment, than they would answer a person.

The word processor

Until mass-produced silicon-chip technology dawned, there had been little innovation in the typewriter world since the 'golf ball'. But in 1980 the electronic typewriter changed the situation dramatically because it led to the addition of various extras, particularly interfacing, which transform it into the

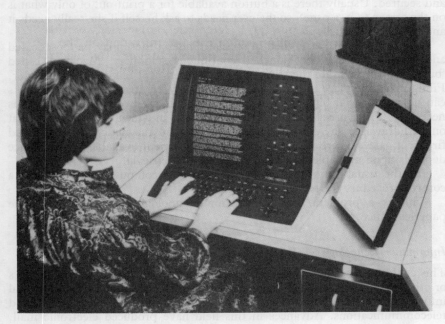

Fig. 13.7 Coding data for analysis.

nucleus of the modern office. Interfacing matches the 'senses' of all computers and related equipment so that the typewriter can be linked to microcomputers, other typewriters, to Telex and to word processors.

Basically, there are two types of word processor.

1 The dedicated machine can record, store, edit and print the text typed in, and with its 'Move', 'Block', 'Edit' keys it is simple to use.

2 The microcomputer with a software word processor package is more versatile, as it performs all the usual computer functions, as well as word processing.

The software varies from machine to machine so the operator must learn the appropriate system in order to give commands, such as 'Delete', 'Insert', 'Print', etc., via the keyboard.

Storage. This, too, varies with the machine and may be on disks, magnetic cards or cassette tapes. Hard disks are built into the equipment in many cases. Floppy disks are inserted into disk drives at the word processing station. Disks are like records and spin round, storing characters in tracks. They are made from magnetically treated circular sheets of flexible plastic in protective vinyl jackets. They come in three sizes, 3 in (76 mm), 5¼ in (134 mm) and 8 in (203 mm) and with various capacities, such as double-sided (storage on both sides) and double density (double the storage capacity on one side only), in addition to single-sided and single-density. The small disks are usually used on portable computers.

Floppy disks must be treated carefully. Their paper jackets must never be removed because dust and finger-marks, as well as magnetics and heat, can spoil, even destroy, the text.

Hard disks are more expensive, faster, have greater storage capacity, and are useful when working with lots of data.

Equipment. Similar to that of a computer, the basic word processor station comprises a typewriter keyboard (for input), a VDU, the CPU (with a memory storage ranging from 5000 characters (5 K) to 80-million characters (80 megabytes), and the printer; the disk for storage may or may not be incorporated into the CPU.

The stand-alone system

This is a self-contained single work-station with a keyboard, VDU, printer and CPU together usually with a disk drive unit for two disks.

The screen size varies; the automatic printer generally uses a daisy wheel and produces any number of perfect copies, all amendment and corrections having been organized beforehand. A small dedicated stand-alone system could deal with a certain amount of the work in general practice.

The shared logic system

This has a keyboard, a VDU and printer but the CPU is shared, sometimes being a large or main frame computer, so that a greater volume of work and more complicated text is carried out by a number of work-stations in different locations.

Shared resources

These have the keyboard and VDU but share the CPU and printer(s). The smaller units of both shared logic resources systems may be found in hospitals.

Proofreading is always important, and never more so than when work is displayed on the screen and is about to be committed to print. In some large organizations the more intensively used printing facilities are housed separately from the work-stations (to remove noise etc.).

Uses

As everyone is now aware, the word processor is ideal for handling documentation that is comprised of repetitive matter.

Examples of hospital usage could include admission and discharge paperwork, patient letters, lectures, drafting research papers and curriculum vitae. But the possibilities are enormous, making a definitive list difficult.

In a small survey conducted by the author it appears that not all hospitals possess the equipment, although those administrators and medical record officers who were approached declared a wish for it; some hospitals have a limited facility—not used by *medical* secretaries—and others are well-endowed. What seems certain, however, is that from now on all secretaries must be prepared to add word processing operations to their skills.

Memory typewriters

These are also capable of storing and reproducing words. The words may make up, for example, commonly used sentences such as letters making appointments, requests for investigations or lists of names and addresses. Storage capacity can vary from less than 5000 characters (a character is a single letter or digit) to 500 000 characters, and the machine can be upgraded to display small amounts of texts for editing.

THE DATA PROTECTION ACT, 1984

This Act pertains to personal information that is held and processed by computer-type equipment. Its main points are:
1 Data users must register details of personal data with the Data Protection Register.
2 They must adopt appropriate security measures to prevent unauthorized access, alteration, damage, loss, accident and destruction.
3 Data subjects have right of access to their own data.
4 Data subjects can insist that the information is amended if incorrect, or even erased.
5 Financial compensation may be awarded if a subject suffers damage or distress as a result of inaccuracies.
6 Those data users found guilty of offences will be fined.

Diploma Questions Set in the Examination for the Diploma of the Association of Medical Secretaries

⋆Denotes an incomplete question

1 Write short notes on word processing equipment.⋆
2 The versatility of a word processor makes it ideal for use in all branches of health administration. Discuss this statement.

III

The Secretary/Receptionist in the Hospital

III

14

Staffing

The person who is intending to become a medical secretary might look around a general hospital and wonder, 'Who are all these people? What on earth do they all do? And where could I fit in?'

The first thing to understand is that a hospital is a conglomerate body, comprised of very many groups, all aspiring to the same goal yet working in markedly different ways to achieve it.

These groups are: doctors, nurses, scientists, technicians, educators, therapists, dieticians, caterers, cooks, porters, cleaners, engineers, experts in law and finance, administrators, secretaries, clerks and receptionists, chaplains, and a body of voluntary workers.

Some deal directly with the patient and some work on his behalf behind the scenes, while others make supportive or maintenance contributions. However, one line of demarcation is clear and cuts across all specialities and seniorities; that is, some staff are privileged to *handle* patients physically and some are not; the medical secretary is in a 'caring' position but she belongs to the latter group.

THE MEDICAL STAFF

The Consultant

Nowadays, with the advance of technology and research, there are all kinds of highly-trained professional people associated with the medical profession who are not doctors per se, particularly in the teaching hospitals. But at the top of the tree of immediate concern to the secretary is the *Consultant*, a specialist in a particular branch of medicine. He is salaried and works full- or part-time. He may or may not have a private practice. (The secretary's involvement when he does depends upon individual arrangements; her first loyalty is to the hospital employing her.)

The medical care of a patient attending a hospital as an in-patient or an out-patient is the sole responsibility of the Consultant in charge of the case.

Consultants are appointed by the RHA or, in the case of teaching hospitals, by the health authority concerned. The appointment can be a joint appointment between two regional authorities or jointly with a university, and the Consultant may either devote himself to a single hospital or divide his time among a Group—the grouping of hospitals, with a sharing of staff, resources and responsibilities is common nowadays.

A Consultant whose name is on the Domiciliary Visiting Register, circulated to general practitioners in the neighbourhood, will sometimes examine in the home patients who, for medical reasons, cannot travel to the hospital. (As this is a provision of the NHS, the secretary will see that his claim for a fee and mileage is submitted.)

There are some Consultants, however, who rarely see patients. These are the specialists in charge of the radiography or anaesthetic departments or the pathology laboratory. Sometimes, in such departments, one Consultant may act as a director exercising overall control of the organization of the department. (In the United States and some continental countries it is the practice to have directors and superintendents of clinical departments, such as surgery or medicine, who exercise clinical control over the work of other specialists, but this is not the practice in the United Kingdom. Here, once a doctor has attained Consultant or specialist rank, he has complete clinical charge of his patient and his medical independence is assured. However, in many hospitals specialists working within a particular discipline may organize themselves into divisions. Thus there may be a medical division, a surgical division, a paediatric division and so on. Each of these will elect its own chairman for administrative purposes. The committee representing all these hospital doctors is known as the Medical Executive or Medical Staff Committee.)

While it is the Consultant who carries total clinical responsibility for his patients, they are also likely to be attended by more junior medical staff.

Other medical staff

The grades into which hospital staff are divided are, in descending order of seniority:

- Consultants
- Medical Assistants
- Senior Registrars
- Registrars
- Senior House Officers
- House Officers

These posts recognize experience and responsibility and are the normal steps by which specialists or GPs are trained to exercise full and independent clinical responsibility. As a rule, the team of Consultant, Registrars and Housemen devoted to one speciality is called a 'firm'. (The well-trained person might be appointed as secretary to a 'firm' or group of 'firms'.) Specialists are either physicians or surgeons, and by tradition in the UK the latter are addressed as 'Mister' rather than 'Doctor' (see Chapter 4).

The precise duties of doctors vary from hospital to hospital. The *Senior Registrar*, who has been qualified for four or more years, can be regarded as a Consultant in training. He usually holds a higher qualification than the *Medical Assistant*, a new grade which in part replaces the Senior Hospital Medical Officer (SHMO) grade. This post may be full- or part-time and is filled by doctors who are trained in a speciality but have not got Consultant status. It may be a step towards a Consultant post and yet is a career grade in itself. The posts may be occupied by suitably experienced GPs on a part-time capacity.

Clinical assistantships are part-time posts where the doctor does not exercise full clinical responsibility for patients. They are often occupied on a sessional basis by GPs and the work done will depend very much on the experience of the particular doctor. In some cases they will be regarded as a training post, designed to act as 'a refresher course', but in others they will exercise a degree of responsibility, under the Consultant, which may be considerable. They bring a contact between two branches of the medical profession, which can be valuable to both.

The *Registrar* is a qualified doctor who is now undergoing further specialist training. *House Officers (or Housemen)* are fully trained young doctors, but under the Medical Act of 1956 their official registration is provisional until they have practised for 12 months in an approved hospital or institution. The Housemen working under the jurisdiction of a Consultant will, naturally, be involved with the same speciality, but only so long as the association lasts; afterwards they may branch off into different specialities or go into general practice, industrial medicine, local health authority medicine, or may decide to practise abroad. In some hospitals, posts at Senior House Officer levels are occupied by doctors undergoing vocational training for general practice, where they spend part of their time in hospital and part in selected general practices as a 'trainee'.

While the precise duties vary according to the hospital, in general, Consultants see patients on their first attendances at the out-patient department, once or twice a week on the wards and, of course, at any other times deemed necessary; day-to-day responsibility is delegated to the Registrars, and routine care to the Housemen.

Many of the junior posts are resident ones; that is, the doctor resides in the hospital and is thus in close attendance on the patient. The senior surgical resident occupies the position of Resident Surgical Officer (RSO) and the senior medical resident that of Resident Medical Officer (RMO). Their particular responsibilities are the organization of the residents' mess, off-duty periods and the admission of emergencies. Again, the actual duties and responsibilities of each of these posts will vary from hospital to hospital, depending principally upon staff numbers, and the medical secretary must soon acquaint herself with the medical organization inside the hospital. It may be, for example, that in one hospital the discharge letters are all done by the RSO, in another it may be the responsibility of the House Surgeon to write these letters to the patient's own GP, and in yet another hospital it may be the Consultant who dictates them.

Teaching hospitals

The secretary working in a teaching hospital will also encounter other members of the medical hierarchy. At the top of the ladder is the Professor, and below him come the posts of First Assistant, Reader and Lecturer. The medical students are just beginning their careers and it is customary in teaching hospitals for some duties to be delegated to students in their last three years of training. This is usually done by a system of attachment, whereby a group of students are attached to a particular Consultant for a period of clinical training. When they are attached to a surgeon or a 'firm' of surgeons they are known as 'dressers' and when attached to a medical 'firm' are called 'clerks'—these names being derived from the old terms referring to apprentices. Their duties are to attend on the patient throughout his stay in hospital, take a careful history of the patient's condition and follow the patient through his course of treatment, observe and make clinical notes.

THE NURSING STAFF

The nursing service within each district may be managed by the District Nursing Officer or a General Manager and the hospital services are part of her responsibility. At a higher level there may be a Regional Nursing Officer who is the head of her profession within the region. However, the Griffiths report has resulted in a wide range of administrative posts and titles. Districts are divided into Units administered by Managers who may or may not be nurses.

The District Nursing Officer may be also concerned with the education of nurses, as there is almost certainly a nursing school within her district, and with the community nursing services.

The titles held by different grades of nurses have been altered. The familiar title of Matron might have been held by the nurse in charge of a thousand-bed teaching hospital or a twenty-bed cottage hospital. The top posts in the profession are held by Regional Nursing Officers. They are usually in charge of a number of hospitals within the district, or a very big district general hospital with a number of separate nursing divisions. Nursing Officers (or General Managers) are in charge of various units within a large hospital or district. The middle grades are often now known as Senior Nurses. Their jobs relate to groups of wards and units such as midwifery departments. The ward Sister (or, if male, Charge Nurse) organizes the nursing care and general administration of a single ward and she will have one or more Staff Nurses under her charge. These are fully trained nurses who deputize for the Sister in her absence and at other times look after specific groups of patients.

Student nurses qualify after three years as a registered general nurse (RGN) or after two years as a state enrolled nurse (SEN).

The titles for nurses may vary from one hospital to another. The medical secretary/receptionist needs to learn individual job titles as they vary from district to district.

CHAPLAIN

The spiritual welfare of patients is provided for by the notification to the hospital chaplains of admissions. Different denominations are visited by the appropriate minister.

VOLUNTARY WORKERS

Supporting the medical and nursing staff is a band of unpaid workers; these include members of the British Red Cross Society and the Women's Royal Voluntary Service. Not only do these people run canteens and library trolleys, etc., they carry patients' suitcases up to the wards and take round menus; they work in out-patients' clinics, receiving patients and weighing them, dealing with attendance lists and, in some of the smaller hospitals, retrieving case notes—and many participate in a car service.

Nor should the *League of Friends* be overlooked—local men and women who organize all kinds of activities in order to raise money with which to make the patients' time in hospital as pleasant as possible.

The secretary will soon learn to recognize these people, for one of their many outstanding characteristics is the unfailing regularity with which they appear, and she can show her appreciation of what they do by helping them in any way possible.

THE ADMINISTRATIVE STAFF

The hospital administrator

The hospital administrator could be described as the chief executive because he is responsible for the overall day-to-day running of the hospital or group of hospitals. It is he who represents the hospital in the outside world, speaks for it and liaises between it and various official bodies. It is he who must ensure that the hospital abides by the law and all bylaws. He is empowered to attend most internal meetings that are not clinical and to convene meetings of his own.

At the same time, he supervises the staff (except those directly responsible to the Chief Nursing Officer or to the senior medical and dental practitioners)—and this includes the secretaries.

His own staff includes the engineers and the following officers: finance, supplies, catering, transport, medical records, admissions, surgical appliances.

In a small hospital, some of these positions may be combined, or not held at all, or they may administer a Group. Some of the officers may have secretaries of their own, even a large clerical staff, and the medical secretary's contact with them is minimal, but she should understand their functions.

The finance officer. Although certain personnel, such as the supplies officer and the surgical appliances officer, check invoices against statements of accounts before submitting them to the finance officer for payment, he is responsible for the accounting systems, all budgets and expenses and all salaries and wages. He reports to a financial subcommittee and controls and organizes the financial side of that committee's decisions. His staff may be large.

The supplies officer. He deals with the purchase of supplies and stores for the hospital or group of hospitals. Acting on the advice of the pharmacists and other experts, he orders drugs and medical equipment. The stores' staff come under his jurisdiction, and he has control of the sale of waste products, such as used X-ray film and kitchen-stuffs. Another of his duties is to advise on tenders and quotations, this being an area of his ·expertise, so it is not surprising that in a large organization he has to delegate various tasks, while retaining ultimate responsibility for them.

The medical records officer. This is another key person in the hospital structure, and may be a man or woman, with tremendous authority and responsibility delegated to him by the hospital administrator. Not only is he in charge of all records, including patients' case notes, it is his job to organize the clerical and secretarial services throughout the hospital or Group.

The surgical appliances officer. He is a member of the medical records department but usually has his own office (like the *admissions officer* who is also a part of the medical records department), where patients are fitted with appliances authorized by their doctors.

The transport officer. He is attached to a large hospital and organizes patient-transport.

These four officials are of particular interest to the medical secretary and will receive a closer study later on.

The chain of command in hospitals is not always clear-cut. There are other professional groups under the jurisdiction of the hospital administrator yet who answer for their work only to the medics. These are:

● *therapists*—physiotherapists, occupational therapists, speech therapists, orthoptists and, in some hospitals, remedial gymnasts
● *radiographers*
● *pathology laboratory technicians*
● *pharmacists* and *dispensers*
● *chiropodists*
● *catering officer* and all *dieticians*

There are also a host of highly skilled people who operate complex diagnostic equipment, etc. Social workers, too, are among the vast army of people manning our hospitals.

15

The Medical Records Department

CONFIDENTIALITY

Anyone who has access to medical records is in a privileged position and must never forget it. Although no express legal obligation to treat them as confidential actually exists, there is no doubt whatsoever that the Courts do everything possible to protect the private relationship between doctors and their patients.

Consequently, information contained in the records may be disclosed only in special circumstances:

1 with the patient's consent
2 where disclosure is the only means of safeguarding the interests of the hospital
3 for clinical reasons (from one doctor to another)
4 when a higher obligation, in the interests of the public, supersedes the interests of the individual

This final provision allows for the notification of infectious diseases, notification of death and industrial poisoning, the compilation of statistics and claims for National Health Insurance benefits.

The medical records officer will require secretaries to sign a form stating that they understand the legal and ethical aspects of confidentiality pertaining to the records; any behaviour contravening this understanding will, undoubtedly, result in the termination of employment.

Discretion, therefore, is essential in dealing with enquiries from people outside the hospital, such as solicitors, insurance company representatives, and relatives and friends of the patients, and it is equally vital when speaking to patients themselves. A delicate path must be trodden, too, when talking to colleagues, so much so that some hospitals advocate the practice of using the patient's hospital number instead of his name—even inside 'privileged' walls—because that 'interesting case', or 'that piece of correspondence' could so easily deteriorate into 'that funny story' related on top of a bus with the accidental use of a patient's name.

A respect for confidentiality, as fastidious as that which she hopes is being given to her own case notes, is the secretary's first prerequisite for membership of the medical records department.

125

STAFFING

Although the medical records officer answers for his work to the hospital administrator he/she is an extremely important person in his/her own right. He is responsible for all the secretaries, clerks and receptionists in the hospital and, in addition, for the surgical appliances officer and administration officer (although these two have their own offices).

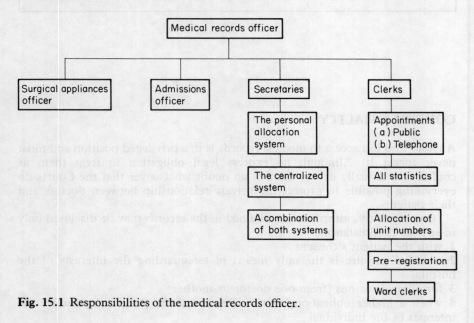

Fig. 15.1 Responsibilities of the medical records officer.

DUTIES

The duties of the medical records officer may be summarized as follows:
1 administration
2 records
3 organization of medical secretarial services
4 the collection and presentation of research and statistical data

RECORDS

Patients' case notes are the most important hospital records and their physical maintenance and protection are the responsibility of the medical records officer. He will not lightly change the system of their filing and indexing but, if necessary, he can devise an alternative because, as a rule nowadays, he is highly-trained in this field. Ideally, the system should be infallible yet so simple that everybody can follow it. The key-word here is 'everybody', for it is not only the medical and nursing staff who handle records. Almost every movement of case notes creates a clerical and/or secretarial job. One of the most difficult yet imperative tasks is that of keeping track of their movements around the hospital and ensuring that they are returned to the filing system.

For the medical records officer integration and control of the record-keeping system is a grave responsibility; for if muddles, and if delays and losses are to be avoided, all procedures must maintain continuity of action.

ORGANIZATION OF THE SECRETARIAL SERVICES

There are two ways in which these may be organized:
1 a centralized system, sometimes called the 'pool' or 'secretariat'.
2 a personal scheme, sometimes called the personalized or the personal allocation system.

The girl who has undertaken a course of training as a medical secretary frequently visualizes herself in the second category but rarely in the first, yet she might be well-advised to start her hospital career in the 'pool'.

The centralized system

This department consists of shorthand and audiotypists with a supervisor. Either the medical staff visit in order to dictate, or they have somebody sent to them. Alternatively, tapes and cassettes are sent for transcription, or there may be a remote-control dictation system whereby dictation is transmitted from a bank of special telephones elsewhere in the building, usually located where most convenient for the doctors.

The advantage to the hospital is that a centralized system is cheaper than a private secretary system because shorthand- and audiotypists without secretarial or high-speed qualifications are engaged at lower salaries. Recruitment is easier because not everyone is able or willing to assume secretarial responsibilities, and it makes part-time work possible, so married women are attracted back to employment when their children attain school-age. Furthermore, absenteeism is a lesser problem when there is a large staff to fill the breach. Finally, the supervisor ensures that the standard of work is high, and the layout of correspondence consistent.

Actually, the supervisor is the strength or weakness of this arrangement; the hospital relies upon her for efficient organization, the staff for job satisfaction. She can impart a sense of involvement to staff, who might otherwise feel out of the main stream, by arranging for them to work always for the same group of doctors. She helps to train not only newcomers but those who want to increase their shorthand-typing speeds or knowledge of medical terminology. At the same time she ensures that the workload is evenly spread. (Even with the introduction of word-processing equipment she will remain a key figure.)

After a comparatively short time, the technical competence of her shorthand-typists can become very broadly based, not merely confined to a single speciality, so the more competent staff are encouraged to apply for positions within the personal scheme.

Word processing may or may not take place in the 'pool'; at present it is used mainly in administrative sections, although not exclusively so.

The personal allocation system

A secretary is assigned to a Consultant, to a 'firm' or to a group of 'firms'. Sharing an office with another secretary or even having one to herself, she becomes a focal point for 'her' doctors. Identified with their interests, she can smooth their paths, answer inquiries on their behalf and generally coordinate as only a secretary can. As a result of this involvement, she is rarely a clock-watcher and often volunteers extra service.

Inevitably, her terminology and shorthand for 'her' doctors' speciality reaches a high standard. In addition, she will be able to utilize all of her secretarial training, by drawing on her specialized knowledge, making travel arrangements, convening meetings, taking minutes, handling financial matters, appointments, correspondence, and human relations.

A combination of the central and personal system

This scheme is operated in some hospitals side by side with a full-scale 'pool'. Secretaries are accommodated in small groups, with one acting as the senior, providing help and supervision and organizing the workload.

THE COLLECTION OF RESEARCH AND STATISTICAL MATERIAL

The medical staff may ask the medical records officer to retain information for their individual research purposes; he will devise an appropriate method of compilation and presentation, and probably delegate the task to one of his clerks (except in those very large hospitals with coding and indexing sections). Otherwise, data of all kinds are demanded of the hospital by various official bodies, annually, quarterly or monthly, and this will include the following.

1 In-patient statistics relating to the length of time patients are required to wait for admission; waiting lists are the medical records officer's responsibility (although, of course, he has nothing to do with the decision to admit). These statistics might be based on the bed states—a daily return filled in by ward Sisters about the number of beds occupied and the number vacant.

2 In some areas the DHSS will ask for a 10% random analysis of all admissions. This is known as HIPE (hospital in-patient enquiry)—a return is made on every tenth patient.

3 Out-patient statistics relate to the length of time people wait for appointments.

4 A treatment index involves the recording of treatments for various conditions.

5 In addition to registers for other diseases, a Cancer Register is often maintained, and malignancies reported to the Cancer Registration branch of the Office of Population Censuses and Surveys.

6 Birth and morbidity rates are required from time to time. (It should be noted here that—in addition to producing overall statistics—the hospital is responsible for notifying the local Medical Officer of Health of all births within 36 hours of delivery and for certifying all stillbirths. Death Certificates are sent to the Registrar of Births and Deaths within five days of expiry, signed by the doctor who attended the final illness.)

7 Hospital activity analysis (HAA) is a computer-based scheme in which many hospitals are participating in order to compile a national store of administrative and clinical information; it will be examined more closely later on.
8 The diagnostic index; this, too, needs to be studied in detail.

The diagnostic index

Responsibility for this function of the medical records department is delegated to a clerk so that its maintenance receives undivided attention.

The diagnoses of all cases handled by the hospital are listed according to the code numbers based upon the Manual of International Statistical Classification of Diseases, Injuries and Causes of Death; operations are classified by the Code of Surgical Operations.

Unit No.	Age	Sex	Specialist	Discharge Date	Results	Other Diseases by Code Nos.	Operations Code Nos.

Fig. 15.2 One version of the diagnostic index.

Doctors enter the final diagnosis on the identification sheet (HMR 1) of case notes so that the person responsible can code and record it. The index has two purposes:
1 It enables doctors to investigate diseases and/or treatments that interest them. By using the unit number allocated to each patient in a centralized filing system, they can retrieve the relevant case notes. This is particularly important in teaching hospitals and institutions where research is carried out.
2 Statistics, such as hospital morbidity rates, can be compiled to facilitate hospital administration, i.e. to estimate the number of beds and other resources needed for specific conditions.

Format of the index

The diagnostic index may consist of cards filed according to the code numbers of the diagnoses, edge-punched cards or a visible-edge system.

Alternatively, in a very large hospital or Group, it may be computerized. This may take place 'on line', that is, through a keyboard connected directly to the computer so that immediate print-outs are available, or it may involve microfiche, or both. A great many hospitals rely on HAA alone for their diagnostic index; just how this is accomplished will be explained shortly.

Problems

Sometimes there are difficulties surrounding the maintenance of a central index; these can be summarized as follows.

Busy doctors fail to play their part in its compilation, so that it is incomplete, or they neglect to make use of it so that the time and effort devoted to it is wasted. The secretary can help the situation with diplomatic reminders about:

1 the recording of proper and complete diagnoses and the final diagnosis on the identification sheet HMR 1.

2 the siting of entries in the case notes in their proper place so that the clerk in charge of the index does not overlook them.

3 not delaying summaries on patients so that the diagnoses cannot be included.

Above all, she can ensure that case notes are not filed before the final diagnosis has been indexed. Some hospitals have a department devoted to the job of indexing statistics. Whoever is responsible, however, should rubber-stamp the records with the words 'coded' or 'indexed'.

Hospital activity analysis

This national bank of data is stored at the hospital computer centre under patients' unit numbers so, outside the particular hospitals those people attended, it cannot be linked to their names; not only are computer staff subject to the same discipline of confidentiality as hospital employees they have the further constraints of the Data Protection Act.

The information falls into two classes:

1 Information for the use of administrative staff inside and outside hospitals, such as the deployment of facilities, workloads, the 'blockage' of beds and the pressure on operating theatres, etc.

2 Information for the use of doctors, such as the outcome of clinical problems, the waiting-time for admissions, and a full diagnostic index of the unit numbers of patients with certain diseases.

Collection of the data

The secretary need not worry unduly about this, the customary hospital forms are used, but consist of no-carbon-required (NCR) paper so that copies can be detached and sent to the hospital computer centre. (For example, under HAA the identification sheet, HMRI, in the case notes becomes HMR 1 (1P).

Details are completed by the medical records department (HAA clerks). The information covers three areas—admission, discharge or medical data—and once a sheet is complete it is ready to be sent to the computer centre in the weekly batch.) This takes place on the admission and discharge of patients and on completion of the medical data coding.

Distribution of the data

Some results of HAA are issued monthly, some annually and others on request. They range from admissions, bed-usage and surgery to the distribution of religious denominations among patients—this is to calculate payment of hospital chaplains.

HAA does not cover everything, however (see below).

SH3

This is filled in annually by the medical records officer and sent to the DHSS and the RHA.

(a) *Part 1*—private and amenity beds, private patient consultations, beds used by non-in-patients (mothers, relatives)

(b) *Part 2*—specialities and departments. Workload, beds, in/out attendances and new patients, waiting-list statistics

(c) *Part 3*—available maternity services and their use and specialist services such as: radiography, physiotherapy, occupational therapy

(d) *Part 4*—any changes in the hospital since the last return

Other methods of presenting statistical information

Economic considerations rest upon the compilation of many of these statistics as well as reviews of the incidence of disease, treatments, and the allocation of resources to aid those treatments. The hospital service employs some sophisticated techniques to help it to expand and realize its potential, yet the medical secretary's contribution is simple; once the criteria have been defined and the methods of display established, she applies herself to the process of maintenance regularly, with care and precision—even if the method is one of the simple ones she learnt at school or college, for the simpler means of presentation are often the best (see pages 101–103).

Diploma Questions

*Denotes an incomplete question
ˣA question to be answered after further reading

1 Describe the responsibilities of the medical records officer.

2 List the categories of staff one might expect to find working under the supervision of a medical records officer, and describe the duties likely to be assigned to staff in three of the categories.

3 Write short notes on the clerical duties involved in connection with the diagnostic index.*

4 Describe the major records kept by the medical records department outlining the importance of their accuracy and dependability.[x]

5 What use can be made in the medical records department of
   (a) visible indexing[x]
   (b) remote control dictation equipment?

6 How may a medical secretary in hospital be involved with in-patient statistics?

7 Produce a graph (on the paper provided) to show comparisons for the following operations:

1978	Hysterectomy
January	8
February	6
March	7
April	10
May	8
June	5
July	9
August	5
September	10
October	6
November	8
December	9

8 Draw a line graph showing the in-patient statistics in a hospital:

	1974	1975	1976
July	100	125	145
August	75	80	100
September	100	100	100
October	100	140	180
November	100	140	180
December	70	100	120

9 The doctor for whom you work is writing an article for a medical journal. Describe in detail the various steps to be taken between the manuscript being handed to you and the final proof being returned to the printer, bearing in mind the special considerations for typing scientific material.

10 Describe the advantages and disadvantages of adopting a centralized department for medical secretarial services in a hospital.

11 Describe the advantages and disadvantages of the personal secretarial system and the central secretarial system in hospitals from the points of view of all concerned.

16

Case Notes

STANDARDIZATION OF MEDICAL RECORDS

Medical records were standardized when the NHS was instituted, in order to ensure uniformity of record-keeping procedures and continuity of action, and to facilitate the compilation of statistical and research material. By setting down a national standard, the health service provides a safeguard for itself.

This is not to say, however, that as the medical secretary moves from one hospital to another during her career she is going to find herself handling exactly the same forms and following exactly the same procedures. There is a central supply of forms to hospitals but some find it necessary to alter and adapt them, even to print their own if they have the allocation of funds, in order to meet their particular needs. Some have the benefit of computerization and microfilming, some do not, and others are about to have it. Some participate in HAA and some do not. And some hospitals are large and some are small! All of these factors influence the physical appearance and purpose of the forms the secretary will be handling, not to mention the amount of them, so she has to be flexible.

The more hospitals she works in, the more clearly will she see that standardization overall does exist but without rigidity.

CASE NOTES

Basically, these follow the same pattern everywhere, contained in folders of A4 size and consisting of four sections:
   (a) identification
   (b) medical
   (c) nursing
   (d) correspondence

The identification section

This sheet is classified as HMR 1 unless the hospital is participating in HAA when it becomes HMR 1(1P) and, because of its NCR paper (no-carbon-required) must be filled in on a typewriter or with a ball-point pen (see Figs 16.1 and 16.2). It has spaces for:
   1 the hospital's name and code number, which is usually printed
   2 the patient's name, address and telephone number
   3 unit number
   4 status

IDENTIFICATION SHEET   UNIT No.

.... Hospital ....

No.HO106/12

SURNAME	ADDRESS
FIRST NAMES	
	TEL. No.
N.H.S. NUMBER	CHANGE OF ADDRESS
MAIDEN NAME	OTHER PREVIOUS SURNAMES
	TEL. No.

D of B	Day	Mth	Yr	Age	Male	Female	S	M	W	Not known
					1	2	1	2	3	4

EMPLOYER

| OCCUPATION | RELIGION |

Name and address of G.P.	Next of kin............ Relationship:...............
	Name.. Tel.:............
Tel. No.	Address...
Change of G.P.	Change of kin............ Relationship:...............
	Name.. Tel. No.:..........
Tel. No.	Address..
Blood Group Rh	Other Records
Drug Sensitivities	
Steroids	

Date of Admission / /	CONSULTANT			CODES	Date of disposal DISCHARGE / /
Date entered on W/L / /	WARD DEPT.	Provisional diagnosis			DEATH
SOURCE OF ADMISSION 1. Waiting List 2. Booked 3. Immediate 4. Other 5. Trans. other Hospital 6. Born in Hospital 7. R.T.A. 8. Home Accident 9. Accident at work 10. Other accident 11. Not known	Type of Bed 1. Priv. 2. Staff 3. Pre-C. 4. Con. 5. Other	Discharge diagnosis—principal —other	Operation Date / /		1. Trans. this/other Hosp. 2. Trans. pre-con. bed 3. Trans. con. bed 4. Trans. other 5. Home/other 6. Died autopsy 7. Died other G.P.s Notice

Date of Admission / /	CONSULTANT			CODES	Date of disposal DISCHARGE / /
Date entered on W/L / /	WARD DEPT.	Provisional diagnosis			DEATH
SOURCE OF ADMISSION 1. Waiting List 2. Booked 3. Immediate 4. Other 5. Trans. other Hospital 6. Born in Hospital 7. R.T.A. 8. Home Accident 9. Accident at work 10. Other accident 11. Not known	Type of Bed 1. Priv. 2. Staff 3. Pre-C. 4. Con. 5. Other	Discharge diagnosis—principal —others	Operation Date / /		1. Trans. this/other Hosp. 2. Trans. pre-con. bed 3. Trans. con. bed 4. Trans. other 5. Home/other 6. Died autopsy 7. Died other G.P.s Notice

GMR 1

Fig. 16.1 An example of the identification sheet.

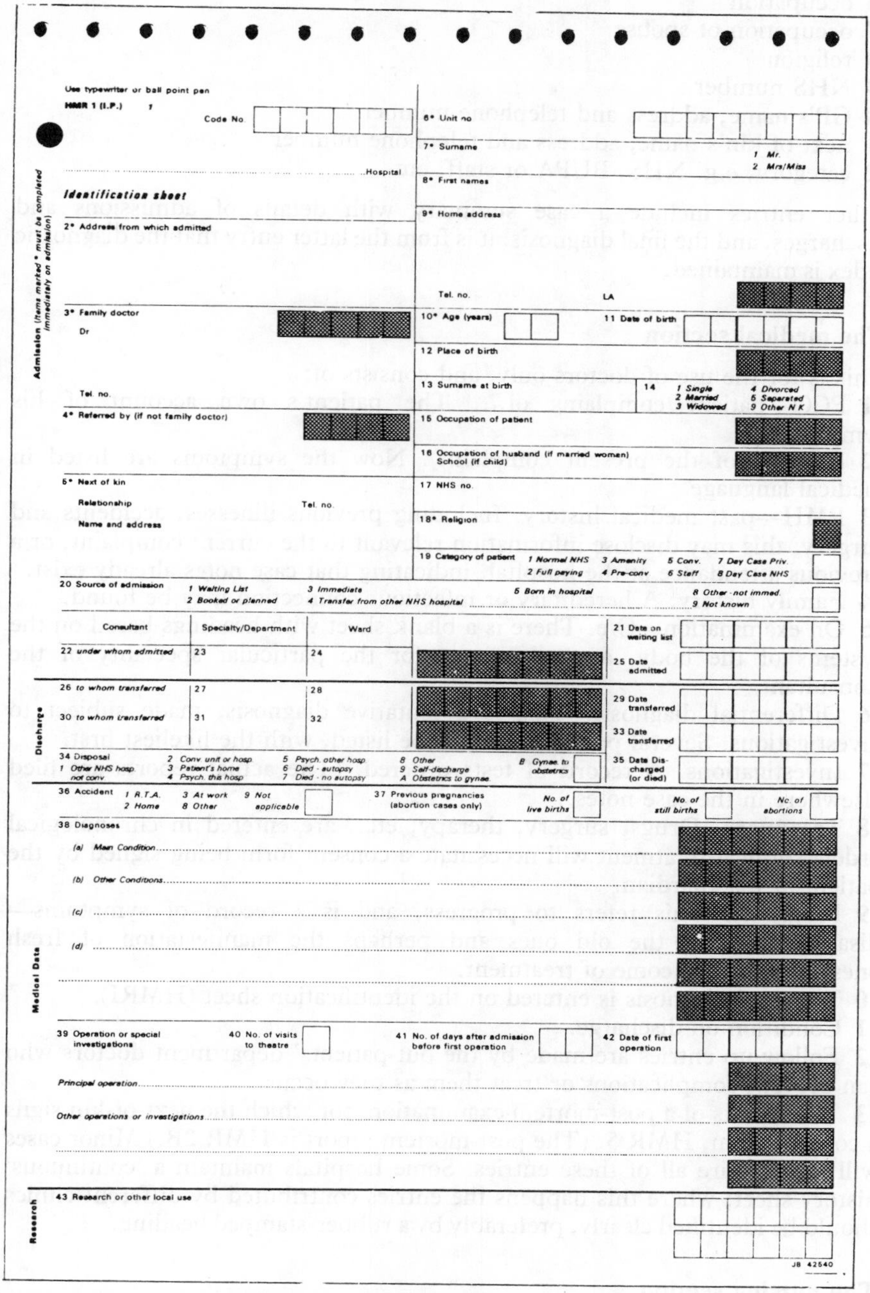

Use typewriter or ball point pen
HMR 1 (I.P.) 1
Code No.
6* Unit no
7* Surname
1 Mr.
2 Mrs/Miss
.... Hospital
8* First names
Admission (Items marked * must be completed immediately on admission)
Identification sheet
9* Home address
2* Address from which admitted
Tel. no.
LA
3* Family doctor
Dr
10* Age (years)
11 Date of birth
12 Place of birth
Tel. no.
13 Surname at birth
14 1 Single 2 Married 3 Widowed 4 Divorced 5 Separated 9 Other N.K.
4* Referred by (if not family doctor)
15 Occupation of patient
16 Occupation of husband (if married women) School (if child)
5* Next of kin
17 NHS no.
Relationship
Tel. no.
Name and address
18* Religion
19 Category of patient 1 Normal NHS 2 Full paying 3 Amenity 4 Pre-conv 5 Conv. 6 Staff 7 Day Case Priv. 8 Day Case NHS
20 Source of admission 1 Waiting List 2 Booked or planned 3 Immediate 4 Transfer from other NHS hospital 5 Born in hospital 8 Other - not immed. 9 Not known
Consultant
Specialty/Department
Ward
21 Date on waiting list
22 under whom admitted 23 24
25 Date admitted
Discharge
26 to whom transferred 27 28
29 Date transferred
30 to whom transferred 31 32
33 Date transferred
34 Disposal 1 Other NHS hosp not conv 2 Conv. unit or hosp 3 Patient's home 4 Psych. this hosp 5 Psych. other hosp 6 Died - autopsy 7 Died - no autopsy 8 Other 9 Self-discharge A Obstetrics to gynae. B Gynae. to obstetrics
35 Date Discharged (or died)
36 Accident 1 R.T.A. 2 Home 3 At work 8 Other 9 Not applicable
37 Previous pregnancies (abortion cases only) No. of live births No. of still births No. of abortions
Medical Data
38 Diagnoses
(a) Main Condition
(b) Other Conditions
(c)
(d)
39 Operation or special investigations
40 No. of visits to theatre
41 No. of days after admission before first operation
42 Date of first operation
Principal operation
Other operations or investigations
Research
43 Research or other local use
JB 42540

Fig. 16.2 HMR 1 (IP)—the identification sheet according to HAA.

5 date of birth
6 occupation
7 occupation of spouse
8 religion
9 NHS number
10 GP's name, address and telephone number
11 next of kin's name, address and telephone number
12 category, e.g. NHS, BUPA or staff, etc.

Other entries include a case summary with details of admissions and discharges, and the final diagnosis; it is from the latter entry that the diagnostic index is maintained.

The medical section

This is for the use of doctors only, and consists of:

1 PCO—patient complains of.... The patient's own account of his symptoms.
2 History (of the present complaint). Now the symptoms are listed in medical language.
3 PMH—past medical history. Including previous illnesses, accidents and surgery; this may disclose information relevant to the current complaint, or a previous attendance at the hospital, indicating that case notes already exist.
4 Family history. A hereditary or infectious connection may be found.
5 On examination—O/e. There is a blank sheet with headings based on the systems of the body, as well as one for the particular speciality of the Consultant.
6 Differential diagnosis. This is a tentative diagnosis, made subject to investigations. Several possibilities may be listed, with the likeliest first.
7 Investigations. A record of tests ordered. (The actual reports are filed elsewhere in the case notes.)
8 Treatment. Drugs, surgery, therapy, etc., are entered in chronological order; surgical treatment will necessitate a consent form being signed by the patient or his guardian.
9 Prognosis. This refers to progress, and is a record of symptoms—disappearance of the old ones and perhaps the manifestation of fresh ones—and the outcome of treatment.
10 The final diagnosis is entered on the identification sheet (HMRI).
11 Condition on discharge.
12 Follow-up entries are made by the out-patients' department doctors who can prevent complications or treat them as they occur.
13 The results of a post-mortem examination, for which the next-of-kin signs a consent form, HMR 5. (The post-mortem report is HMR 2B.) Minor cases will not require all of these entries. Some hospitals maintain a 'continuous' history sheet; where this happens the entries contributed by different clinics should be identified clearly, preferably by a rubber-stamped heading.

The nursing section

Observations by the nursing staff, HMR 7, are recorded only when patients are admitted.

1 The nursing record. Concerning treatments, this may be written on visible-edge cards (filed alphabetically or according to bed numbers on the ward) and recorded in the case notes only when the patient is discharged.

2 Intake and output charts record all fluids taken orally or by transfusion, all fluids lost by micturition, defaecation, vomiting or drainage.

3 Graphic records are specially printed sheets for TPRs (temperature, pulse and respiration), blood pressure, micturition and bowel-function. Entries might be made every 15 minutes or just twice a day, according to the nature of the case.

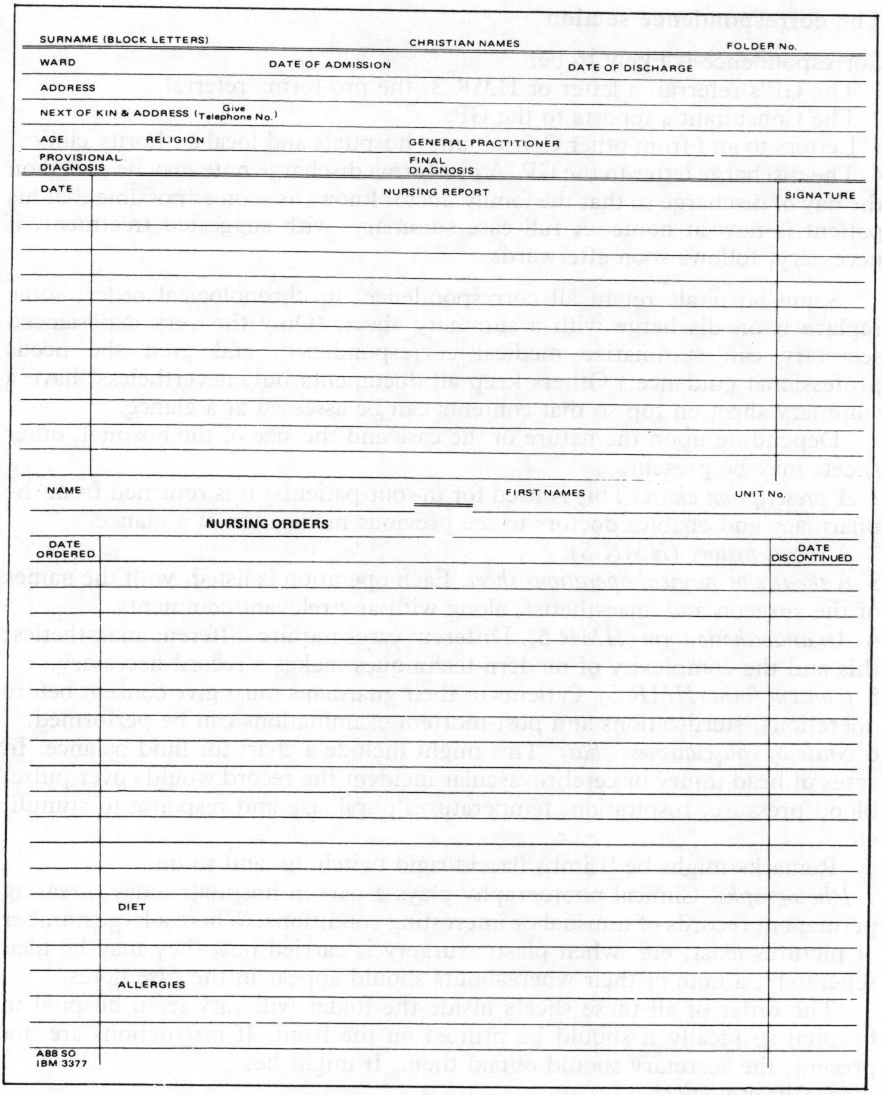

SURNAME (BLOCK LETTERS)	CHRISTIAN NAMES	FOLDER No.
WARD	DATE OF ADMISSION	DATE OF DISCHARGE
ADDRESS		
NEXT OF KIN & ADDRESS (Give Telephone No.)		
AGE	RELIGION	GENERAL PRACTITIONER
PROVISIONAL DIAGNOSIS	FINAL DIAGNOSIS	

DATE	NURSING REPORT	SIGNATURE

NAME _____ FIRST NAMES _____ UNIT No. _____

NURSING ORDERS

DATE ORDERED		DATE DISCONTINUED
	DIET	
	ALLERGIES	

A88 SO
IBM 3377

Fig. 16.3 The nursing record—visible-edge card system.

The nursing section carries Sister's signature or, in her absence, that of the Staff Nurse.

Often a visible-edge system is used, perhaps mounted on the bed rail (see Fig. 16.3).

Some hospitals retain all these records and some substitute a summary sheet once the case ceases to be current, while others do not keep the nursing section at all after discharge. (The bulkiness of records creates space problems in the filing system.)

The correspondence section

Correspondence is likely to be:
1 The GP's referral, a letter or HMR 3, the pro-forma referral.
2 The Consultant's reports to the GP.
3 Letters to and from other Consultants, hospitals and local authority clinics.
4 The discharge letter to the GP. A pro-forma discharge note may be issued on the day of discharge so that the family doctor knows as soon as possible that his patient is now at home. A full case summary, with suggested treatment, if necessary, follows soon afterwards.

Some hospitals retain all correspondence, in chronological order; some replace it on discharge with a summary sheet. (Only the very experienced secretary can summarize medical correspondence, and even she needs professional guidance.) Others keep all documents but, nevertheless, have a summary sheet on top so that contents can be assessed at a glance.

Depending upon the nature of the case and the size of the hospital, other sheets may be present:
1 *A prescription chart*. This is used for in-/out-patients; it is returned from the pharmacy and enables doctors to see previous medication at a glance.
2 *A social history (HMR 8)*.
3 *A theatre or surgical operations sheet*. Each operation is listed, with the names of the surgeon and anaesthetist, along with any relevant comments.
4 *An anaesthetic form (HMR 6)*. Different cases require different anaesthetics; this and the complexity of modern techniques makes a record necessary.
5 *Consent form (HMR 5)*. Patients or their guardians must give consent before operations, sterilizations and post-mortem examinations can be performed.
6 *State of consciousness chart*. This might include a chart for fluid balance. In cases of head injury or cerebrovascular incident the record would cover pulse, blood pressure, respiration, temperature, pupil size and response to stimuli, etc.
  Remarks might be 'Limbs flaccid/rigid/twitching' and so on.
7 *Photographs*. Clinical photography plays a part in hospitals today, creating permanent records of unusual or interesting conditions. Where a large number of pictures exist, e.g. when plastic surgery is carried out, they may be filed separately; a note of their whereabouts should appear in the case notes.

The order of all these sheets inside the folder will vary from hospital to hospital so ideally it should be printed on the front. If instructions are not present, the secretary should obtain them. It might be:
  (a) Chronological
  (b) With a division of in-/out-patient attendances

(c) With separate folders for in-/out-patient attendances, reports and correspondence

(d) Occasionally psychiatrists and venereologists will keep very private notes in their own hands in order to make patients feel totally secure.

As always, the golden rule is that when case notes are split up a clear and prominent note of their location must be made on the main folder.

The order of all these sections inside the case notes may vary from one hospital to another, but within the organization it should be uniform.

Case notes follow patients to wards and operating theatres.

Problem-orientated records (PORs)

POR is a subject receiving considerable attention at the moment. PORs contain a comprehensive description of cases with contributions from all the personnel involved, so that there may be medical and surgical notes, psychiatric notes and entries from various social workers.

The dermatologist who knows of no psychological reason for Mrs Smith's stubborn skin condition might find the psychosomatic indication in the social worker's report; namely that young Tommy Smith is about to appear in the Juvenile Court!

Unfortunately, the disadvantages of POR are equally obvious; files will become bulkier and require more space.

OWNERSHIP OF RECORDS

Physically, case notes belong to the NHS, yet the clinical information obtained in them belongs to the doctor who wrote it. But this information is personal to the patient and would appear to be his property. In fact, neither doctor nor patient has a right to them. *Nominal* ownership is vested in the hospital and the hospital retains possession always in normal circumstances, sending only summaries to other hospitals, doctors, convalescent homes, etc.

If a patient wishes, the opinions expressed in the notes may be passed to a solicitor. Should a solicitor want possession of reports or the folder itself, however, he must apply to a Court. Courts possess the power to overrule doctors' disinclination to disclose information or to produce case notes. It must be concluded, therefore, that ultimately ownership of NHS records rests in the hands of the Secretary of State for Health.

Diploma Questions

*Denotes an incomplete question
ˣA question to be answered after further reading
1 Write notes on the standardization of medical records.
2 As a secretary in a busy hospital, you are asked by a patient to have his case notes forwarded to a doctor at the factory where he works. How would you explain the situation?

3 A set of case notes is normally divided into four sections. What kind of information would you expect to find recorded in each section. Give examples.
4 Write short notes on case summaries.*
5 Write briefly on the secretary's duties in hospital in relation to case notes.*x
6 Write notes on the hospital's legal obligations regarding medical records.*

17

The Filing of
Medical Records

A centralized filing system is considered ideal, but generally the system depends upon the design of the hospital; if it consists of scattered buildings, centralization—with every record in one room—is impractical. The alternatives are unpopular with medical records officers for very good reasons but until they are abandoned completely the medical secretary needs to understand them.

Departmental attendance

A set of notes is started when a patient attends a medical clinic, and a number is allocated to them. Should he be transferred to a surgical clinic, however, they will be closed and fresh notes opened.

Obviously, clinical information can be exchanged between clinics, but this is time-consuming, and often the patient is obliged to tender his basic details more than once. Another disadvantage is that unless the medical records officer is able to maintain rigid control of the situation, departments may adopt the particular filing system that suits them and only them so that all continuity is lost.

Hospital attendance

Records are commenced on the first out-patient attendance or admission, and closed on discharge. A fresh set is started at the next series of attendances.

The three-department system

The out-patients, in-patients and the casualty department are regarded as three separate units, each one starting records on the first attendance and closing them on discharge.

There are risks inherent in each of these systems. The one which is therefore officially advocated, and which takes precedence wherever possible, is the unit system.

The unit system

Its main features are:
1 The patient is allocated a hospital or unit number, and regarded as a separate unit.

2 Case notes are created at his first visit to the hospital and, unless he transfers to another general hospital, could be used throughout his life, from birth to death, no matter how many different specialists he has to consult.
3 The case notes are filed according to the unit number which, as stated, is retained permanently.
4 Thus, the folder contains a complete medical history.
5 The system depends upon the existence of a centralized filing system.
6 As the filing is numerical, a master index is essential.

CLASSIFICATION OF RECORDS

Numerical filing

As every student of office practice knows, this is capable of infinite expansion and so is appropriate for very large systems. But dealing with long numbers is not easy for some people, so useful variations might be:
1 Each batch of one thousand unit numbers has different coloured folders.
2 Each speciality or department has its own colour for folders. This is expensive when cases are referred to other specialists, unless the cover is a temporary one, easily slipped on and off the basic folder; the self-adhesive labels containing the identification details usually peel off without causing damage.
3 More economically, each department is given tags in its own colour to affix, temporarily, to the folders. Colour classification enables the filing clerks or other staff visiting the library or filing room to 'spot' their quarry more quickly than by trudging from shelf to shelf.
4 Each speciality is allocated a set of consecutive numbers. Familiar with their particular range, staff soon learn where to look for the records. New case notes, thus, tend to be grouped together, making filing easier but causing concentrated activity in one section of the main system.
5 *Terminal digit filing.* Under this method of filing lengthy numbers are broken down into pairs from the right (a nought being added to the beginning if there is an uneven amount of digits, so that 12345 becomes 01 23 45). The system is broken down into 100 sections with 100 sub-sections; each sub-section holds approximately 100 sets of files. Case notes with a unit number of 234567 will be taken to a main section of the system marked '67'. Here a middle section is marked '45', and the notes are filed according to their first part of digits '23'. This is an oversimplification when describing a system consisting of an enormous number of files to which thousands more may be added each week. It is true to say, however, that not until another ten thousand sets of case notes have been created will any join number 234567 in its sub-section. Thus, new records are dispersed throughout the system, avoiding simultaneous activity in one area.

Terminal digit filing has other advantages. Staff have only two digits to think about at a time; pre-sorting is easier, therefore, and there is less risk of misfiling. Retrieval is simpler, too.

Microfilming

Microcopying of case notes is not widespread among hospitals. Some confine it to records that are 10 years old; some combine microfilming with computerization, while others use it for certain tasks only, e.g. maintenance of the master index.

Not only is microfilming a secure method of filing, it occupies approximately 5% of the space used by traditional filing; this is a major advantage when the high cost of floor-space is considered.

The film comes in various shapes and sizes, and a whole subject can be viewed chronologically.

Roll film. This is suitable for the archives or inactive records where insertions are not required. Two-to-three thousand documents can be stored cheaply in a hundred-foot reel but, as the reel is continuous, updating presents problems. Roll is available nowadays in cartridges which dispense with conventional lacing and rewinding.

Of course it serves a purpose as a teaching aid.

Microfiche. Approximately a hundred documents can be stored on a piece of film the size of a postcard, in standardized rows, which is usually brought up to date by refilming. It is, nevertheless, often used for the master index.

Jackets. These are an extension of the roll method but film is fed into a unit which cuts each file or document recorded. The pieces are then inserted into 'jackets'—transparent holders or slots set in channels on a backing about the size of a postcard. Material can be brought up to date either by inserting films into vacant slots or by starting another jacket.

Aperture cards. These are punched cards mounted with microfilm. The punched holes represent the contents of the film and its indexing. When the film has to be viewed or a paper copy made, the holes lend themselves to electronic scanning so that sorting and retrieval is speedy.

Edge-punched cards. Microfilm is also mounted on edge-punched cards. As office practice students know, the point of edge-punching is that it facilitates very quick sorting. Each hole represents an item of information, e.g. sex. To retrieve all the cards belonging to males it is merely necessary to pass a steel rod or needle through the appropriate hole and lift them out. The hole representing females is in a different part of the card.

Computerized film. Microfilm can originate from a computer (CIM) but is expensive.

Computer output on microfilm (COM). This is a fast and efficient way of handling vast amounts of data. The microfilm is output directly, with no intermediate paper print-out. Copies for normal reading, without the aid of a viewer, are made, as required. Computer information on magnetic tape can be converted into microfilm at rates of up to 90 000 characters per second.

COM is often used for the master index. When the Group index is housed in the main hospital, microfiche or print-outs are issued to the others.

Viewing

The projector and screen have their place but they have to be safeguarded and take up space and time. In order to view easily and quickly documents which have been microfilmed a machine called a reader or viewer is necessary. This projects an enlarged image on to its own screen, and need be no bigger than desk-top size. There is one suitable for cartridges, and it can be partly dismantled in order to become a projector.

The viewer/printer will even produce a paper copy of a selected frame at the press of a button. Some also have a keyboard attachment on which the number of the required document can be tapped out prior to its projection on to the screen.

The preparation of documents for microfilming

First of all, only authorized persons may decide which records—or part of records—are to be filmed; the medical records officer will be working in close liaison with a microcopying department or officer.

In the large hospital with a filing staff much of the preparation, etc. will be carried out in the library or central filing room, but the secretary needs to understand what is involved.

All staples or treasury tags must be removed once details, including the unit numbers, have been noted. Sheets should be arranged in their correct sequence before being sent to the person in charge of the operation.

In the smaller hospital with no specialist filing or coding staff it may be necessary for the secretary to enter the whereabouts of originals on an absent card or tracer and insert the card into the appropriate place in the filing system. Once filming has taken place code numbers will be entered in a major record book; the tracer card can then be removed.

The film itself has to be indexed. Colour coding is possible, and so is classification by the terminal digit system. However, clear guidelines will be laid down about both filing and indexing procedures.

Filing of microfilm

1 Reels can be filed in indexed cannisters which stand on racks or roll-out shelves, ideally in fireproof units.
2 Various storage units for cartridges are available, some with spring-loaded mechanisms which eject the one required. Again fireproof humidity-controlled cabinets are necessary after processing.

For speedier access or a smaller system, storage books can be used.
3 Microfiche, jackets and aperture cards can all be lodged in card-index equipment, in labelled envelopes if required, or with interleaving to prevent scratching. In addition, the jackets with their index slips lend themselves to drawers or shelves, while microfiche can be slipped into plastic panels, on a rotary stand (see Fig. 17.1). Alternatively, units are available where the microfiche is slotted into panels on one 'page' with indexing on the other (see Fig. 17.2).

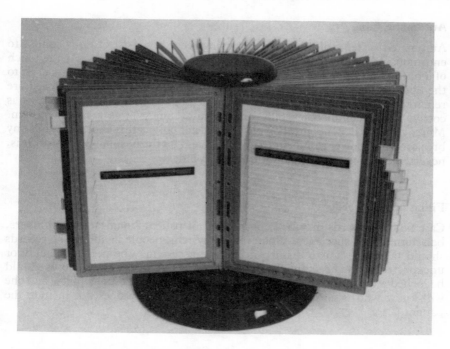

Fig. 17.1 Monodex microfiche system.

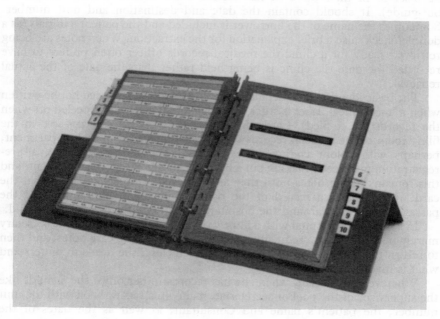

Fig. 17.2 Microfiche storage.

Automatic filing

Automated systems of filing and retrieving records consist of units similar to enormous metal cabinets containing boxes or drums on shelves. At the touch of a button or switch the shelves rotate until the one required presents itself to the operator; some work on the conveyor-belt principle. Ease and speed are remarkable but this sophisticated equipment has some disadvantages. It is costly, and accommodates only one operator unless it is a rotary system. Moreover, it is dependent upon electricity; not only is this expensive, but any breakdown of power results in an extra demand on the hospital generator. It is, nevertheless, sometimes used for the master index.

Filing on the wards

Case notes on wards may be kept in order of patients' names, unit numbers, bed numbers or speciality. Whatever the system, people handling the records should take care not to disturb it because access may be needed quickly or unexpectedly, and speed might be crucial. When not in use, case notes should be locked away. While on the ward they are the Sister's responsibility, and she will know who is allowed to read them; this certainly does not include the patient.

The retrieval of records

Whenever case notes are retrieved from the filing system an absent card should be inserted in their place (it has various other names: tracer, out-card or out-guide). It should contain the date and destination and unit number. Sometimes the name of the borrower is included and the patient's initials (as a double-check) also a brief explanation for the extraction. When notes are being retrieved ready for a clinic the medical records officer often prefers to have recorded the date the clinic is being held rather than the date of the actual retrieval.

The basic identification details, including unit number, need not be written when a 'mechanical' label is stuck onto the absent card (to be peeled off when the records are re-filed). Cards may be stored somewhere accessible in the filing room or the medical records officer may issue a set to each department, perhaps with colour coding. Alternatively, some hospitals follow a pre-registration practice of making out a personal absent card for each patient, and this remains in the notes until they are retrieved. One advantage is that the card, thus, carries a record of the patient's personal programme and the passage of his notes around the hospital, which is useful if they are mislaid.

In a very large hospital with a library or filing staff, sometimes the secretary merely needs to fill in a requisition slip in order to obtain case notes, and then to return them as quickly as possible. Nevertheless, she needs to understand what is involved.

Whatever the system, when she has records in her office she should, like the supervisor of the pool or secretariat, maintain a record book with the unit number, the patient's name and Consultant, as well as the dates of the borrowing and the return.

Lost case notes

However deplorable it may be, it is futile to deny that records are lost from time to time. There are a number of steps the secretary can take:

1 Recheck thoroughly—in the office, the secretariat, the main filing room and in all likely departments. (This is where the personal absent card is very useful, assuming that it is not inside the missing notes! Even if the last person to use it has neglected to make an entry, the programme recorded on it might contain a vital clue.)

2 Collect a new manila folder.

3 Using the master index card, write the patient's name and unit number on the outside, and all identification details on fresh case-sheets.

   (a) In bold letters mark the file 'Temporary'.

   (b) Collect such information as is available. The X-ray department and pathology laboratory will have file copies of any reports they have issued. Where computerization is taking place print-outs can be obtained of these, the identification details and perhaps other useful information.

4 Keep in a prominent place a note about the need to continue searching for the original notes.

5 When they reappear it is worthwhile to study the manner of their disappearance in order to avoid a repetition.

6 Ensure that the doctor receives an apology for any inconvenience to which the loss puts him.

7 By every means possible, spare the patient knowledge of the error lest it undermine his confidence in the hospital.

Diploma Questions

1 What do you understand by
   (a) terminal digit filing
   (b) automated systems in the medical records department?

2 In a general hospital a numerical system of filing is the complete answer to the problems of storing and retrieving medical records. Discuss.

3 Outline the method of filing and retrieving case notes using the unit system.

4 A number of important decisions need to be made when introducing a microfiling system for the first time in a hospital.
   (a) Identify these decision areas, and
   (b) state the factors which need to be considered when they are being resolved.

5 Describe the advantages and disadvantages of running an alphabetical filing system. Give reasons why this method of filing might be considered unsuitable for the filing of patients' records in a large hospital and suggest alternative methods.

18

The Out-patient Department

The out-patient department can make or mar a person's view of the whole hospital and, as more people pass through it than through any other department, the new medical secretary will understand why the correct attitude and procedures are particularly important.

The DHSS has stated that 75% of out-patients should be seen by doctors within half-an-hour of their appointment times, so the aim is clear—adequate preparation and a steady flow of patients into the consulting rooms. Although it is usually full of people, the out-patient department nearly always seems quiet and orderly. This smooth running is aided by nurses, secretaries, clerks, receptionists, voluntary workers, porters, ambulance drivers and technicians, as well as systems of buzzers and bells or flashing lights and a series of notices, directions and arrows (and sometimes even cups of tea and magazines) so the outsider could be forgiven for assuming that organization is easy.

But patients have to be 'squeezed' in onto a full list. Half way through sessions doctors are summoned urgently elsewhere. Films are delayed because the radiographers are under pressure, and although that 'path. lab.' report is on its way it has not yet reached the clinic. That patient is due back at his office, and this lady has to collect her child from school in 10 minutes time. There are at least two patients who do not fully understand English, and the ambulance driver has to wait while old Mrs Smith, who is enjoying her only outing of the week, has a chat with a friendly fellow-patient.

And this is not all! No patient should come to the out-patient department without being referred by a GP, but in some large cities certain sections of the populace do not understand or do not bother to register with GPs and, therefore, rush in with what they deem to be emergencies. Occasionally, these cases can be re-educated or deflected in some way if they are not eligible for treatment in the casualty department, but it is not for the secretary to turn people away. In those hospitals where patients without GP referral form part of the regular scene a policy of handling them will be set out for her to follow.

PURPOSE OF THE OUT-PATIENT DEPARTMENT

Not only does this department provide treatment without withdrawing people from their homes, it has other advantages:

1 It forms a channel of communication between the GP and the specialist. The GP who does not specialize and who lacks the diagnostic facilities available in a hospital can have a diagnosis made or confirmed and, if necessary, specialized treatment can be given to his patient.

2 Follow-up treatment and/or supervision by the out-patient department is possible.
3 Accident and emergency cases can be dealt with promptly by the casualty department.
4 The provision of out-patient care costs less than that of in-patient treatment.
5 Casualties and emergencies are the sole official exception to the regulation that people can receive out-patient attention only when referred by their family doctors. The advantage of this rule is that when treatment is over or can be continued at home, patients are referred back to their GPs. This ensures continuity of care, the maintenance of comprehensive records by both the hospital and the GP and the preservation of the relationship between the patient and his family doctor. It also ensures that the consultation principle is operating, whereby the GP is able to advise the patient in the light of the opinion the specialist has proffered, and the patient is free to decide whether or not to accept that advice.

REFERRAL

This is done by a letter or a pro-forma (HMR 3) specially printed and supplied to GPs by hospitals (see Fig. 18.1). In shape and design the pro-forma resembles a Post Office airmail letter-form, so the doctor can write a letter one side, fold it and seal it by moistening the gummed edges, leaving a section where the patient can add the following information:
(a) Name, address and telephone number

GMR3. PATIENT REFERRAL LETTER

______________________ Hospital

Please give my patient an appointment to attend

______________________ clinic.

The patient has had X-ray/Pathology investigations in connection with this appointment at ______ Hospital on ______ (date)

(PLEASE DELETE INAPPROPRIATE)

Please arrange for an URGENT
EARLY
ROUTINE
FOLLOW-UP APPOINTMENT

For an urgent appointment this form must be accompanied by a letter.

ADDRESS:

G P's Signature ______________

Date ______________

FOR HOSPITAL USE ONLY

CONSULTANT:

DATE TIME

HO106/11

TO BE COMPLETED BY THE PATIENT
(Block Capitals)

Surname or Family Name	Date of Birth: Place of Birth:
First Names	Religion: Occupation:
Address: Telephone No.:	Please tick: Male ☐ Female ☐ Single ☐ Married ☐ Widowed or other ☐

Any Hospital Attendance in this District:
Hospital: ______ Date ______
Hospital No. if known ______
Doctor ______
Previous Address or Maiden Name if changed since last attendance

THIS FORM WHEN COMPLETED MUST BE SENT TO THE HOSPITAL

Fig. 18.1 The general practitioners' pro-forma letter of referral.

(b) Status
(c) NHS number
(d) Occupation
(e) Details of last hospital attendance in the district; this includes a request for the hospital number, if known

The GP can request that the case be seen by a specified Consultant or, otherwise be given the first available appointment in a particular speciality, and, if necessary, he can request transport for the patient. It is useful if he mentions the date of any connected X-ray or pathology investigations.

From this it will be seen that the referral, whether by letter or by pro-forma, is necessary not only for new out-patients but for any subsequent series of attendances.

PRE-REGISTRATION

A patient's first attendance at hospital necessitates a considerable amount of documentation but, as a consequence of GP's referral, this can be accomplished before the patient appears. Then, not only is he spared tedious form-filling but the doctor is not obliged to set up the case notes and take identification details or to wait while a clerk does so. In any case, the time a person has to spend in the out-patient department must be kept to a minimum.

The larger hospitals have a registration section to which new patients are directed, but little work is necessary when pre-registration procedures have been followed efficiently.

Procedure

1 The patient's name is written on an A4 manila folder.
2 The unit number is written prominently beside the name; usually a clerk is in charge of the allocation of hospital numbers.
3 As the case notes are going to be filed numerically, a master index card must be made out; various entries might be made on this, but none as important as the patient's unit number.
4 Case sheets are inserted—identification, medical, nursing and correspondence. (Later, when others are stuck by their tops over these first ones they are often called mount sheets.)
5 Using the information on the GP's referral, the identification sheet is filled in.
6 The name and unit number is written on all the other sheets unless a 'mechanical' label bearing these details, is used.
7 Where computerization is being carried out details can be 'keyed' in later to be recalled, as required, on the VDU, by tapping out the unit number; print-outs are available, if necessary (see Chapter 13).
8 Where the absent card is personalized, it will be made out at this stage (or created by the library filing staff when the notes are received by them for the first time).

THE MASTER INDEX

All filing classifications, except alphabetical, rely on the support of a master index, itself filed alphabetically according to patients' surnames (see Fig. 18.2a,b). Not only does the unit number appear on the case notes and on the appointment card handed to the patient, *it must go against the name in the appointment book.* If it is omitted, the person who has to retrieve the records can locate them only by consulting the index and noting the number.

NAME		
	UNIT No.	
ADDRESS		
AGE	DATE OF FIRST ATTENDANCE	
		MR.
		MRS:
		MISS
CONSULTANT		
IBM 1112		Form A.12.KS

Fig. 18.2a An example of a simple master index card.

RELIGION		WARD			
MOTHER'S No.		MARITAL STATUS Married - Widowed - Single - Other			
WARD	DATE OF ADMISSION	SEC 4&5 R.T.A.	CONSULTANT	DATE OF DISCHARGE	ADMISSION REGISTRAR No.
A.2P St.A.H. IBM 1465					

Fig. 18.2b The larger version of a master index card.

Thousands of new cards are added every year, and daily references to the index amount to hundreds so access should be easy and the facts should be displayed clearly:
- the unit number displayed prominently at the top
- surname and forenames
- status
- address
- date of birth
- sex
- name of GP, and his address

In a Group with computerization the main hospital houses the index, and sends microfilmed copies or print-outs to the others.

There are two golden rules:

1 The details recorded on the card should be checked from time to time; apart from sex and date of birth, they can all change.

2 The card should stay where it belongs, information being 'lifted' or added to/from it *in situ*. Computerization avoids this problem because the tapping out of the unit number produces the details on the VDU screen, and amendments can be keyed in.

The larger index card

Some hospitals employ a bigger card in order to record on it additional information, such as:
- occupation
- religion
- next of kin
- date of first out-patient attendance
- Consultant
- date admitted
- ward
- duration of stay
- date of transfer or discharge

Like the smaller version, this card is useful for the compilation of statistics. Some hospitals follow a practice of extracting it from the system when a patient is admitted. When relatives telephone they can be told the ward without delay, and chaplains can visit admissions of their particular denomination. But the practice is falling into disuse in hospitals where multidocumentation is possible, because it infringes the rule about keeping the card in the filing system. Where lists can be reproduced easily, information about ward-cases can be lodged with the switchboard operators, and chaplains told about denominations (via their pigeon-holes) when the admissions officer distributes her records.

Filing of the master index

As stated, filing is alphabetical but a very large system may require further classification:

1 'F' for female or 'M' for male is written above or below the unit number.

2 Quicker retrieval is possible, however, when the cards for males and females are filed separately.

3 Male cards are one colour, female another.

4 Identical surnames with identical forenames are filed according to the date of birth:

SMITH, John.   12.4.24
SMITH, John.   8.7.39
SMITH, John.   19.1.80

Alternatively, the second Christian name is the guide:

SMITH, John Andrew
SMITH, John James
SMITH, John Maurice

Filing equipment varies according to the size of the index.

1 It may consist of drawers with primary and secondary (and even tertiary) guide cards.

2 A strip index set inside metal frames is suspended from a spindle so that the frames can be opened like the pages of a book. Expansion is limited, however (see Fig. 18.3).

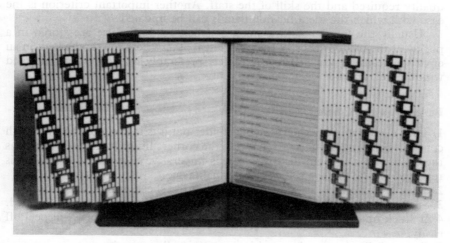

Fig. 18.3 A Bankdex strip index system.

3 A wall-mounted strip index has good visual impact but, again, expansion is restricted.

4 Also unsuitable for the really large system is the rotary unit whereby cards are attached to a wheel which is turned until the required section comes to the top.

5 The carousel—or roundabout—has a central pivot supporting boxes which swing out, providing access to several users at once. Units with big boxes are available so this system is economical of space.

6 The index may be computerized and/or microfilmed.

THE MECHANICAL RECORDING OF IDENTIFICATION DETAILS

This is the production of self-adhesive labels bearing the identification/ registration details, as recorded on the master index cards; the first requisite is a 'master' which can be made on various machines:

1 A spirit 'master' is created by typing (or writing with a ball-point pen on a hard level surface) on a piece of art paper, one side of which is coated with china clay, laid against a sheet of hectographic carbon paper; labels can then be run off on a spirit duplicator, manual or automatic. As the carbon paper is manufactured in several shades, colour-coding is simple.
2 A small stencil is inserted into the typewriter, and typing is carried out with the ribbon disengaged. Alternatively, a stylus pen can be used. Labels are produced on an ink duplicator.
3 An embossed metal plate is made on a special machine, then fed into an imprinter which transfers the information automatically onto the labels, or onto multi-sets of documents.
4 A plastic plate can be created in a similar way.
5 A foil plate is made on the typewriter.
6 The labels can be computer-produced.

The choice of method depends on the existing equipment, or on the cost, the quality required and the skill of the staff. Another important criterion is the ease with which the identification details can be updated.

Usually the 'master' and a stock of labels ready for use are stored in a pocket at the front or back of the case notes; otherwise, they can be kept in an envelope securely attached to the folder, preferably by staples, and marked with the unit number.

Purpose of the labels

1 They *can* be stuck to the case notes folder but it is inadvisable because with constant handling, filing and retrieving the corners lift or wrinkle. Where it is the custom to use them in this way it is imperative that the unit number is repeated on the folder itself in the normal fashion.
2 They are extremely useful for heading up the sheets inside the folder.
3 Specimen containers being sent to the pathology laboratory can be labelled.
4 If stuck onto the absent cards used in the filing system, they will peel off easily.
5 Occasionally they are inserted into operation 'bracelets'.
6 They can be used on waiting list cards.

As GPs receive a great many reports from the hospital, 'masters' with their names and addresses are time-saving.

THE APPOINTMENTS SYSTEM

Appointments can be made in a number of ways: where possible, postal charges to the hospital should be avoided.
1 Patients may telephone. This is straightforward when they are booking follow-up appointments; it is helpful if they can quote the unit number on

their hospital card. When making a first appointment they will either state that their GP is sending a referral letter or, if it is in their possession, be asked to forward it promptly.

2 Patients call at the hospital and deliver the referral.

3 The GP refers the case by post.

These three methods work well because the clerks in the appointments section are skilled in the technique of making appointments and are normally within easy reach of the master index.

4 During clinic sessions, however, the appointment books may be in the out-patient department so that the secretary there will make the bookings. She has the advantage of being able to consult the doctor about dates and times, if necessary.

5 Follow-up appointments may be booked from the wards for patients who are being discharged.

Once an attendance list has been drawn up the clerk in the medical records department may rule a line, perhaps in red, across the page. If the medical secretary is instructed to slip in a last-minute appointment this line will remind her to inform all the staff involved with lists and case notes.

Usually, there is a separate appointment book for each clinic or Consultant. It may consist of:

1 A loose-leaf book in which each page is headed by the Consultant's name. The date may appear at the top, depending upon whether one page represents a day or a month.

2 A visible-edge system. Cards are mounted on a tray or in a book, each overlapping the other but leaving visible the edge bearing the key factors, such as the Consultant's name or the clinic, and the day on which the session is being held (see Fig. 18.4).

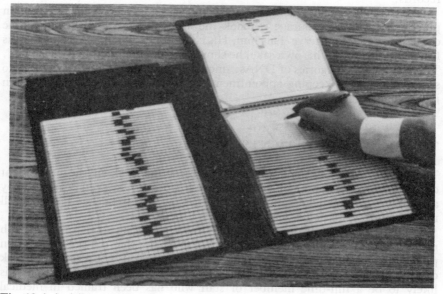

Fig. 18.4 A visible record unit.

3 One doctor or a small department might use a diary.
4 An NCR (no-carbon-required) system is useful. The back of the top sheet and the front of the bottom sheet are chemically treated so that a ball-point pen creates copies which can be distributed to any other departments or personnel involved, and one copy can serve as the attendance list.

The secretary making appointments should observe the following points:
1. The unit number must be written beside the name.
2 Patients should be offered the first available time. It is, nevertheless, sensible to make sure that the results of any investigations ordered will be ready on that date.
3 As a rule, new cases are allotted more time than old ones.
4 No urgent request should be refused without reference to a doctor, even if the session is fully booked and even if it is the patient himself making the request with a seemingly unjustified sense of urgency.
5 Urgent appointments need a distinguishing mark placed against them, e.g. an asterisk, so that if any rearrangement is necessary staff can see at a glance which attendances may be postponed and which may not.
6 When patients neglect to cancel appointments yet do not appear, 'DNA' (did not arrive) is written beside their names in the appointment book, and the doctor running the clinic is informed. He will decide what action is to be taken. Sometimes a 'DNA' rubber-stamp is available. This will imprint on the case notes various alternatives for him to tick:

    (a) No action
    (b) No further appointment but inform GP
    (c) Send further appointment
    (d) Letter to GP (often this is a standardized document)

The secretary follows the particular instruction marked before filing the records.

A history of 'DNA' against a name could be significant. The patient often plucks up sufficient courage to book the appointment, yet when the time comes to keep it his 'nerve' fails him. His condition may not be serious but his fears could be so; for his own sake, he should not be permitted to 'slip the net'. There are other categories of DNAs, among whom is that group of people who seem incapable of keeping appointments; it is not for the secretary to sit in judgement on them.

THE ARRIVAL OF PATIENTS

The smaller hospitals tend to have one reception desk in the out-patient department to which both old and new cases report. It may even be manned by a voluntary worker who simply ticks names on the attendance list while all related matters are being dealt with behind the scenes.

At the other end of the scale there is the registration section to deal with new patients; this should consist mainly of checking that the pre-registration procedures have been properly conducted. There will also be a reception desk or area to which other patients are directed. In this case the receptionist is likely to be a full-time member of staff who has been trained in medical reception duties. She will:

1 Mark arrivals on the attendance list
2 Note DNAs
3 Handle case notes
4 Perhaps date-stamp the case sheets
5 Take the appropriate action when identification/registration details have changed
6 Check that the results of investigations are present before the patient is called in to the doctor
7 After the consultation she will ensure that any request forms are properly completed, direct patients to other departments, procure wheelchairs when necessary, and organize transport and follow-up appointments

PREPARING AND RUNNING AN OUT-PATIENT CLINIC

Running the clinic needs flexibility and diplomacy. Not only do procedures vary from clinic to clinic, but the unexpected tends to be routine. Nerves become frayed when patients, already worried, have to wait for what seems to them to be an undue length of time. Delays should always be explained, and an apology works wonders! After all, most medical secretaries derive immense satisfaction from contact with patients, especially when secure in the knowledge that they have made the best contribution they can towards the preparation and running of the clinic. The precise details of this contribution will vary from clinic to clinic and hospital to hospital, depending upon the complexity of the institution and the existence of other staff, e.g. receptionists and clerks, so the following is merely a guide to what *may* be expected of the medical secretary:

1 The appointment book is collected from the medical records department; it may or may not be accompanied by an attendance list.

2 Case notes may have to be retrieved and absent cards/tracers inserted in their place.

3 All reports and relevant X-ray films must be present, and the doctor's attention drawn to them. If a report is delayed and the patient is due, the secretary has three options. She can—

   (a) go and fetch it
   (b) take the dictation over the telephone and type it, securing a signature later on
   (c) type a summary and receive the proper report later on

4 When a patient has not attended for some time, identification details should be checked, and any changes noted on the identification sheet. If access to the master index is not possible, a note for the medical records department should be pinned to the folder. Obviously, the only exception to this rule is when the details have already been checked at the registration or reception desk.

5 When it is the secretary's job to usher patients into the consulting room she announces them by status and name. She will have to judge whether a child is at the stage to like, 'Here is Jenny to see you, doctor' or to prefer, 'Miss Smith'.

6 Instead of showing in patients, she may be 'sitting in' on the clinic and taking dictation. In this situation the physical examination of the patient takes

place behind a screen. The highly qualified medical secretary, trusted implicitly by the Consultant, may have the actual clinical notes dictated to her. Otherwise, during or after the clinic, correspondence could be:
    (a) replies to the GP's letters of referral
    (b) reports to GPs on investigations and/or recommended treatment,
    (c) letters to Consultants of different specialities, seeking guidance in the management of a case or actually referring the patient.

7 The secretary may be instructed to enter a name on the waiting list.

8 When surgery is involved she will give the patient or his guardian a consent form (HMR 5) and make sure that it is signed. It is the doctor's responsibility to explain the form and see that the person understands what he is signing.

9 Investigations may have to be organized, therapy of some kind arranged or a visit to the surgical appliances officer, and patient-transport may be required. Each of these things will have its own correct procedure.

10 When a follow-up appointment is necessary the patient may be directed to the main appointments section; if the appointment book is in the clinic the secretary must write the unit number against the same.

11 Before the doctor leaves the clinic he must be shown any reports that have arrived, even if they concern a patient who has not attended that particular session, because action may be necessary before filing, e.g. a letter to the GP.

12 He is informed about any DNAs and will issue appropriate instructions.

13 The appointment book is returned to the medical records department; the lists will, no doubt, also be required for statistical purposes.

14 Any necessary alterations to the master index cards may be made now, or the attention of the staff responsible drawn to the fresh details, ideally, in writing.

15 Letters will be typed without delay. Meanwhile, the unit numbers of case notes in the secretary's possession will be entered in her record book, along with the date.

16 Once the letters have been signed, carbon copies filed and any necessary statistics recorded, the case notes can be filed and absent cards removed.

17 The date the notes are returned to the main system will be written in the secretary's record book.

CONTRACEPTIVE CLINICS

These are run in some hospitals. The main point for the medical secretary to note is the use of the cooperation card (as in maternity work, see page 290). Usually this carries brief details of the general medical history and a full record of the contraceptive prescription and check-up. Weight and the results of pathological tests might be included, along with a note that the patient smokes.

The card is in the patient's keeping, to be presented to any doctor she sees.

Diploma Questions

*Denotes an incomplete question
*A question to be answered after further reading
1 Write short notes on
    (a) pre-registration of patients in hospital
    (b) mechanical recording of identification details.

2 Explain the importance of the master index card.*

3 Write short notes on clinic appointments.*

4 What duties might a medical secretary expect to undertake during a busy out-patient session? Describe the subsequent secretarial and clerical work these duties might involve.

5 How may the medical secretary be involved with the following:
  (a) reports on clinical investigations[x]
  (b) follow-up of out-patients who fail to keep their appointments?

6 Compare the duties of the medical secretary at a routine surgery in general practice with those of a medical secretary in attendance at an out-patient clinic.

19

Other Departments

CASUALTY—THE ACCIDENT AND EMERGENCY DEPARTMENT

This department might be called 'casualty' or just 'A and E'. Organization varies from one hospital to another; in some of the smaller towns two hospitals may share casualty duties over a mutual area on a rota basis, so that details of dates and locations have to be publicized on posters, etc. and in the local newspapers. The secretary must familiarize herself with such arrangements until such time as the 'powers-that-be' can rectify the situation.

The large department is in the charge of a Consultant, with a Registrar and a rota of Senior House Officers. The doctor on duty may be referred to as the Casualty Officer. There may be clerical assistance for the nurses, and there may be voluntary help when there is no receptionist. However the casualty department is organized, its primary function remains the same—to provide care for accident and emergency cases; these tend to fall into the following categories:

1 Minor injuries, treated at one or two attendances; there could even be a minor dressings department, e.g. for sprains, lacerations, etc.

2 Casualties, given instant emergency treatment and then admitted; an accident area will be manned day or night. Sometimes there is a medical area for heart attacks, faints, pneumonia, etc.

3 Minor surgical cases which can be treated 'on the spot' but which, for various reasons, the GP cannot handle.

A substantial part of the population is not registered with a GP, and research has shown that some prefer to use the 'A and E' department anyway, so the secretary should be armed with the telephone number and address of the local FPC, not to mention a persuasive manner!

Disposal of casualty cases

1 The patient who has wrongly referred himself might be treated, or might not, depending upon the size and busyness of the department. He might be told to call on his GP or, if he is a temporary resident in the area, he will be told that GPs are empowered to treat visitors who are staying from 24 hours to three months. (The GP will claim payment for this consultation from the FPC.) Furthermore, the patient's own GP at home will receive clinical details about the episode.

2 The patient is treated and discharged; a report is sent to his family doctor.

3 Alternatively, after treatment he may be referred to his GP, to a district nurse or to his works' medical department.

4 He is sent to an out-patient clinic, his casualty card acting as the letter of referral.

5 Admission takes place, with normal documentation.

6 He is referred to another hospital, with a full clinical report.

7 He is brought in dead (BID) (or dead on arrival [DOA]), usually by ambulance, and is taken to the hospital mortuary, but the casualty department carries out its usual documentation.

8 Patients involved in vehicular episodes are of special interest. According to the Road Traffic Accidents Act in 1960, hospitals treating such cases are entitled to claim compensation from the users of the vehicles involved and their insurance companies.

(a) An emergency treatment fee is payable by the user of the vehicle from which the patient is taken to hospital. (Vehicles belonging to the hospital, to the civil service or the army are excepted.)

(b) The cost of further treatment, either in the out-patient department or on a ward, may be claimed by the hospital against the insurance company of the person held responsible for the accident, provided that the company has agreed that payment to the injured party is warranted.

Documentation

1 Details about each case are recorded in the casualty register (see Fig. 19.1); these tend to differ from hospital to hospital, as does the physical appearance of the register, but generally the details include: name, address, age, GP, date and time of arrival, the nature of the injury and where it occurred (e.g. at home or work, in the street, etc.), and any relevant remarks. Usually each entry is

No.	Date	Time adm.	Time dis.	Name	Address	Age	RAT (yes or no)	X-ray		

Own Doctor	Seen by	Treatment	Nature of Complaint	Disposal

Fig. 19.1 Pages from the casualty register (ledger) used in some hospitals.

numbered; the running total that this provides and other information recorded may be needed for the compilation of statistics.

2 Instead of case notes of the usual kind the patient has a casualty card; sometimes this consists of an A4 sheet and sometimes it is NCR, producing copies for GPs.

(a) If the patient is to return, the casualty card is put in the current file. Visits to this department must be in the short-term; otherwise, the patient can be referred to the out-patient department. (Sometimes the casualty card has a 'flimsy' attached to it, to be detached and sent to the GP as automatic notification of his patient's attendance—see Fig. 19.2a.) Another version has two 'flimsies', one for the GP and the other for details of treatment given to a child under five years of age—for use in those areas serviced at different times by the casualty departments of two hospitals. This copy is sent, as a matter of routine, to the Principal Nursing Officer (child health) so that the risk of overlooking non-accidental injuries is eliminated (see Fig. 19.2b).

(b) When attendance ceases the card goes into the secondary file.

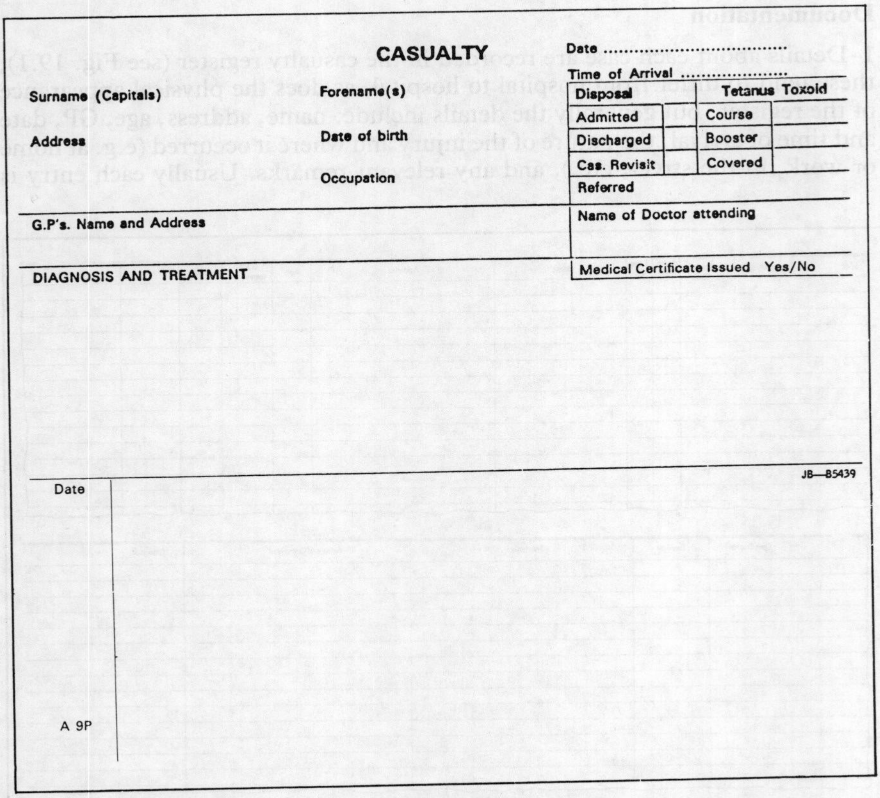

CASUALTY				Date ....

		Time of Arrival	
Surname (Capitals)	Forename(s)	Disposal	Tetanus Toxoid
		Admitted	Course
Address	Date of birth	Discharged	Booster
	Occupation	Cas. Revisit	Covered
		Referred	
G.P's. Name and Address		Name of Doctor attending	
DIAGNOSIS AND TREATMENT		Medical Certificate Issued Yes/No	

JB—85439

Date

A 9P

Fig. 19.2a An example of a casualty card with an NCR slip for general practitioner notification.

```
┌─────────────────────────────────────────────────────────────────────────────┐
│                              CASUALTY            Date .........................│
│  CHILDREN UNDER 5                                Time of Arrival ..............│
│  Surname (Capitals)        Forename(s)          ┌──────────────┬──────────────┐│
│                                                 │ Disposal      │ Tetanus Toxoid││
│  Address                   Date of birth        ├──────────────┼──────────────┤│
│                                                 │ Admitted      │ Course        ││
│                                                 ├──────────────┼──────────────┤│
│                                                 │ Discharged    │ Booster       ││
│                                                 ├──────────────┼──────────────┤│
│                                                 │ Cas. Revisit  │ Covered       ││
│                                                 ├──────────────┴──────────────┤│
│  G.P's. Name and Address                        │ Referred                     ││
│                                                 ├──────────────────────────────┤│
│                                                 │ Name of Doctor attending     ││
│  DIAGNOSIS AND TREATMENT                        ├──────────────────────────────┤│
│                                                 │ Medical Certificate Issued   ││
│                                                 │                      Yes/No   ││
│                                                                                 │
│  Date │                                                             JB—85439    │
│       │                                                                         │
│       │                                                                         │
│       │                                                                         │
│       │                                                                         │
│  A32P │                                                                         │
└─────────────────────────────────────────────────────────────────────────────┘
```

Fig. 19.2b An example of a casualty card used for children under five years of age.

   (c) It might be filed alphabetically or, in the large department, numerically, with a master index.

   (d) Should the patient be admitted, the card accompanies him to the ward where it is lodged in the case notes.

   (e) On his discharge it is removed from the case notes and returned to the casualty department, there to be filed permanently in the secondary file.

3 After treatment the patient is given a printed form on which clinical details of the episode have been written, and he will take this to his GP (alternatively a letter is sent).

Often the police bring cases to the casualty department, and the number of the particular officer may be recorded, if there is a box for it, on the casualty card or register. Police enquiries are not uncommon so the secretary should be clear in her own mind about her public duty and her responsibility to the hospital and, above all, she should seek instructions as to whether her involvement is necessary and, if so, in what particular aspect of the situation. Although in no way shirking her obligations as a member of the public, she refers questions elsewhere usually because, as a rule, the contribution she can make is limited by the peripheral nature of her position.

THE MOBILE ACCIDENT UNIT

Not all hospitals have a 'flying squad' but when they do it is a part of the accident and emergency department and incorporates some or all of the following features.

The medical and nursing staff perform the duties they normally perform in the department, assessing, resuscitating and treating. But when they go out with the mobile accident unit they may wear a special uniform, often marked 'Doctor' or 'Nurse' so that the public can recognize them quickly; it may have to consist of protective clothing. Helmets, boots and oxygen breathing apparatus, etc., for a major emergency is stored at the hospital, usually in a special equipment room which is easily accessible.

The unit carries a radio so that extra equipment or personnel can be summoned. Sometimes a multi-channel radio set in casualty connects with the ambulance service. There may be a direct telephone line bypassing the hospital switchboard for use in a large-scale crisis, or even a direct line to the police or fire brigade.

Some hospitals have an obstetric 'flying squad'.

Secretarial duties

These depend upon circumstances so it is the responsibility of those in charge to issue instructions. Medical secretaries will probably be required to do nothing more than carry out their normal duties as unobtrusively as possible or to work late in order to man telephones, run errands or send out urgent reports, etc. Perhaps they can help by seeing that a medical bag is ready, appointments cancelled quickly and courteously and then rebooked; all sorts of people may need to be informed of the doctor's involvement: his family, a committee, another hospital, for example. The admissions officer might need help in handling a rush of admission-documentation; in a small hospital, without a 24 hour admissions service, the secretary may be capable of taking over this task, or just helping the ward Sisters—it depends on the type and size of the emergency. She should never overlook the fact that her most effective contribution could be to keep out of the way!

Large-scale crises tend to produce leaders and heroes but, more often than not, it is the properly planned, well-drilled procedure that is most successful.

THE X-RAY DEPARTMENT

This section of the hospital is run by a Consultant who is a specialist in radiology. A senior radiographer supervises the radiographers (some qualified, some in training) and the secretaries, clerks and/or receptionists and porters, as well as 'dark'-room staff.

Some departments are closed units, working only for staff doctors: others are open or direct access units to which local GPs can make referrals without first sending cases to the out-patient department.

Requests

1 Patients are given appointment cards, the department keeping its own appointments book.

SURNAME (capitals)	FORENAME(S)	X-RAY DEPT.	X-Ray No.
Mr. Mrs. Miss		HOSPITAL	
Reg. No./Address	Date of Birth	Report Required By :-	Ward/Dept.
		Consultant:	
		G.P.:	
TEL. No.		Examinations Required	
PREVIOUS X-RAYS DATE HOSPITAL			
10 DAY RULE	Ignore/Observe*	APPOINTMENT DATE	
DATE OF L.M.P. .... * delete as required			
Clinical History and Diagnosis			
Signature	Date	Radiographer's Initials	
JB—83866			Code A85P

Fig. 19.3 An example of an X-ray request form.

2 The out-patient department refers cases, either by telephone or by sending them, to X-ray with some kind of authorization, containing instructions about the type of film needed.
3 On medical instructions, ward Sisters and secretaries request films for in-patients.
4 Requests from the accident and emergency department tend to be urgent.
5 When the unit is one of direct access, the GP will contact it by letter or request form; the hospital keeps him stocked with an assorted supply of these.
6 Request forms are specially printed, often NCR, and vary according to the kind of radiography required; they include spaces for an indication of the patient's condition, e.g. walking, sitting or wheelchair or stretcher, and main medical findings or provisional diagnosis (see Fig. 19.3).
7 Labels bearing identification details may be used to head up the forms.
8 According to the nature of the film, the patient is given instructions about diet and any other necessary preparations; ideally, these are printed.

Reports

The radiologist dictates a report to be typed either on its own form or on the bottom or reverse side of the request form, and it will accompany the plate to the person who requested it. The exception is the GP, who receives only the report. Films stay in clinics only long enough for doctors to view them and on wards for the duration of the patients' stay, and are ultimately returned to the

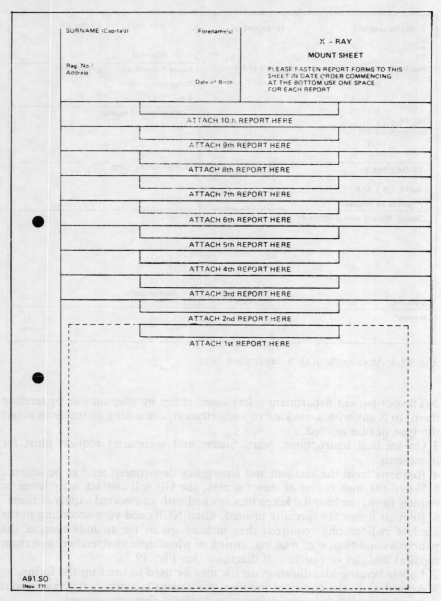

Fig. 19.4 An example of X-ray reports in the case notes.

radiography department. (Only after a certain period of time will they end up in the library or central filing room; they may even be microfilmed.)

Inside the case notes the reports could be affixed to a card marked with the name and unit number. When the card is full another is stapled to it, thus—because the order is chronological—the latest report is on top and a continuous record of all X-ray findings is at hand (see Fig. 19.4).

Filing of X-ray plates

The medical records officer is responsible for the filing of films wherever they are stored. As a rule, current or 'active' films are kept in the X-ray department itself, usually with a file copy of the report attached, and in an envelope.
Classification varies:
(a) Alphabetical filing, best suited to small systems.
(b) Numerical according to the unit number, not ideal because there are gaps in the sequence caused by the fact that not every hospital patient has films taken.
(c) Numerical, perhaps terminal digit, with a master index.
(d) Subject filing according to the parts of the body filmed. The primary guide cards are labelled 'Chest', 'Leg' and so on, and within these are secondary guide cards marked with the alphabet; again, a master index is vital.
(e) Microfilming requires coding and indexing, of course.
(f) Chronological filing, except in the smallest of systems, is at best temporary unless it is subdivided into other classifications, and a master index employed.
(g) A combination of methods might be used, incorporating the separation of large plates from small. As usual, an index is required.
(h) The patient's date of birth is used as an indexing unit in some hospitals, also colour coding for the year the film is taken.

When films are removed to the main filing room or library a record is made.

The points system

The secretary attached to the radiography department will discover that each type of X-ray film is evaluated by points, the complex ones receiving more than the others. These are recorded according to a code in order that the department's workload can be measured and resources allocated.

Ownership of X-ray plates

As a private patient pays to be X-rayed, the film is his property, although it is usually practical for his GP or specialist to store it for him.

For NHS patients the situation is much the same as that of their case notes. Physically the plate belongs to the NHS but the facts yielded by it are personal to the patient, while what is contained in the report would seem to be the property of the writer. In practice, nominal ownership rests with the hospital.

It is the doctor's prerogative to disclose to the patient only what he deems to be necessary or advisable about what has been revealed by the picture.

THE PATHOLOGY LABORATORY

In some teaching hospitals where very advanced diagnostic systems, treatments and/or research are being carried out there may be highly qualified persons—of a status at least equal to that of the Consultant—who are not medical practitioners; they may be in the employ of universities or the DHSS.

In the average general hospital the pathology laboratory is run by a Consultant pathologist with the assistance of other pathologists. Technicians, supervised by a senior, might be specializing in biochemistry, the study of living things, or histology, the study of organic tissue, etc., and might be trained or undergoing training. Although not medical doctors they are very skilled people, carrying out a wide variety of investigations. Helping them is a third tier of staff, the laboratory assistants. In addition, there are mortuary attendants and porters. The large department has a secretary and/or clerical team and, occasionally, a nurse is attached to the staff.

Like the X-ray department, the pathology laboratory may be a closed unit, carrying out work only for the hospital or an open unit to which GPs have direct access.

Requests

1 As with radiography, requests are made by doctors or by nurses and secretaries acting on medical instructions and, in areas without a public laboratory, by GPs.

2 Certain investigations necessitate a period of notice being given.

3 Specially printed forms are used and vary according to the nature of the test (see Fig. 19.5a,b,c). Secretaries should note when mechanical labels cannot be used to head up the forms; this may be due to their small-box design or to the fact that they are NCR and/or a part of HAA. Sometimes the embossed plastic

SURNAME (capitals)		Forename(s)			☐		☐	G.P. ☐
						☐ Other (specify)		
Address				Sex	Ward		CLINICIAN/G.P.	Signature
Unit No.		Date of Birth		Date collected		Time collected		Lab. No.
CLINICAL SUMMARY				INVESTIGATION REQUIRED				
FOR LABORATORY USE ONLY								

| Date received | Date of report | Signature | | MISCELLANEOUS |
| A10150   JB—B2690 | | | Haematology Department | HAEMATOLOGY |

Fig. 19.5a Request form for investigation by the Pathology Laboratory.

SURNAME (capitals)	Forename(s)	☐ ☐ G.P. ☐ ☐ Other (specify)			
Address		Sex	Ward	CLINICIAN/G.P.	Signature
Unit No.	Date of Birth	Date collected		Time collected	Lab. No.

TO BE COMPLETED BY CLINICIAN

CLINICAL SUMMARY

Blood group if known ABO......... Rh......... Antibodies YES/NO

Previous transfusion YES/NO Date ....

ALL previous pregnancies YES/NO Dates ....

Miscarriages, early YES/NO
late YES/NO

Neonatal jaundice YES/NO

BLOOD REQUIRED FOR: put ✓

a) Group and retain serum (maximum 5 days) ☐

b) Urgent transfusion TIME ....

c) Transfusion DATE .... TIME ....

(Blood/packed cells) UNITS ....

1) 10 ml of clotted blood FULLY labelled with patients forenames, surname, date of birth, Hospital number (or home address) must accompany this request.

2) A minimum of 24 HOURS notice is required for all routine grouping and crossmatching.

3) Blood will be kept for 24 hours ONLY after indicated time of transfusion.

FOR LABORATORY USE ONLY	Group	ABO	Rhesus	Atypical antibodies	Date	Signature

BLOOD CROSSMATCHED — METHODS OF COMPATIBILITY TESTING

Date	Test No.	Blood Unit No.	ABO	Rh	Sal 20°C	Sal 37°C	Enz	ALB	Coombs	Comments	Fate	Signature

Date received Time received	Date of report	Signature	Haematology Department	BLOOD TRANSFUSION SEROLOGY

A102SO JB—82506

Fig. 19.5b Request form for investigation by the Pathology Laboratory.

Please use a Ball-point pen

SURNAME (Capitals)	Forename(s)	☐ ☐ G.P. ☐ ☐ Other (specify)			
		Sex	Ward	CLINICIAN	Signature
Reg. No./ Address	Date of Birth	Date collected		Time collected	LAB. No.

CLINICAL SUMMARY including ALL DRUGS please

BLOOD SAMPLES ONLY

TICK PRIORITY TEST(S) TO COVER SMALL SAMPLES OR MACHINE FAILURE

SMA PROFILE

Prior arrangements must be made for Urgent Requests

Electrolytes Urea ☐ Calcium Phosphate ☐ Creatinine ☐ Proteins ☐

Date received	Date of report	Signature PATHOLOGY SERVICE	CLINICAL CHEMISTRY / SMA

A107 SO
XXXXXX
(Oct. 78)
JB—86832

Fig. 19.5c Request form for investigation by the Pathology Laboratory.

card can be used to imprint identification details. Labels can be used on most containers, however.

4 Out-patients are often sent to the laboratory, either with their specimens or with some kind of authorization (usually the request form itself). Where this occurs somebody will be acting as a receptionist and making the customary entries in a record book.

5 Ward specimens and request forms are usually collected by a porter, both he and the ward maintaining a record of what is given and received.

6 Requests are not valid unless signed or initialled by a doctor.

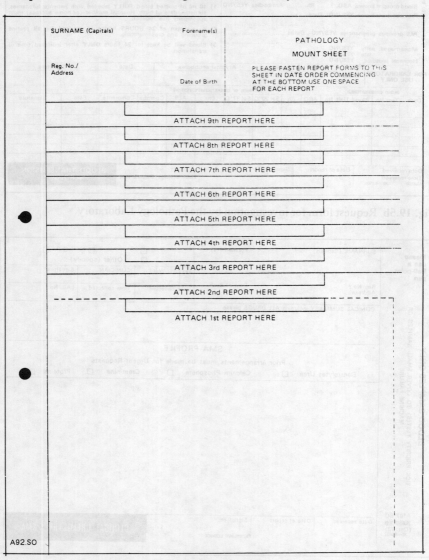

Fig. 19.6 An example of a mount sheet for pathology reports in the case notes.

Reports

These may be written at the bottom of request forms or on the reverse side, or the request forms may contain boxes for the results. File copies are retained, filed alphabetically or numerically, sometimes according to unit numbers, sometimes not, or with subject classification etc. They may be stored and/or analysed in a computer, with print-outs as necessary or VDU display. They may be affixed to mount sheets in the case notes, similarly to X-ray reports (see Fig. 19.6).

Reports are often delivered to wards by the porter who collects the samples. A book or folder may be used, and receipt is acknowledged by a signature.

Where computerization exists the patient's unit number must be tapped out along with a 'password' and the kind of report wanted, e.g. 'M' for microbiology, 'H' for haematology, etc. A list of results appears on the VDU, starting with the first test recorded, perhaps some years before, if necessary.

THE OPERATING THEATRE

In a Group, surgery may be carried out in one hospital and not at another, or one kind of surgery here and another there. In a very small hospital there may be only one theatre, possibly with a recovery room where patients on trolleys' 'come round' from anaesthetics before being taken to wards. Large organizations have several operating theatres with a Sister in charge of each and one, sometimes senior, in overall charge. Where the theatre suite is extensive the permanent nursing staff can specialize.

Roughly speaking, there are two kinds of surgery:

1 Emergency cases at any time of the day or night. These are organized by the Surgical House Officer and the theatre staff, and patients are taken directly

---

CONSENT FOR OPERATION

_____ Hospital

I _____ of _____
_____ hereby consent

to the submission of my child/ward* _____

to undergo the operation of _____
the nature and purpose of which have been explained to me by Dr./Mr.* _____

I also consent to such further or alternative operative measures as may be found necessary during the course of the above-mentioned operation and to the administration of general, local or other anaesthetics for any of these purposes.

No assurance has been given to me that the operation will be performed by any particular practitioner.

Date _____ Signed _____
                                          Patient/Parent/Guardian*

I confirm that I have explained the nature and purpose of this operation to the patient/parent/guardian*

Date _____ Signed _____
                                          Medical/Dental* Practitioner

*Delete as appropriate

St.A.H.IBM 2396   A15SO JUNE 1977

Fig. 19.7 A consent for operation form.

into the theatre. The identification section of the case notes may not be filled in until afterwards, and in certain circumstances the regulations about the consent form may have to be waived; as with all matters relating to the consent form, ultimate responsibility rests with the surgeon (see Fig. 19.7).

2 Non-emergency surgery falls into three groups:
  (a) cases admitted from the waiting list.
  (b) those admitted as emergencies but found to be in need of a period of ward-care prior to surgery.
  (c) minor surgery for which only a few hours' ward-care is necessary or even none at all; such cases are normally entered on a separate waiting list.

The operations list

The decision about who is to receive surgery at a particular time is taken by the surgical team in consultation with the theatre staff; the availability of beds is shown on the beds states return made that day to the medical records department.

Ideally, the order in which operations are going to be performed is entered in a diary or register from which the medical secretary can type a circulation list. The secretary who finds herself in any doubt about the order of this list must seek advice. No theatre Sister welcomes a mixture of long and short operations, complex and simple or 'clean' and 'dirty'; in any case, a surgeon of a particular speciality may be needed, and neither he nor the anaesthetist welcomes a 'staggered' programme.

Declining to accept responsibility for the order until it has been professionally approved, the secretary will type the details (usually on a specially-printed list) and, if she is wise, delay this until she has been informed that the patients have been admitted and declared fit for surgery. Then the list is circulated to:
  (a) the surgeon, Surgical Registrar, House Surgeon (a Senior House Officer) and the anaesthetist
  (b) the theatre Sister, Principal Nursing Officer and ward Sister
  (c) the pathology and radiography departments
  (d) the physiotherapy departments
  (e) perhaps the medical social worker, and any other interested parties about whom she will be notified. The latter could include people responsible for student training, special equipment, photography and so on.

THE PHYSIOTHERAPY DEPARTMENT

The Consultant in charge of the physiotherapy department is a specialist in physical medicine. He has a staff of physiotherapists, trained or undergoing training, working under the supervision of a senior, possibly with clerical assistance. In contrast to this, the small department could be manned solely by the physiotherapists and their superintendent, acting on medical instructions.

Treatment includes massage, muscle-stimulation by heat or electricity, remedial exercise and various physical measures; all kinds of equipment is used but drugs play no part in physiotherapy. Postoperative physiotherapy is an integral part of treatment in a great many cases so a copy of the operations list facilitates the planning of schedules.

Appointments

Occasionally GPs have direct access to the department and will book appointments in the customary way. Otherwise, patients are referred from the wards or from the out-patient department and afterwards may well make their appointments direct. The appointment book may be:
- (a) centralized, with several pages for each day, headed by the name of the physiotherapist, or
- (b) one book for each therapist.

Sometimes the unit number is used, sometimes not. Record-keeping systems follow the usual options, depending on the size of the department. The actual case notes will have to be retrieved whenever doctors are in attendance.

Reports

1 In some cases no written report is required. The doctor orders a course of physiotherapy, and when it is finished the patient reports back to him.
2 When a specialist in physical medicine is in charge of the department he will see patients at regular intervals, making the usual entries in their case notes; when the referring doctor is a hospital colleague, this may be all that is necessary. Otherwise, the Consultant sends reports to GPs and, when appropriate, other hospitals.
3 In the small department the superintendent physiotherapist keeps staff doctors informed, as necessary; sometimes they will see their patients in the department.

Secretarial duties

Unless the medical secretary is assigned permanently to the physiotherapy department or is working for the Consultant, her main duty is liaison. She directs patients to the department, ensures that appointments are made, reports passed to and fro, etc.

MATERNITY—THE OBSTETRIC DEPARTMENT

Hospital confinements have taken precedence over home-deliveries; in the Group, maternity cases may be referred to one particular hospital only. But there are cases where three agencies are involved, i.e. the hospital, the local authority, the GP.

The situation is further complicated by the fact that antenatal care may be undertaken by the hospital or by the GP irrespective of where the confinement is to take place. Under these circumstances the *cooperation card* is invaluable, as the patient takes it with her to each consultation, no matter where it is being conducted or by whom, so that each party can make an entry for the other(s) to

CONFIDENTIAL   Ambulance Depot Tel. No._____

Mrs._____

_____

_____

IF FOUND, PLEASE RETURN TO ABOVE

IMPORTANT NOTE: This card must be kept in YOUR POSSESSION.

Please show it to the doctor or midwife at each examination
or on admission to hospital.

B. 40P

Fig. 19.8 One kind of envelope in which the cooperation card is kept.

read. On the principle that patients do not have access to their medical records, this card may be returned to the woman in a sealed envelope each time. This precaution is dispensed with, however, by some doctors who have observed that the recorded information is of tremendous interest to the mother-to-be and stimulates healthy discussion, the voicing of worries and queries. After all, she is not ill and the better she understands what is going on inside her the more relaxed she will be. Unfortunately, there may be clinical and other circumstances contraindicating such a practice, so the medical secretary receives instructions about whether the envelope (see Fig. 19.8) is to be sealed or not.

After the birth, the *cooperation card* is retrieved by the GP and is summarized or placed in the woman's medical records envelope; the secretary can offer a timely reminder about this.

Integrated maternity care

Although less and less confinements are taking place in the home nowadays, the community midwife still has an important contribution to make in antenatal and post-natal care; in many hospitals she is able to participate in the maternity service, including delivery, as they run a GP maternity unit or welcome her into the consultant obstetric unit.

There are several ways in which obstetric care can be integrated. When the patient makes the initial booking for her confinement she could be seen not only by her GP but the midwife and a health visitor. Then at the next appointment when she sees the GP and the Consultant Obstetrician a scheme of management is evolved for her. Assuming that everything is normal, she is from then onwards attended by the GP and the midwife.

The secretary knows that antenatal attendances are commonly monthly up to the 26th week of pregnancy, fortnightly to 36 weeks and then weekly until delivery. General care might be shared by the GP and the midwife, with the patient visiting the obstetrician only when necessary. (Both the hospital and GP's secretaries will be on the alert for DNAs.) The cooperation card accompanies the patient when she enters hospital for her confinement.

The advantages of controlled integrated care are as follows:

1 The obstetrician's workload is reduced yet he is monitoring the case with optimum responsibility.
2 The GP–patient relationship is not interrupted.
3 He is more easily accessible than the hospital doctor.
4 She spends the minimum time in unfamiliar surroundings.
5 The midwife is a known figure from the beginning to the end of the pregnancy.
6 The involvement of the health visitor adds to the strictly medical/nursing care. Her notes, combined with those of the midwife, and the GP's long-standing record, facilitate the best management of mother and child once they leave hospital (and constitute a limited kind of patient-orientated case history).
7 Nonetheless, all the specialized resources of the hospital are available throughout for problem cases.

Secretarial duties

The secretary may be working for a Consultant Obstetrician or a 'firm'. She must be familiar with the way the maternity service operates not only within the hospital but in the catchment area as a whole so that it functions smoothly through all the channels of communication with which she is involved.

Whether obstetric care is limited, shared or integrated, referral must contain certain details:

1 name, address, age and marital status. (If the records show that the patient is unmarried yet calls herself 'Mrs', the secretary calls her 'Mrs'.)
2 Primigravida—first baby
3 Multigravida—the patient has had more than one pregnancy
4 LMP—last menstrual period
5 EDD—expected date of delivery

The secretary will see that all communications are despatched as promptly as possible, that investigation request forms are filled in promptly (invariably the date of the last menstrual period is required, whatever the nature of the test) and that reports are received on time and, where applicable, copies distributed.

If required, she can advise the patient about maternity benefits, exemption from prescription charges, etc., the forms involved and the address and hours of the local DHSS and she can ensure that any ambulance-booking is arranged. When the mother is discharged from hospital, usually within 48 hours of delivery, it may be the secretary's job to see that the GP and/or midwife receive the standard notification.

When the post-natal examination takes place at the hospital the questions of cervical cytology and contraceptive advice may arise; forms may have to be completed and appointments booked. The patient will also be advised about the baby's immunizations; if these are administered by anyone but the GP he must be informed. Some hospitals give the mother a booklet of forms to use as a kind of 'cooperation' record for the child until he is sixteen. In it doctors enter details not only of immunizations but infectious diseases, injuries, allergies, etc.

Statistics may need to be recorded at each step, or the necessary information relayed to the clerk or department responsible (possibly coding and indexing).

THE INTENSIVE CARE UNIT (ICU)

The ICU is not a part of the hospital with which the medical secretary has close contact, but she is familiar with its main features and she is in a position to enlighten those people who confuse it with the operating theatre's recovery room!

Staff

The ICU is run by a specialized team headed by a Consultant Physician and including anaesthetist, pathologist, Senior Registrars in medicine, surgery and anaesthetics, as well as a Senior House Officer (medical). When a patient has been admitted by a particular 'firm' that Consultant, his Registrars and Housemen become members of the team for the duration of the stay. The nurse–patient ratio might be as high as 4 : 1.

The unit is characterized by complex medical and nursing procedures, allied to sophisticated equipment—the operation and maintenance of which often relies on the expertise of other disciplines.

Cases

The aim of the ICU is the provision of constant medical and nursing attention for the critically ill. Cases may be graded, however, as requiring intensive, medium or minimal care and the length of stay varies accordingly.

Typical cases are those who have undergone major surgery, and others who need continuous monitoring, the maintenance of an airway, the control of toxaemia, the relief or prevention of shock, cardiac cases and those with multiple injuries, particularly to the head.

The secretary may become involved if her Consultant or 'firm' is on the team for the duration of a particular case, or she may work permanently for the Consultant in charge of the unit; whatever her position, she observes meticulously all the regulations concerning the ICU.

CENTRAL STERILE SUPPLIES DEPARTMENT (CSSD)

The purpose of this department is to provide packs of clinical instruments and materials (some disposable and some for re-use), all sterilized and packed under controlled conditions for use on wards, in operating theatres, and all departments.

Clinical responsibility is customarily in the hands of a Consultant who is, generally, a pathologist. His is in no way a managerial role, but he will monitor tests of equipment and the standards of sterilization.

FOLLOW-UP DEPARTMENT

Some special cases need following-up, possibly on a life-long basis, in order to achieve the following objectives:

1 results of treatment
2 provision of further treatment if the need arises
3 research

Where such a department exists the categories most likely to be dealt with are malignancies or tuberculosis and—possibly for lesser periods—eye conditions and progressive disease of the central nervous system.

Procedure

1 A control card is created bearing the patient's names and address, unit number, and date of first treatment. A note is made also—perhaps on a separate card—of the GP, next of kin, and a second responsible relative.
2 The card is inserted into a tickler system.
3 Case notes have a special mark, such as a coloured flash which indicates that the follow-up department and/or GP must be told about DNAs, admissions and deaths, also any change in identification details. (When the really efficient medical records officer issues a form for this purpose, the department will be on the circulation list.)
4 Departments dealing with the patient make regular reports to the follow-up department, e.g. radiotherapy.
5 Secretaries report the names of patients with malignancies treated by 'their' Consultants; again, there should be a special form.
6 Ward Sisters report any admissions of appropriate conditions.
7 Copies of relevant discharge summaries are issued to the department.

Types of follow-up

1 Out-patient attendance
2 Written follow-up may be feasible where attendance is unnecessary or impossible. For example, in the case of a patient:
    (a) who is remaining well, having responded to treatment
    (b) where, after all possible treatment, the condition is taking its course
    (c) where attendance is impossible for reasons unrelated to his condition, i.e. another disability or distance

Keeping in touch

Even assuming that full identification details are recorded originally, that a good relationship is established with the patient, and that case notes are *never* lost, keeping in touch can be difficult, but there are various possibilities.
1 In order to establish that the patient is still alive, he can be approached directly, providing he was well when last seen. A printed form may be used.
2 GPs are sent a printed form.
3 In addition to next-of-kin, another responsible relative can be asked if the patient has moved without informing the hospital.

4 A next-door neighbour or occupant of the patient's house can be approached when letters are returned marked 'Gone Away', but ordinary hospital note-paper must be used, without clinic or department headings, because no indication of the condition should be made.

5 Any other hospital involved in follow-up will send information.

6 The health visitor or social worker may be able to persuade patients to attend when examination is necessary.

7 The local Registrar of Births and Deaths will supply notification of deaths from a registered disease.

8 The Office of Population and Censuses and Surveys will produce date and cause of death if application is made on its own form.

THE PERSONNEL DEPARTMENT

Although she does not work in this department, the medical secretary will come into contact with it and may well have been recruited by the Personnel Officer.

Size and structure vary but, generally, its responsibilities are as follows:

Recruitment of staff. This will involve the drafting of advertisements, job descriptions, job specifications and interviewing.

Training and promotion. Like staff selection, this will entail liaison with senior personnel in other departments.

Staff welfare. Any social and sports facilities come within the terms of reference, as does counselling of staff and contact with those on sick leave.

Legislation. The department must be familiar with all Acts of Parliament and codes of practice pertaining to employees and be able to handle disputes and grievance procedures, receive Trade Union representatives, and also deal with matters relating to resignations, retirement and redundancy.

Documentation. Typical of this department are personnel records, advertisements, job descriptions (details of the job) and job specifications (details of the person required to do the job), job evaluations and appraisals.

Diploma Questions

*Denotes an incomplete question
ˣA question to be answered after further reading

1 Describe documentation in the casualty department, without admission.*

2 Write short notes on
(a) the documentation for patients needing radiography.
(b) and outline the various methods of filing X-ray films.

3 Describe the function and organization of the X-ray department with reference to filing and ownership of records.

4 Describe the organization of the following in hospital, outlining the duties of the staff who work there and the procedures followed:
the X-ray department.*

5 Describe the documentation involved in the following:
investigations by the pathology department.*

6 Write notes on the medical secretary's duties in relation to pathology reports.*

20

Some Important Personnel

THE MEDICAL SOCIAL WORKER

It is accepted without question nowadays that if the social and psychosomatic aspects of illness are overlooked the prognosis may be affected adversely so the number of cases handled by the medical social worker has increased dramatically.

Hospitalization can cause all kinds of problems ranging from a pet left untended to loss of earnings, and often the illness has been aggravated or even produced by conditions prevailing before admission, so, unlike most of the other staff, the medical social worker's terms of reference are very closely linked to the home/work environment from which the patient has come and to which he must return. Bound by the British Association of Social Workers' code of ethics, however, she passes on information only as necessary and with the patient's approval.

Casework

1 She records the social history, HMR 8, for the doctor, and an assessment is made of the help she can contribute.

2 Her role may be advisory, helping the patient and his family to understand the nature of his condition, to accept it and adjust to it.

3 She can arrange for the care of children and other physically dependant relatives.

4 When patients are to be discharged she can mobilize resources within the community and organize the following: convalescence; home-help; meals-on-wheels; the provision of equipment such as wheelchairs, cradles and pulleys; the installation of ramps to facilitate a wheelchair in the house, and so on.

5 By interceding with the local authority, she may be able to bring about the structural changes necessary to the house of a patient requiring, for example, renal dialysis.

6 She is able to inform patients about their entitlement to pensions and other financial benefits.

7 The hospital patient may then pass from her care to that of the medical social worker on the GP's team.

8 She is informed not only of all admissions and discharges but of all deaths in the hospital. Not only can she comfort and offer counsel about the problems of bereavement but she can also give practical advice about funeral arrangements and death certificates; often the Registrar of Births and Deaths attends the larger hospitals, making the documentary side of this situation easier.

THE PSYCHIATRIC SOCIAL WORKER

The treatment of the mentally sick is controlled by the Mental Health Act of 1959 which is based upon the premise that admission for psychiatric care should be the same as that for physical care, i.e. voluntary. Consequently, there are a great many more out-patients and, although this is laudable, the structure for dealing with them has yet to be fully implemented.

There is a lack of training schemes, rehabilitation centres, day-care centres and hostels. Meanwhile, psychiatric clinics are pressurized by the sheer weight of numbers. Under the guidance of Consultant Psychiatrists, the psychiatric social workers (or mental welfare officers), appointed by the local authority, help to relieve this situation.

Case work

1 The psychiatric social worker is skilled at taking histories. Not only do these uncover areas where practical help can be given, they contain valuable pointers to the nature of the illness. Frequently the mentally sick find it difficult to speak about their problems, and certainly cannot be hurried.
2 Like the medical social worker, she undertakes counselling.
3 She can mobilize local resources and intercede with other agencies in the community, e.g. adult training centres and special schools, etc.
4 Another important part of her work is home-visiting. Not only can she make things easier for the patient, she can provide advice and support for his family.

The secretary working in a psychiatric clinic cooperates with the social worker in the normal way. She will, however, make a point of *demonstrating* the confidentiality of the case notes because, obviously, this is an extremely sensitive area. As stated earlier, some psychiatrists keep certain notes in their personal possession in order to retain the patient's trust and make him feel more secure; when this occurs there should be a cross-reference in the main record.

The medical secretary should also be particularly solicitous towards relatives accompanying patients because they are often labouring under considerable stress themselves.

THE SURGICAL APPLIANCES OFFICER

Male or female, this officer is a member of the medical records department, but has his own office where records are kept and where patients are advised and/or fitted by the representatives of firms who supply the appliances.

Duties

1 He orders surgical appliances and supplies them to both in- and out-patients.
2 Renewals and replacements are his responsibility.
3 He must, therefore, maintain patient-records and a follow-up system; their format depends on the number of cases he handles. The follow-up system may consist of:

(a) A diary containing entries about which patients should see him again and on what dates. A standardized letter may be sent to them (a duplicated circular or a 'personalized' communication produced on a word-processing machine).
(b) A file or drawer contains twelve sections, marked with the months of the year, each subdivided for weeks or days. Appointment cards or reminder letters can be inserted at the appropriate date, making allowance for postage-time.

4 He must check all invoices and statements of account before submitting them to the finance officer.
5 He is usually 'on call' to certain wards and clinics.
6 He may have his own secretary. Any other secretary will telephone to make appointments and/or direct them to his office.

THE TRANSPORT OFFICER

The ambulance service is under the control of the health authority. In order to arrange patient-transport the secretary will either contact the service's headquarters or, in a large hospital, the transport officer. This may be done on behalf of:
1 A GP who wants a patient brought to hospital from home and taken back.
2 A hospital doctor who recommends transport for a follow-up attendance, discharge or transfer.

Members of the public may dial 999 and ask for the ambulance service in cases of emergency and, in certain circumstances, for women in labour.

Procedure

The secretary may contact the transport officer by telephone when authorized to do so but the efficient method is for him to receive a completed form (see Fig. 20.1). Whichever way requests are organized, the following information is required:
1 Twenty-four hours' notice so that routes and time-schedules can be planned.
2 When a patient is going to need regular transport, planning is helped by future times and dates.
3 The name, age, and address of the patient.
4 Full details of the destination—the department as well as the hospital—and the time the case is expected there.
5 Information about the patient's condition enables the transport officer to decide his priorities:
(a) He must be told if it is a stretcher case; when a patient is able to sit, a different kind of vehicle can be used.
(b) When it is an emergency he needs to know if the patient is unconscious or delirious, in labour or suspected of suffering from a condition like appendicitis.
(c) When a patient is to be accompanied by a relative or a midwife this must be stated.

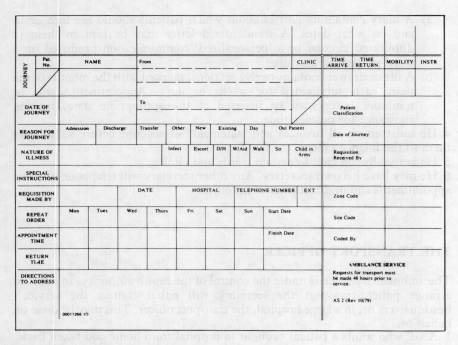

Fig. 20.1 An ambulance request form.

(d) Where infectious conditions are involved, the transport officer should be informed; in some cases the ambulance service may decide to use a special 'isolation' vehicle.

6 Finally, he will need to be given the name of the person authorizing transport.

Secretaries, doctors and patients have an obligation to use this costly service with care because annual wastage runs into thousands of pounds. One survey listed the following reasons for abortive journeys:

1 The transport officer is not informed when out-patients are being seen for the first time.

2 Patients are too ill to travel or have even died.

3 Patients are out when the ambulance arrives or have changed their minds.

4 Ambulances arrive at wrong addresses.

Other methods of transportation

The ambulance service, like so many other services, is working under pressure and its regulations have to be stringently observed. Often transport is wanted for reasons not covered by those regulations, and, so long as the reasons are not frivolous, the secretary can refer people to the British Red Cross Society and the St John's Ambulance Association. Their charge is per mile, and often a trained escort or first aider can be provided.

THE WARD CLERK

Working at the grade of Clerical Officer and responsible to the medical records officer, the ward clerk may carry out the following duties providing clerical and receptionist duties to ward staff:

1 (a) Check case notes before the patient's arrival to ensure that sheets are in correct order, paying particular attention to completion of the identification sheet (HMR1).
   (b) If case notes or X-ray plates have not been retrieved, inform Sister.
   (c) Set up bed boards for TPR charts, etc.
2 Before case notes are produced for the doctor, check that there are sufficient continuation sheets and file outstanding investigation reports. Note which reports and X-ray plates are required and collect them if there is any delay in their arrival.
3 Take patient's personal property to the designated place (General Office) if required.
4 Ensure all private patients' agreement forms are signed.
5 Maintain and replenish records for the nurses' observation.
6 Complete diet sheets.
7 Order stationery.
8 Answer the telephone.
Other routine tasks may be allotted to the ward clerk by the Sister or MRD.

Diploma Questions

*Denotes an incomplete question
ˣA question to be answered after further reading
1 Write an account of the work of the surgical appliances officer.
2 As a medical secretary to a 'firm' in hospital, describe the duties you might be expected to perform for patients requiring transport.*
3 Write short notes on the following personnel in hospital and describe how their work might involve the medical secretary:
(a) The medical social worker
(b) the radiologist
(c) the pathology laboratory technician.*

21
Admissions

THE ADMISSIONS OFFICER

The registration of all admissions to hospital is carried out by the admissions officer. He/she is a member of the medical records department, although she has an office in which to create records and interview ambulant patients when they arrive. In a large hospital she has assistance and a 24-hours' service is maintained. Assigned to her office may be a receptionist, a voluntary worker or a porter, and whichever of them escorts patients to the wards should be able to answer questions about the disposal of clothes and suitcases and the visiting hours.

In the smaller hospital, where a round-the-clock service is impossible, each ward has its own admission book; the top copy is detached and sent to the admissions officer, so that as soon as she returns on duty she can carry out her documentation. (As this tends to occur out of office hours, the admissions are likely to be of an emergency nature so that the ward may also set up case notes from its own stocks. The medical section could well be the first to be completed, and the Sister may or may not fill in the identification sheet. A full set of notes is assembled during office hours in the normal way, a unit number allocated and a master index card made out.)

THE AVAILABILITY OF BEDS

The decision to admit is a medical one; the decision about *when* to admit has to be based upon the bed states, the daily return the ward Sisters make to the medical records department about the number of beds occupied and the number unoccupied. These returns are made on printed forms, perhaps separate sheets or perhaps in books providing several copies. They are collated in the medical records department; sometimes a control board (the bed board) is used to provide instant visual impact of the overall beds situation. Alternatively, bed states information can be computerized, so by checking that there is a bed free on an appropriate ward selection from the waiting list can be made.

DOCUMENTATION

The TCI letter

As well as a booklet about pyjamas, etc., shopping trolleys and other facilities, the patient receives a TCI (to come in) letter/card. Sometimes the secretary

184

sends it, using a TCI diary, but sometimes it is issued by the admissions officer.

The admissions form

An admissions form might also be sent to the patient to complete and bring in with him; to be of real use it should contain a section marked 'For hospital use only' so that other details can be added, and it needs to consist of NCR paper so that more than one copy is created (see Fig. 21.1). Different hospitals follow

```
........................... Hospital

                    ADMISSION SHEET

   You are requested to complete this form and hand it in on your admission.
```

SURNAME (block capitals)	MAIDEN NAME	Please tick as appropriate :-
		MARITAL STATUS
FIRST NAMES		Married / Single / Widowed / Other
Home Address		Telephone No.
Postal Code		
Date of Birth	Age	Religion	County or Country of Birth

Next of Kin		Relationship
Address		Telephone No.
Name and address of Family Doctor		
Please tick if you receive :-	Retirement and/or Supplementary Pension Benefit	Please indicate if you are a member of H.M. FORCES YES/NO

FOR HOSPITAL USE ONLY

Date Admitted	Time a.m. p.m.	Hospital No.	Ward
Please tick as appropriate	SOURCE OF ADMISSION W.L. IMMED. CAS. ROAD DATE ON W.L. TRANSFER O.P. ACCIDENT		
Admitted from (if different from Home Address)			
Please tick as appropriate	CATEGORY OF PATIENT: N.H.S. SEC. 1 SEC. 1V DAY CASE MEDICAL NECESSITY		
Consultant in Charge on Admission :-			

A69SO

Fig. 21.1 An example of an admissions form.

different customs—sometimes the form is filled in by the admissions officer when the patient arrives—but in either case she must receive full information about all patients who are expected.

The form contains:
- the patient's identification details
- the date of admission
- the time of admission, useful with emergency cases
- the Consultant and the ward

Occasionally additional information is included:
- date and place of birth
- surname at birth
- status
- occupation
- religion
- date that the patient's name was entered on the waiting list and grade of priority given
- diagnosis

All of these facts aid distribution of copies and the compilation of statistics.

Distribution of the admissions form

Copies might be sent to the following:

1 The ward—to be filed there as part of the ward register.
2 The medical records department where it can be checked against the waiting list and the name removed.
3 The switchboard operator—she can pass authorized messages to the next of kin and inform others about the ward and visiting hours. For the same reason, the person manning the reception desk might receive a copy.
4 The chaplain—he has a pigeon-hole somewhere so that he is kept informed about admissions of his particular denomination. In our multiracial society representatives of other religions make regular calls and receive the same courtesy. Secretaries should make a point of finding out as tactfully as possible how they should be addressed.
5 The medical or psychiatric social worker—either of these may receive a copy where special cases are involved.
6 Computerization and word processing facilitate the creation of further copies that can be distributed usefully to other people and departments.

Hospital activity analysis

HAA will probably require its own forms to be produced at this point.

The register

As a part of the medical records department's statistical function, admissions and discharges are often recorded by the admissions officer in a register or ledger (see Fig. 21.2). It is commonly referred to as the 'A and D' book, although admissions may well be recorded separately from discharges. Where

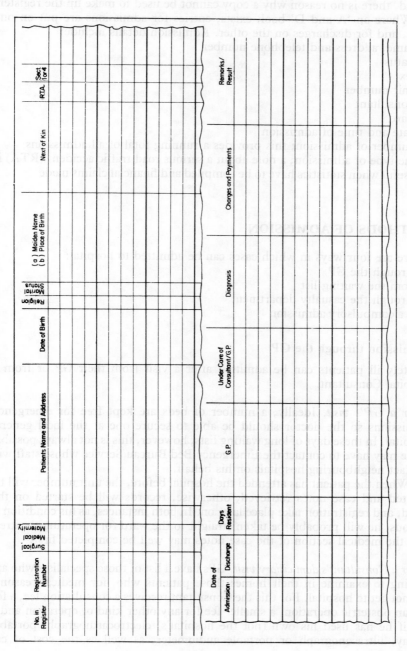

Fig. 21.2 Pages from an admissions register (ledger) used in some hospitals.

the admissions form is comprehensive, with space for discharge details to be added, there is no reason why a copy cannot be used to make up the register.

Where an 'A and D' book exists, entries for admissions are put on one page, and for discharges on the other. Admission details include:
- name, address and telephone number
- status
- sex
- unit number
- Consultant
- ward
- date and time of admission
- number of admission; this provides a running total of all admissions
- the type of admission; a note about a serious road traffic accident (RTA) is useful when statistics have to be compiled and financial claims made

METHODS OF ADMISSION

There are four ways in which cases can be admitted to hospital:
1 through the GP
2 from the waiting list
3 through the casualty department
4 as a compulsory admission

Admission through the GP

Acutely ill patients can be admitted after a visit from their GP or from a hospital Consultant.

After a GP's visit. Ideally, a number of beds are kept free for emergency admissions so the doctor should be able to secure one at the local general hospital. In these days of long waiting lists, however, this is not always possible so he may have to contact the Emergency Bed Bureau/Service whose staff will contact neighbouring hospitals on his behalf.

When the patient has attended the hospital before, the unit number will be elicited and case notes retrieved; otherwise, records will be started on the ward, and registration take place later on. In both instances, as his condition is serious, he will probably be taken straight to the ward (or operating theatre), and the medical section of the case notes may well be completed first.

After a Consultant's domiciliary visit. GPs have a list of those specialists who are willing to examine in their homes those patients who, for medical reasons, cannot get to hospital. For this the Consultant receives a consultation fee, a fee for an obstetric operation, a smaller fee for any other kind of operation and a fee if he has used his own (not the hospital's) electrocardiograph, portable X-ray, ultrasonograph or portable audiometer, as well as the cost of car mileage.

In this context the word 'home' means the patient's residence for the time being and may include an old people's home, a hotel or a residential school; it may also include a private nursing home when it is a permanent residence and in the event of an obstetrical emergency.

On receiving the GP's request for a domiciliary visit, the Consultant's secretary obtains full details, including the degree of urgency, then enters the time, date, etc. in the diary. Afterwards she checks that the claim form has been filled in and signed. The GP fills in Part I, whether he attended the consultation or not, and when the patient lives permanently in a private nursing home, he must add the endorsement 'Permanent Resident'. Part II is completed by the Consultant who, being the claimant, will expect the secretary to forward the document to the RHA.

Secretaries should note that admission does not follow automatically; instead the patient's name may be put on the waiting list. On the other hand, admission via the GP or a domiciliary visit may necessitate an ambulance.

Admission from the waiting list

The list

This may be kept:
1 Departmentally, with one for each speciality; this could be more convenient for the Consultant, his 'firm' and his secretary.
2 Centrally, with each department/speciality submitting names. It will be housed in one office with a staff who are adept at maintenance, answering questions and generally dealing with all the complications of additions to the list and deletions, including those caused by death.

Occasionally patients attend the out-patient department of one hospital while their names are on the waiting list of another; this is legitimate so long as the hospitals are part of a group or the patient is involved with both.

The list may take the form of a book, a card index, a strip index or a planning board, and it may be computerized but the information recorded is the same:
- name and status; address and telephone number
- unit number
- usually the GP's name and address
- name of the Consultant
- date of entry onto the list
- diagnosis
- degree of urgency; sometimes a grade is allotted, e.g. A, B, C.
- dates when a patient is unavailable e.g. on holiday or working out a necessary period of notice to his employers.
- the TCI date

The waiting list in book form. As a rule, a TCI Book is used only in small departments. After ward-care has been ordered, the Sister or medical secretary enters the details, in duplicate or even triplicate. The waiting list clerk will be sent a copy or will examine the book after each clinic.

The waiting list in card form. These might be visible-edged cards on which the doctor writes the medical details and the nurse or secretary adds the social

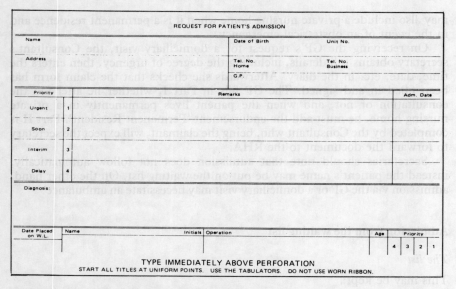

Fig. 21.3 An example of a visible-edge waiting list card.

details such as holiday dates or the need for transport, etc., depending on the design of the card (see Fig. 21.3).

'Mechanical' labels or the embossed imprinter can be used to head up most versions. Some hospitals use blue cards for male patients, and pink for females.

The waiting list as a strip index. This is useful when several names have to be recorded after a clinic, because the sheet of perforated strips will fit into the typewriter easily and can then be inserted into the metal or plastic frame. Although they can be removed from the system without disturbing continuity, this is an advantage only in a small system, however, as some medical records officers do not consider them ideal for the wear and tear suffered by the centralized list.

The waiting list on a control/planning board. Based on the information provided by conventional lists or cards, etc., the board or chart might be headed up by the names of wards or specialities, with the numbers waiting for admission represented by coloured signals or magnetic studs. The aim is to convey an immediate visual impression of the whole waiting list situation.

A variation is the bed board which displays the beds in use, with the names of wards, patients and Consultants; up-dated daily, it shows the beds available for emergency admissions and can also incorporate a forward-planning system for expected admissions with, say, a seven-day period.

These boards, like so much equipment, require forethought. They should suit the situation, not vice versa, and they should not be so high as to need a step-ladder or so complex that maintenance demands the total working hours of people who have other duties. The really good ones improve control and decision-making.

Computerization. Selection for admission can be made by matching waiting list demands against the bed states data.

Selection from the waiting list

Secretarial responsibility for calling patients in from a waiting list should be confined to acting under orders. In those circumstances where this is not so, hopefully rare, she should shoulder the burden only under the most rigid guidelines.

Once the decision to admit on a particular date has been made (on the basis of the bed states and possibly the availability of an operating theatre), a TCI letter, a standardized printed document, is sent to the patient, together with the pamphlet about facilities. He may also need to be instructed about special preparations, such as diet, during the 24 hours before admission. In urgent cases a telephone call could be substituted for the letter; when this occurs, the secretary can ensure that he or his next of kin receives the useful pamphlet as soon as possible.

All departments and personnel likely to be involved with the case are informed of the pending admission: admissions officer, ward Sister, theatre Sister, physiotherapy department, surgical appliances officer, and medical social worker, and maybe many more. Again, the computer/word processor is time-saving.

At some point in the procedure a check should be made against the waiting list in case the lady waiting for a routine appendicectomy has already been admitted as an emergency or even died from other causes.

Unless the name was entered on the list after a domiciliary visit, out-patient attendance has been made so case notes already exist and are sent to the ward, with X-ray films, before the patient arrives. His name is not removed from the list until he appears.

Should he not appear, 'FTCI' (failed to come in) is written against his name while inquiries are made, usually through the GP. Should he inform the hospital that he is unable to accept the admission his name is placed at the bottom of the list. He must understand that his waiting time now 'dates' from this 'second' entry, not the first.

Secretarial duties. The extent of the secretary's involvement with waiting list procedures depends upon her position in the hospital; in any case the following points should be kept in mind:

(a) In an ideal world a waiting list would not exist, so when entering a name on it the least the writer can do is to ensure that all details are accurate.

(b) For most patients hospitalization necessitates considerable preparation so the TCI letter should be issued as far in advance as possible.

(c) Any special instructions included with it should be clear.

(d) Before case notes are sent to the ward the results of all investigations should be collected and inserted, and the latest films should go with them, so that the House Officer has as much clinical information as possible when he conducts the initial interview with the patient.

(e) It should never be assumed that the consent form (HMR 5) has been signed by the patient or his guardian; this must be checked.

Table 21.1 The summary of admissions.

via waiting list	via GP	compulsory	via casualty department
Central or departmental list	Emergency or domiciliary visit	The Mental Health Act, 1983	Casualty register
Book/cards/strip index/visual aid/computer	Case notes retrieved or made up	Mentally-sick or infirm	Casualty card
Contains usual details, plus	Patient sent direct to ward	Section 2—assessment and treatment (28 days)	Sent to ward with case notes
Consultant, diagnosis, degree of urgency, remarks and date sent for	After a domiciliary visit he may have his name entered on the waiting list	Section 3—admission for treatment (6 months)	Case notes retrieved or made up
(TCI letter/diary; consent form)	Diary-note of meeting place, date, time, etc.	Section 4—emergency admission for observation only (3 days)	Patient direct to ward or theatre
Reports collected; case notes and X-ray films sent to ward	Claim form for fee and mileage and use of private equipment	Application forms	
Patient's name left on list until his arrival	Ambulance for either type of case		
FTCI—GP is notified. Name put at bottom of the list			

Admission through casualty—the accident and emergency department

The attendance will have been noted in the casualty register and a casualty card issued. The decision to admit may be taken by the Casualty Officer alone or in consultation with another doctor; there is bound to be some degree of urgency about the case.

When the admissions officer is informed, she makes the customary entry in the admissions and discharges register and distributes the usual copies of the admission form. Case notes are either retrieved or set up. The casualty card accompanies the patient to the ward and is inserted into the case notes where it remains until he is discharged; then it is returned to the casualty department to be filed.

Compulsory admission

Approximately 5% of patients in England and Wales are detained in hospital under the Mental Health Act, 1983; the aim of the law is to have voluntary admission wherever possible. Every effort is made by General Practitioners, psychiatrists and social workers to persuade patients to enter mental hospitals informally; only when this is out of the question is the formal application made, according to the following provisions of the Act:

Section 2. The patient is admitted for up to 28 days in order that his mental condition can be assessed and, if necessary, treated. The nearest relative or social worker may make the application, with the support in writing of two medical practitioners.

Section 3. Admission here is for a period up to 6 months, which may be followed by a further 6 months and thereafter by annual renewal—and the patient's condition must be treatable. If the next of kin is opposed to admission the social worker may apply to the County Court for the function of consent to pass elsewhere, e.g. to the Local Authority, another relative, or the social worker himself.

Section 4. An emergency admission up to 72 hours, with one medical recommendation.

Section 5. This grants holding powers to certain doctors so that they can detain a hospital in-patient for a limited period. It applies to cases who have entered voluntarily but who wish to leave prematurely. A nurse may detain a patient for up to 6 hours when the attendance of the medical practitioner in charge of treatment cannot be secured.

Diploma Questions

*Denotes an incomplete question
ˣA question to be answered after further reading

1 Describe four methods by which a patient can be admitted to hospital and describe the documentation involved with one of these procedures.

2 Describe the documentation of the casualty department with and without admission.

3 Write briefly on the medical secretary's duties in hospital in relation to the waiting list.*

4 Describe the various methods by which patients can be admitted to hospital, outlining the procedures and paperwork.

5 Write short notes on:

(a) the admissions and discharge register

(b) information found in the waiting list

(c) the filing of the waiting list.

6 Describe the additional sources of income available to the Consultant.*

22
Discharges

BASIC PROCEDURES

1 As soon as the doctor announces the date on which the patient may leave the hospital, the ward Sister sends a discharge note to the medical records department; this can be dispensed with if the bed states form is the type that includes a space for the patient's names (see Fig. 22.1).

2 It is not always possible or practical in busy hospitals to write to the GP on the actual day of discharge but, as he must assume clinical responsibility for the case, a pro forma, HMR 2A (Fig. 22.2), is posted to him or handed to the patient to deliver (see Fig. 22.3). This contains information about the diagnosis and treatment and anything else he needs to know immediately. Shortly afterwards a case summary follows, containing all or some of the following information:

(a) symptoms
(b) investigations
(c) results
(d) diagnosis
(e) treatment
(f) prognosis

A carbon copy of this report is placed in the correspondence section of the case notes (or summarized), a dated entry already having been made about the sending of the pro forma.

3 The admissions officer makes the discharge entry in the admissions and discharges register:

(a) the discharge number
(b) the date of discharge or death
(c) name
(d) unit number
(e) ward
(f) A note may also be made of the fact that a pro forma summary has been issued, and any relevant comments.

4 Films are returned to the X-ray department.

5 If there is a casualty card this is extracted from the case notes and sent for filing in the casualty department's secondary file.

6 The presence of all reports is checked.

7 The necessary statistics are recorded, e.g. the diagnostic index, etc. and any forms required for HAA and HIPR are completed (in the coding and indexing section, if there is one, or by designated clerks in the medical records department).

195

RETURN OF PATIENTS

PATIENTS
REMAINING PREVIOUS
RETURN

WARD

DATE

IN

ADMISSIONS

HOSPITAL NUMBER	NAME OF PATIENT	HOSPITAL NUMBER	NAME OF PATIENT

INTER-WARD TRANSFERS IN

HOSPITAL NUMBER	NAME OF PATIENT	WARD TRANSFERRED FROM

OUT

DISCHARGES (Forms attached)

HOSPITAL NUMBER	NAME OF PATIENT	HOSPITAL NUMBER	NAME OF PATIENT

DEATHS (Forms attached)

HOSPITAL NUMBER	NAME OF PATIENT	TICK HERE FOR P.M.

TRANSFERS TO OTHER HOSPITALS (Forms attached)

HOSPITAL NUMBER	NAME OF PATIENT	HOSPITAL TO WHICH TRANSFERRED

INTER-WARD TRANSFERS OUT

HOSPITAL NUMBER	NAME OF PATIENT	WARD TRANSFERRED TO

NUMBER OF PATIENTS REMAINING

Signature ——— (Nursing Officer)
——— (Nurse-in-Charge)

Fig. 22.1 An example of the bed state form.

8 Case notes are returned to the central system and the absent card/tracer removed. (Where there is a library, any requisition slips will be 'cancelled'.)
9 All departments and personnel who had to be informed of the admission must be informed of the discharge.
10 A follow-up appointment may have to be booked with the out-patient department.
11 Transport may be needed for this and to take the patient home.
12 Other procedures depend on the nature of the discharge.

HMR 2A (90-615)
(GP Copy)

*Please do
not enter
details in
this margin*

DISCHARGE NOTIFICATION

FROM

HOSPITAL
TEL No   EXT
(For this matter only)

UNIT No

SURNAME
(Block letters)
MR /MRS /MISS

FIRST NAMES

ADDRESS

POSTCODE

Dear Doctor
Your patient admitted under the care of...
will be discharged/transferred + on...................................to.............................

Diagnosis:

Treatment given:

Fold →

Treatment recommended:

Drug sensitivity:

NOTE
If any of this
information
requires to be
known urgently
by the GP
it should be
communicated
by telephone
— the discharge
form should be
completed
to follow
subsequently.

Community services arranged following discharge:
  + Home Nurse
  + Health Visitor
  + Social Worker
  + Other (please specify)
               has
Medicine has not + been supplied (for.................. weeks/days +)

Information given to the patient:

                      has
+ An appointment has not + been made for attendance as an outpatient on........................

                    have
+ Arrangements have not + been made for attendance as a day patient on.............. days a week,

commencing

Fold ←

+ The patient should be fit to return to work on .... ⎫ A certificate
                                                                                                        ⎬ has been
+ The patient's fitness for work will be reviewed in out-patients/day hospital ⎬ issued
                                                                                                        ⎭ accordingly
+ The patient has been advised to see you within...........days/weeks +

+ A summary of the notes will follow   Yours sincerely

*(Continue
overleaf
if necessary)*

                              Date: Position held:

Fig. 22.2 One kind of discharge notification sent by hospitals to general practitioners prior to, or accompanied by, a consultant's letter.

There are four kinds of discharge from hospital—to the home, to a convalescent establishment, to another institution and by death (see Table 22.1).

DISCHARGE TO THE HOME

In addition to the procedures outlined, after-care and rehabilitation may have to be organized. Perhaps domestic help is needed, the services of the district nurse or the obtaining of a wheelchair, a bedpan or air-ring. Sometimes a hospital liaison officer is appointed to a district and can help to organize this

```
                                    ┌──────────────┐
                                    │ Name         │
                                    │ and          │
                                    │ Address      │
                                    │ of the       │
                                    │ Hospital     │
                                    └──────────────┘

                                          Date_____

Dear Dr. _____

      Your patient _____

  (Address)        _____

                   _____

  under the care of _____

  will be discharged on _____
  _____

  is being transferred to _____

  Diagnosis:



  Treatment and / or Recommendations:



  Information given to the patient  :



  An appointment has / has not been made for further attendance
  as an out-patient.  A summary of the notes will follow.

                              Yours sincerely


                              _____
                              House Physician / Surgeon
```

Fig. 22.3 A discharge pro forma.

kind of aid for the newly discharged patient but, as she is attached to more than one hospital, discharge pro formas do not always come to her attention. Similarly, a health visitor can mobilize resources, but only if she knows that the patient is at home.

The medical secretary can help by ensuring that everybody who should know about a discharge is informed, outside the hospital as well as inside. (This applies even when the patient has discharged himself against medical advice and signed a form releasing the hospital from all clinical responsibility.)

She can also help by liaising with the hospital's own social workers, or simply by carrying out whatever instructions she is given about contacting the community and local authority services. The British Red Cross, the Women's Royal Voluntary Service and other voluntary bodies may be asked to play a supportive role by providing meals-on-wheels, etc.

Table 22.1 Summary of discharges.

Basic procedure	Discharge to the home	Transfer to a convalescent home	Transfer to another hospital	Death
Discharge note sent to medical records department, details entered on daily bed states	Organization of after-care and rehabilitation via:	A case summary is sent. Query follow-up arrangements	A full case summary is sent	Normal discharge documentation
Pro forma discharge to GP	medical social worker hospital liaison officer the primary health care team local authority services WRVS British Red Cross Society nursing home-help meals-on-wheels equipment adaptation of the home financial help		The second hospital may be specialized, so query the patient's return and need for follow-up arrangements	Death Certificate signed by 'last' doctor
Case summary to GP				Cremation Certificate completed by two doctors and next-of-kin
Films returned to X-ray department				Consent form necessary for post-mortem examination
Casualty card filed in secondary files in casualty department				Post-mortem report in case notes
Presence of reports in case notes checked				Copy of report sent to GP
Statistics recorded				
Case notes filed; tracer removed				
Interested parties informed of discharge				
Follow-up appointment booked in out-patients' department				
Transport organized for this and maybe journey home				

DISCHARGE TO A CONVALESCENT HOME

Again the basic procedure is followed, but a summary of the case will be sent to the convalescent home as well as to the general practitioner. Once the patient is at home some of the care mentioned above may be required.

DISCHARGE TO ANOTHER HOSPITAL OR INSTITUTION

Patients can be transferred to mental hospitals, geriatric and chronic hospitals or to hospitals dealing with specialities only, such as dermatology, ophthalmology, etc. or with women and children only. A detailed summary of the case is sent, and a follow-up appointment may or may not be necessary.

DEATH

Clerically, death is treated as a discharge, with all the usual documentation. In addition, the Registrar of births and deaths must receive a death certificate completed by the doctor who attended the fatal illness. In the event of cremation a different certificate has to be completed by two doctors; there is also a section for the next-of-kin which must be witnessed.

The next-of-kin must provide written consent before a post-mortem examination can be carried out by the pathologist. The secretary may be required to do no more than to see that the consent form, as well as the certificate, is available and remain discreetly in the background but if she is further involved, say, with the filling-in of the cremation certificate, she will be sympathetic and quietly helpful.

The post-mortem report is lodged in the case notes, and a copy sent to the GP.

Diploma Questions

1 Describe the documentation and procedures involved in the various methods of admissions and discharges in hospitals.
2 What would you expect to find in a set of case notes for a patient who has been seen in the out-patient department, admitted to hospital for an operation and discharged to a convalescent home? Outline the duties of the medical secretary as far as these case notes are concerned.

23
Communication

SPEECH

There are times when the simplest form of communication, speech, is the most complex and the least reliable. Even when two people are standing face to face, the mental distance between the sender and receiver can be vast; this is often the case in hospital when one is sick and the other is not. The medical secretary, therefore, must not only speak with forethought, she must balance on the extremely fine line between ensuring that people understand what she is telling them and making them feel simple-minded!

With experience she will become skilled in the art of receiving and dealing with people, develop a friendly approach and a willingness to listen, however busy she may be. At the same time she will acquire the ability to recognize the time-wasters and, tactfully, to deflect them.

TELEPHONE

All the basic office practice rules for efficient use of the telephone apply with some additions:

1 The life of the hospital switchboard operator is busy, and she has only two hands and so many lines.

2 A ringing telephone is disturbing anywhere, particularly near wards or clinics so answer it promptly, announcing clearly the department or designation.

3 The good secretary should have a pencil and note-pad on her at all times because the message pads near corridor telephones tend to disappear. Unless the hospital provides message sheets, she should type a 'master' of appropriate design and maintain a stock of duplicated copies for other telephones.

4 The rule about repeating messages of any length to the caller is particularly important when clinical details or drugs are mentioned.

5 When addressing a patient the secretary tries to obtain his unit number, explaining that it is written on any appointment card he holds.

6 She may have to familiarize herself with two telephone attachments:

(a) An ordinary handset may be attached to an electronic jotting-pad which will transmit the written word, sketch or diagram. After dialling the necessary number, the caller presses a switch and then, using a special pen, writes a message which is reproduced on another electro-writer at the receiving end.

Thus verbal and typing errors are eliminated, as well as the physical effort of leaving the place of origin. It is particularly useful for transmitting prescriptions from the wards to the pharmacy.

(b) 'Fax'—facsimile telegraphy—transmits all kinds of handwritten, typed or printed matter over any distance. The original is placed in a tray in the facsimile transceiver, the telephone number is dialled, a button is pressed and a replica emerges from an identical machine at the receiving end, whether or not an operator is there. This is useful in a Group where so much information has to be relayed from one hospital to another, with complete accuracy and without delay.

Intercom

The hospital switchboard may be automatic or manual. Private Automatic Branch Exchange (PABX) enables extension-users to dial one another and to make outside calls, but the switchboard operator has to receive and route all in-coming calls. With a Private Manual Branch Exchange (PMBX) she handles everything. Those hospitals with this kind of exchange usually supplement it with an internal system, generally a Private Branch Exchange (PBX).

The obvious advantage of an intercommunication system is that it does not block the direct-exchange lines. As a rule, the hospital's internal telephone is a handset or a wall-mounted unit with a dial or numbered buttons. But to contact somebody like a doctor, whose exact location in the building is unknown, by ringing each extension in turn is time-consuming, so an alternative system is necessary.

British Telecom technology is advancing apace. The commercial world enjoys the benefits of the electronic switchboard, with its economical call-barring and logging facilities. Hospitals will make the change-over when finances permit, presumably, and doctors can look forward also to tuning television sets into remote brain-scanners and having pictures of their patients transmitted to them in seconds over telephone lines.

The public address system

This consists of a microphone, an amplifier and a series of loudspeakers placed strategically throughout the hospital. The broadcast messages are, of course, heard by everybody who is within range of the loudspeakers. Another disadvantage is that they operate in one direction only; the person being paged cannot explain that he is going to be occupied for the next 10 minutes.

Bells, buzzers and lights

These are inexpensive and provide a simple means of summoning patients into the consulting room, and are still used here and there for informing doctors that they are needed. The lights system is the most common of the three.

Lights, sometimes with colour coding, sometimes on a numbered board, are situated all over the premises, and their flashing sends the doctor indicated to the nearest internal telephone. As it is noiseless, this method disturbs nobody, but it is slow, and often the flashing is overlooked.

Paging

By far the most effective and most popular method is the 'bleep'. Doctors are issued with small transistorized radio-receivers which are carried or clipped to pockets. When a call is transmitted from the switchboard a signal or 'bleep' is heard on the receiver and does not cease until the doctor goes to a telephone. The noise is not so loud that it upsets other people or prevents the doctor from continuing with anything important he is doing at the time; on the other hand, he cannot ignore it indefinitely, although, of course, the switchboard operator uses her discretion about continuous paging.

British Telecom's radiopager is programmed to operate so that the distance at which it is useful is no longer restricted to one building or group of buildings. By arrangement, it can 'bleep' from one end of the country to the other. Another variation is that the pattern of the 'bleeps' denotes the origin of the call, and a numerical display is possible for spelling out messages in code—and, of course, there is two-way speech.

Closed circuit television

Those large hospitals which have closed circuit television as a teaching aid also use it to locate people's whereabouts before contacting them on the internal telephone. (It plays an important part, too, in those big city areas where hospitals require safeguarding against trespassers.)

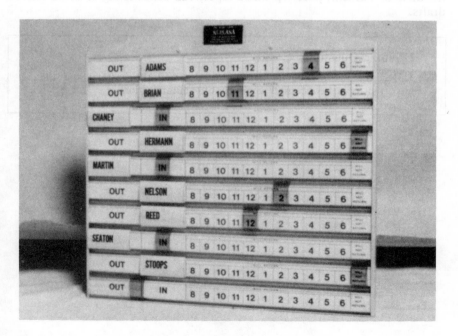

Fig. 23.1 An example of an in and out staff control panel.

Control boards

These form part of the intercom network when they are used as in/out or on/off duty panels. Of any size, they are used to indicate that important personnel are on the premises or off, attending meetings, holding clinics or in theatre, so there could be several of them in the hospital. They are useful in a Group when people are moving from locale to locale, and they serve a purpose when stationed at main doors so that visitors like the chaplain can mark their comings and goings.

Names are typed or printed on cards which are inserted into plastic tabs; these are mounted on the board and can slide over the word 'in', leaving the word 'out' exposed; the returning time is marked by a smaller transparent tab (see Fig. 23.1).

LETTERS

The supervisor of the centralized secretariat or pool will standardize the layout and style of typed correspondence, while the medical secretary follows the doctor's preferences.

When precise wording is important they will dictate to her; otherwise, she should be capable of composing letters and drafting replies while keeping in mind the image she is projecting of the hospital. With good spelling, fast, sound shorthand, both general and medical, and familiarity with reference books and dictionaries and, of course, experience, she will not be daunted by the dictator's accent, poorly planned tapes, bad handwriting or much-altered drafts.

Diploma Questions

1 Describe the intercommunications systems in the hospital and the important points concerning any form of communication.

24
The Office

Hospital offices differ in size, design, decoration and equipment so the secretary has to adapt to whatever working environment presents itself. Some aspects will be beyond her control; some will yield to her influence so she must do her best to create a cheerful atmosphere; personality can achieve a great deal.

Personal possessions must never clutter up an office but some flowers, a plant or a picture can lift morale without getting in the way.

Tidiness is essential, and never more so than when case notes and confidential reports are in the office. It can be managed easily enough when ample drawers, cupboards and shelves exist, which happens rarely and in any case often involve physical effort. A neat desk can be achieved not only by an orderly mind but by various pieces of equipment:

1 Trays labelled 'In', 'Out' and 'Pending' accommodate loose papers, folders, post, etc.
2 A sorter of the flap variety enables documents to be classified before filing.
3 Case notes and other large files can be pre-sorted in a portable basket (see Fig. 24.1).

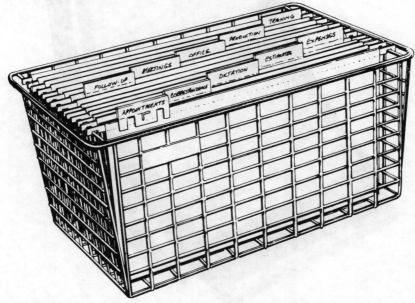

Fig. 24.1 The Busy Bee portable filing basket.

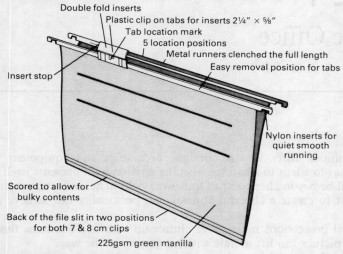

Double fold inserts
Plastic clip on tabs for inserts 2¼″ × ⅝″
Tab location mark
5 location positions
Metal runners clenched the full length
Easy removal position for tabs
Insert stop
Nylon inserts for quiet smooth running
Scored to allow for bulky contents
Back of the file slit in two positions for both 7 & 8 cm clips
225gsm green manilla

Fig. 24.2 The Nuplana Budgetfile.

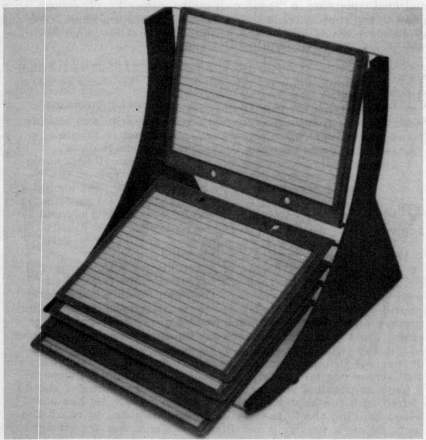

Fig. 24.3 A strip index desk unit.

4 The same basket with its label holder and suspension files with tabs can be adapted to a number of uses in an office (see Fig. 24.2).

5 Strip index units for telephone numbers do away with untidy lists. One could be mounted on the wall out of the way; another type sits neatly on the desk (see Fig. 24.3).

6 A metal waste-paper bin within easy reach.

THE OFFICES, SHOPS AND RAILWAY PREMISES ACT, 1963

This law sets down certain minimal requirements for office working conditions.

1 A temperature of 16 °C (60.8 °F).

2 400 cubic feet (11.3 m^3) for each worker (including furniture and equipment).

3 Proper lighting and adequate seating.

4 Fresh or artificially purified air.

5 Facilities for eating and an adequate supply of drinking water.

6 Lavatories and washing facilities, including hot and cold running water, soap and towels.

7 First-aid boxes must be provided, and all safety measures and fire precautions met.

THE HEALTH AND SAFETY AT WORK ACT, 1974

This law is in addition to the Offices, Shops and Railway Premises Act and places greater responsibilities not only on employers but employees. It is an 'enabling' Act which means that it lays down general principles without detail so that regulations and codes of practice can be drawn up as necessary. Whatever form it takes, all staff must be given a written account of policy. Safety representatives must be appointed from amongst employees by a recognized trade union and the employer notified in writing of their names (but training is needed for some of the functions involved).

Failure to fulfil the duties outlined in the Act is a criminal offence, and the employee is liable to the same penalties as the employer. The secretary, like everybody else in the building (including visitors like window-cleaners, milkmen, etc.), is obliged to take reasonable measures to protect her health and safety and that of others who may be affected by her acts or omissions at work. The law also forbids interference with or misuse of anything provided in the interests of health, safety or welfare so if she sees youths 'having fun' with the sand from a fire bucket she had better warn them that they could be prosecuted.

The prevention of accidents

The Royal Society for the Prevention of Accidents states that over 5000 injuries of a serious nature are sustained annually by office staff (discounting the accidents that keep people away from work for less than three days!). Almost half of these are due to falls, next handling and lifting, followed by stepping on and striking against things, falling objects, machinery, transport, the use of hand-tools, fire and electricity.

It would be particularly ignominious for the medical secretary to add to the number of patients her own hospital has to treat just because she tripped down a flight of stairs on her high heels or did not know how to lift a typewriter.

1 If the siting of furniture and equipment is left to the individual, she should ensure that collision with the sharp corners of desk, cabinets, etc. can be avoided.

2 The contents of cabinet drawers, should, ideally, be spread evenly. Open bottom drawers are a hazard, and leaving the two top drawers open may cause the cabinet to topple.

3 (a) The aisles between desks should be kept clear.

(b) The wires of telephones, electric typewriters, audio equipment and the like should never trail on the floor or cause people to walk into them, but should be kept close to the wall or under special cable covers.

4 When not in use appliances should be switched off and plugs removed from sockets (never by the lead).

5 Breakdowns of electrical equipment should be reported and 'do it yourself' repairs not attempted.

6 Instructions for the use of chemicals for duplicating and copying, etc. should be read with care, containers labelled clearly and kept tightly closed. They can be poisonous, corrosive and dangerous to inhale, not to mention inflammable. The secretary should note that stencil correcting fluid, typewriter cleaning fluid and some thinners for liquid erasers are flammable.

7 Heavy equipment should be moved on a trolley but this still involves lifting. An orthopaedic specialist has said that spinal stress can be avoided by keeping the weight as close to the body as possible, so typewriters should be lifted with the keyboard away from the body. He has also advised bending the knees, rather than the back, to reach the object, taking a firm grip and lifting as the knees are straightened and the head raised.

8 The Royal Society for the Prevention of Accidents advocate keeping pins and razor blades out of offices, and certainly scissors and knives, staplers and guillotines need to be treated with respect.

9 Falls can be avoided by mopping up spilt liquids, using handrails, ensuring that the way ahead is clear, not running or climbing on chairs, and reporting worn flooring when it represents a danger. Also shoes should have heels appropriate to the working environment!

10 The risk of fire can be minimized by placing all waste paper and other combustibles in metal waste bins and not leaving smoking materials in ash-trays.

11 All fire instructions issued by the hospital must be obeyed implicitly but, in addition, the secretary should know where the fire exits are, how to give the alarm and how to use the available fire-fighting equipment in case of an emergency.

BOMB SCARES

The mention of bomb threats is unavoidable in any discussion about safety. Hospitals are not common targets, although they may be in an area where such episodes occur or which is subjected to hoaxes. The Crime Prevention Division issues advice on precautions and emergency action in the area in case of danger and so only general advice is tendered here.

1 Calm is vital. On the other hand, no secretary receiving a warning should be so sanguine as to assume that the incident is just a replay of those mischievous incidents that may have happened at her college or school!

2 When the warning is telephoned ask immediately about the appearance of the device, its timing and its location.

3 Keep the caller talking while relaying this information to where it can be acted upon. Ask why the device has been planted and the whereabouts of the caller.

4 Try to identify his accent and any background sounds.

5 The instant the call is over check that the safety officer or somebody in authority has been informed.

6 Do not delay in notifying the police. The safety officer should ensure that they are met on arrival.

7 If a special evacuation procedure does not exist, the usual fire-drill will be followed. Those responsible for patients will know what they need to do; unless specifically requested to help, others will keep out of the way.

8 A search party will investigate.

THEFT

It is a sad fact of life that some hospitals find it necessary to guard their main entrances from intruders during the day and to have patrols at night; this duty is often performed by outside contractors. Night staff may be issued with 'bleeps' with which to contact the guards.

The most common aim of intruders is theft—not only of drugs, refrigerators and television sets, etc., but even of massive X-ray equipment, which can be broken down and sold. Such stealing, combined with the pilfering which occurs daily, costs the NHS millions of pounds each year. Apart from reporting suspicious behaviour, all that the secretary can do to offset the cost is to adhere meticulously to stock control procedures and be economical in her use of materials.

25

Consultant Private Practice

The part-time Consultant will have a private practice as well as an appointment under the NHS. The amount of private work that he does will depend upon many factors, such as the branch of medicine that he specializes in and the area in which he works, but if his private practice is of any size he will almost certainly find it necessary to have 'rooms' from which to practise and a secretary or receptionist or both. The work done by the secretary in private practice is very different from that she would do as a secretary in hospital practice. She will be employed by the Consultant and her work will vary according to the Consultant. If the volume of private practice that each Consultant does is small, a group may share one secretary.

The Consultant practises from his rooms at set hours by appointment. These appointments will be made by the GP of the patient concerned, or by the patient himself. In the latter case the Consultant would expect, on first attendance, that the patient has a letter of referral from his GP.

After the first consultation the patient may need an appointment for a further consultation or may need treatment. If this treatment is to be carried out in hospital it may be done privately or under the NHS. If there is a waiting list for treatment the patient will take his normal place on this list and be sent for when possible. Accurate liaison with hospital departments is a very important part of the medical secretary's work and must be done in a most conscientious manner.

The work of the Consultant's secretary falls into two groups: (a) reception work and (b) secretarial work.

THE RECEPTIONIST

The first task under this heading will be the making of appointments. The development of a pleasant courteous manner, particularly over the telephone, is of great importance in this type of work. The receptionist will be expected to obtain all the necessary details when the appointment is made.

These details will consist of:
1 The name and address of the GP who is requesting the appointment.
2 The name, address and age of the patient.
3 Whether the patient has seen the Consultant before either at his rooms or at the hospital. (When the patient has been sent before, full details will be needed to enable previous notes to be obtained before the consultation.)

The patient is then given the first available appointment and the name is entered in the appointment diary. Sometimes a card giving details of the appointment is posted to the patient and this card may contain instructions for the patient such as bringing a specimen of urine, or details about preparation necessary before an X-ray or other special examination.

The receptionist will receive patients, as they attend the consultation, at the door. She should take the names and, if the rooms are shared by more than one Consultant, she will make sure that she knows which doctor the patient is to see. This should be done as part of her 'homework' because an important aspect of the job of a receptionist is to make the patient feel that he is expected and welcome. This is particularly important with children and a child should be welcomed by his Christian name.

If the patient has brought the letter from his own doctor she will take this to the Consultant before the patient is seen so that he is aware of the type of problem with which he is faced and the most suitable method of approach.

She will show the patient to the waiting room. This room is her responsibility and she should see that it is warm and well lit, that there are sufficient chairs and clean and up-to-date magazines. There should always be fresh flowers, and if a child is brought a picture book or small toy may be provided to help the mother to amuse or distract him.

When the Consultant is ready to see the patient she will answer his signal (usually effected on an 'intercom' system) and tell him whom she proposes to show in. She will call the patient from the waiting room and precede him to the Consulting room where she will introduce him by name and then leave. After the consultation is finished she will usher the patient out and she must be ready to answer any call from the Consultant as soon as it is made. When a further appointment is necessary it is her responsibility to ensure that this is made before the patient leaves, and if the patient wishes to pay the fee before leaving she should find out from the Consultant how much the fee is, issue an account, receipt it, and do the appropriate bookkeeping, or, if a secretary is also employed, ask her to complete it.

Another task that may occasionally fall to her lot to perform is that of amusing other children of the family whilst the Consultant is seeing mother and child. A small stock of toys in the office will prove invaluable at such times.

It may be part of her duties to look after equipment, to do simple urine tests and to attend to examination rooms, laundry and other matters (see Chapters 26, 35 and 36).

THE SECRETARY

The work of the secretary for the private Consultant may be divided into three categories:
1 Medical correspondence
2 Financial
3 Personal

Medical correspondence. The letter from the GP will be opened by the Consultant. As soon as possible after the session of appointments he will dictate a reply to that letter, either directly to the secretary, or more likely by using a dictation machine. The secretary types the letter and presents it for signature at the earliest possible opportunity; a carbon copy will always be made and filed with the letter to which she is replying. Treasury tags are a convenient method of keeping letters together in chronological order but are somewhat bulky. Some secretaries prefer to staple letters together, but when adding a new letter the old staple should be taken out and a new one inserted to avoid the accumulation of metalwork.

There are several different methods of filing correspondence relating to patients.

(a) They may be filed with the medical notes referring to the patient. In this case they are kept in a suspension file or in a manila envelope, filed alphabetically according to the patient's surname. Letters and notes relating to the current year may be put in a separate file, in which case earlier notes and letters referring to the same patient in previous years will need to be brought forward.

(b) They may be filed separately from the medical notes but, again, alphabetically according to the patient's surname.

(c) They may be filed under the name of the patient's GP to whom the reply has been sent. In this method they may again be subdivided into current year and previous years.

Whichever method is chosen it should enable both the patient's medical notes and the appropriate letters to be found quickly whenever required, and certainly always before the patient is seen for a second time.

Financial. The general principles of sending out accounts are dealt with in Chapter 11. The patient may occasionally wish to find out how much the fee will be before the consultation takes place and the secretary will then have to enquire from the Consultant and either write to or telephone the patient. It will be important to make a note or keep a copy of the letter so that the patient is not told one fee and charged another.

When a patient is admitted to hospital for private treatment it is necessary for the secretary to liaise with the hospital so that she knows when the treatment was given. The responsibility of sending accounts to the patient for the treatment given in the hospital may rest with her and she should get to know the admissions officers of all the hospitals at which the Consultant works so that she can keep a constant check on this matter. This is not quite so difficult as it sounds because, when arrangements have been made for the patient to be admitted to hospital or put on a waiting list for admission, it will be the secretary who will have made these arrangements.

The account should be sent out monthly. If it is not settled by the following month the account is rendered again, this time adding the date on which the original account was rendered. When the account is not paid at the end of the third or fourth month a label may be affixed saying that payment is overdue. If it appears that there is no intention of paying, the Consultant may wish to put the matter in the hands of the protection society of which he is a member.

It is important to note again that there may be many patients that the Consultant wishes to see without charging a fee and these will include other doctors and their immediate relatives. The Consultant will arrange some system of informing the secretary of the fee to be charged, probably at the time when he does his letters.

Personal. Much of the work that may be included under this heading is dealt with on other pages of this book. This includes personal financial matters (page 77), private correspondence (page 67), work relating to committee meetings (page 75), research work (page 74), and the preparation of papers for publication (page 71). Apart from these aspects the private secretary will keep a diary of all her employer's engagements and will see that he is reminded of these in good time and that all arrangements have been made. She should make it her business to know where he should be at all hours of the working day so that she can contact him if necessary. She may keep personal files covering his insurances, arrangements for schools for his children, and any societies of which he is a member.

She should also expect to prepare details and make reservations for any journey he is to undertake. When this is done she should type two copies of the itinerary giving full details of methods of travel, times of departure and arrival, routes and hotel reservations. For the more complicated journeys she will normally be helped by a good travel agency, but it will be her responsibility to check carefully all the details of any arrangements.

This type of work, as in general practice, requires that the secretary should be able to identify her interests with those of her employer and show a high degree of loyalty.

'PAY-BEDS'

Under the NHS Act hospitals are able to set aside private accommodation for people who wish to pay for it provided that the beds are not required for medical reasons for other patients. All Consultants on the staff of the hospital may admit private patients to these beds, and all Consultants may charge a fee for treatment.

Standard charges. These are laid down in DHSS circulars relating to the type of hospital and the service provided. Charges will be made for accommodation, outpatient attendances, investigations, the use of services such as physiotherapy, operating theatres and so on.

Contributory schemes. There are various schemes enabling patients to provide against charges for medical treatment. These are often based on a scale giving benefit according to the amount of the contribution. They may provide for specialist treatment, hospital accommodation or GP treatment, as does the *British United Provident Association* (BUPA, 24/27 Essex Street, Strand, London WC2), or for specialist treatment and hospital accommodation only as in the case of the *Hospital Service Plan* (Tavistock House South, Tavistock Square, London WC1), and *The Western Provident Association for Hospital and Nursing Home Services* (Culver House, Culver Street, Bristol 1).

It is important that a secretary finds out if a patient seeking private treatment in this way is covered by insurance. The claim forms must be accompanied by the appropriate accounts and signed by the GP who advised the specialist consultation.

CONSULTANT SPECIALTIES

There are many different specialties in consultant practice, and the work of the medical secretary in private practice will vary very much according to the doctor for whom she works. Not only are the medical terms used different, but she will also find that there is often a different type of patient attending and that there are many different technical procedures that she will be asked to assist with.

Cardiology

This is the branch of medicine dealing with disorders of the human heart. Patients suffering from these conditions are particularly liable to show anxiety and apprehension, and great care should be taken to put them at their ease. Special examinations that may be required are the taking of blood pressure, X-rays to determine the size, shape and position of the heart, and electrocardiograph (ECG) examination (see Chapter 36). A second ECG examination is often required after certain exercises and the anxious patient should be reassured that this is a normal procedure.

Dermatology

This is concerned with the care of the skin. Patients suffering from skin diseases are often embarrassed by their condition because they feel that it reflects on their personal cleanliness. In fact, however, few skin diseases are contagious or communicable. The specialist will frequently wish to view the whole body surface to determine the distribution of the condition.

Many of the patients will be suffering from allergic reactions. Contact dermatitis may be due to a wide variety of substances, and skin sensitivity tests may be called for. Here a small drop of the substance is rubbed into a tiny scratch and the skin reaction observed. Up to 50 tests may be made at one time. Sometimes a test is made by applying a patch of substance to the skin. Scratch or patch tests may need examination at 24-, 48- or 72-hour intervals and the patient is asked to return for these to be read. Because of the slight possibility of severe reactions, patients should not leave the premises for half an hour after the application of the substances. The secretary may be trained in the performance or reading of these tests.

Gynaecology and obstetrics

The doctor working in these fields is concerned with diseases of the female reproductive system and with the care of the expectant mother.

Pelvic examinations are quite routine and the medical secretary may be called in to assist. She may be asked to assist with the patient's clothing, positioning the patient on the couch, producing the instruments required, and especially with chaperoning. All these important topics are discussed elsewhere in the book. The obstetrician will be very anxious to provide a relaxed and confident atmosphere for his patients, and particular attention will be paid to the comfort and privacy of the consultation.

Close liaison with the hospital or nursing home to which the patient is to be admitted is important, and the secretary should ensure that both she and the patient are kept informed of any arrangements to be made.

Neurology

The neurologist is concerned with disorders of the nervous system due to injury or organic disease.

Many patients who come to see him may have difficulty in walking and will require assistance. Neurological examination is detailed and time consuming, and often requires more time for each appointment than some other specialties.

Sometimes electroencephalograph (EEG) examinations are made, using a machine which measures the electrical currents in the brain and records them for later study, but more commonly the patient is referred to hospital for these because of the complicated nature of the equipment.

Ophthalmology

This specialty has to do with the function and disorders of the eye. A considerable part of the work in private ophthalmology is concerned with refraction (testing of vision and prescription of glasses), and the secretary may be trained to help the ophthalmologist in many ways. Equipment that is used is often complicated and requires special care. The doctor may require drops to be put into the patient's eye—commonly dilators so that the pupil is large enough for examination of the back of the eye to be made with ease. These drops vary both in the length of time needed before they take effect and with the age of the patient. This type of work is exacting, and the secretary will need special training from the doctor if she is to help him in this field.

Otorhinolaryngology

Many minor surgical procedures are performed by the ear, nose and throat surgeon. The secretary in private Consultant practice may be expected to assist with examinations and treatment, and to sterilize, lay out and clean instruments used in diagnosis and treatment.

Paediatrics

Diseases and disorders of children are treated by a paediatrician. Here the secretary will have to learn to deal with both anxious parents and frightened and uncooperative children. Time spent in the waiting room will need to be kept to a minimum, and the secretary may have to learn how to hold a child for examination and to carry out simple measurements of height, weight, girth, etc.

Geriatric medicine

As the proportion of elderly people in the community increases, with their special diseases and problems, the importance of this specialty grows. Patients in this group require special understanding of their possible confusion, fear, poor eyesight and hearing. They have a particular need to have their dignity respected.

Psychiatry

This is a large specialty covering all age groups and working within the general hospital and specialist hospitals.

Other specialties include: general medicine, general surgery, nephrology (diseases of the renal tract), orthopaedics (diseases of bones and joints), radiology, plastic surgery, endocrinology (diseases of ductless glands) and gastroenterology (diseases of the intestinal tract).

Diploma Questions on a Broader Basis

1 Compare the duties a medical secretary performs for in-patients with those she carries out for out-patients.

2 Describe the differences between the medical secretary's responsibilities in general practice and in hospital.

3 How may the secretary help in the field of preventive medicine in general practice and in hospital?

4 With reference to your field-work, write on the most useful areas of your college training, and give reasons.

5 In 1860 Florence Nightingale wrote, 'The material exists but it is inaccessible.' She was referring to medical information.

   Give examples of how this situation has changed in hospitals and of what is being done in this field.

6 As a medical secretary to a hospital Consultant and his firm, outline your likely responsibilities and how you would organize your work.

7 What personal qualities and technical skills would be looked for by members of the panel interviewing candidates for vacancies in a hospital medical secretariat? Give reasons for your choice.

8 You have been asked to speak to a group of school leavers on the duties of a medical secretary in a hospital. Prepare notes which would help you to give your talk.

IV

The Secretary/Receptionist in General Practice

26

The Surgery Premises

THE SURGERY

In Great Britain it is traditional to refer to the accommodation in which the GP works as the 'surgery'. In the rest of the English-speaking world it is usually called the 'office', and it amuses other countries to know that the room in which surgery is performed is called a 'theatre' and the rooms in which it is not done are called 'surgeries'. However, 'office' strikes the British doctor as being too commercial and the phrase 'consulting rooms' has long been applied to rooms in which Consultants practise, and so it will probably go on being called a surgery for many years to come.

In the past, the basic surgery of a GP was usually two rooms: a waiting room and a consulting room. Today the basic surgery consists of three, four or five rooms: the waiting room, consulting room and office, usually an examination room and often a clinical or treatment room. Within this framework the variations are legion. When the NHS Act was drawn up in 1946 it was envisaged that GPs would work from health centres which had been built and staffed by local authorities. For various reasons, principally political, these were never built and practice has continued largely on the lines on which it has been slowly developing during the past 50 years. At first the doctor almost invariably practised from his home. His consulting room and waiting room were two integral rooms of his house and private patients often used his drawing room or dining room to wait in. With the increasing demands upon his time the doctor has felt a need to be able to escape from the pressure of work into the privacy of his own home and there has been a tendency to use accommodation away from his residence. At first this was often a converted private house or shop, but with the development of group practice and more highly organized practice it has been necessary to build accommodation specially designed for the job it has to do. As these developments have occurred slowly over a number of years we find ourselves today with all these various types of building and varied forms of practice existing side by side throughout the country. It is not, therefore, possible to generalize about the accommodation in which the secretary will find herself working, but it is possible to describe the standard approach that she will need to adopt to 'run' a surgery.

THE OFFICE

In modern general practice today the hub of the surgery around which everything will revolve is the office. In fact many of the more modern

219

surgeries, catering for group practice, have recognized this fact and are designed so that the flow of patients from waiting room to consulting room, then on to examination room and way out, is around the office. The experienced secretary should organize the office so that she can perform all the functions required of her efficiently and comfortably. These functions are:
1 The reception and registration of the patients and the control of their movements (see Chapter 30).
2 The storage of medical records, X-rays and all the stationery and forms required (see Chapter 27).
3 The management of the internal communication system and incoming and outgoing telephone calls (see Chaptes 12 and 23).
4 Typing and bookkeeping (see Chapter 10 and 11).
5 Running the appointment system (see Chapter 30).

Details of these duties have been described in other chapers but certain points must be emphasized.
1 The office should always be kept tidy. Notes, papers and equipment not in immediate use should be put away. Here it should be emphasized that it is difficult to do this unless there are enough properly labelled trays or baskets to hold loose papers awaiting attention. The secretary should remember that most of her work is of a highly confidential nature and records and letters must not be left lying about where they can be seen by other people. At the end of the day the office should be left tidy so that work can begin on the next day with the minimum amount of sorting out.
2 Time and motion studies may be somewhat out of place in this type of office, but constant attention should be paid to unnecessary movements and work caused by bad planning. Documents and forms should be stored where they are needed and equipment can often be moved to more convenient positions.
3 The office has to be very accessible for the patient but this is no reason why confidential conversations should be broadcast throughout the waiting room. People have an insatiable curiosity about other people's affairs and the secretary should not gratify this, albeit unintentionally.
4 The office can be kept bright and cheerful with a calendar, picture or small vase of flowers and the secretary can expect a comfortable chair to sit on, good light and a reasonable degree of warmth. She should also have a good desk, typewriter, filing baskets and the usual range of office equipment. Her employer may not be aware of her needs so she should be prepared to tell him what she wants to enable her to do the job efficiently.

THE WAITING ROOM

The traditional 'music hall' picture of the doctor's waiting room is, unfortunately, only too often an accurate one. Nothing is more depressing than waiting for a long time in a cold, cheerless and overcrowded room with nothing to look at but a ten-year-old copy of *Punch*! The secretary can do a lot to improve matters by a little foresight. The object is to keep the waiting room empty. Waiting time is wasted time and makes a patient irritable; overcrowding can lead to the spread of infection and the combination of overcrowding and long waiting plays havoc with chairs, walls and magazines. If an efficient appointment system is run both these evils will be avoided.

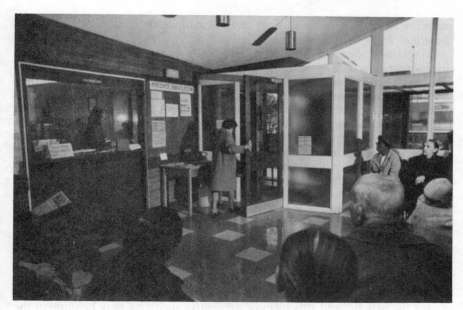

Fig. 26.1 Reception—the patient's view.

The secretary must ensure that every patient registers his attendance with her. If the patient has to wait any length of time before seeing the doctor, the secretary should inform the patient at the first opportunity; this will give him a chance to go away and come back later that day with an appointment, or on another convenient day, and will have the effect of removing any irritation that he might feel at having to wait. When the doctor is late arriving or is called out in the middle of the surgery she should tell the waiting patients. Minor courtesies of this variety will help personal relationships. Sometimes patients are taken ill in the waiting room and she should see that when this occurs the patient is shown in quickly. Some patients have been known to expedite their entrance by being taken ill every time they have to wait! A patient with an irritating cough or a tired and crying child is better out of the waiting room and no other patient will object to the rapid removal of such a problem. No smoking should be the rule in every waiting room and if they must smoke patients should step outside.

In the design of surgeries it is not always possible to have the waiting room in close proximity to the consulting room. This will mean that when the doctor rings or flashes for his next patient there may be a delay of thirty seconds to one minute before they arrive. If the doctor is seeing 20 patients this may easily add up to a quarter of an hour. One or two chairs can often be put in a corridor or small space nearer the consulting room so that the next patient is on the doctor's door-step (it is better to keep them out of ear-shot of the consultation). This chair may then be used for the 'persistent cougher' or crying baby. People will often send for the doctor to see patients with minor infectious conditions such as rubella, who, provided they can be brought to the surgery by car, are otherwise fit enough to attend. These patients should not wait in the waiting room but should be shown straight into an examination room or other suitable 'isolation' area.

Magazines should be tidied after each surgery, and badly torn ones disposed of. Hard covers can often be made for magazines and most doctors (and many patients) are only too anxious to find a home for magazines that they have read. One or two children's books, particularly those with stiff cardboard pages, will help mothers to pacify their offspring. A toy basket with hard and soft toys for children to play with on the floor will stop children getting bored and restless.

Every waiting room should have flowers in it. The provision of out-of-season flowers is an expensive business, but pot plants, foliage or even an arrangement of dried leaves are easy enough and cheap enough to produce and most secretaries will enjoy doing this (in December a Christmas arrangement will not be out of place). Waiting rooms need to be warmed efficiently but this should not be done to the total exclusion of ventilation. The smell produced by a combination of wet mackintoshes and hot bodies is peculiarly lingering and even in cold weather the waiting room needs a thorough airing at the end of each surgery.

One final use that the waiting room is sometimes put to is as a meeting place for patients. Some doctors arrange talks, discussion groups or relaxation classes for patients and this form of preventive medicine may be done in the waiting room. A good notice-board is an essential feature in the waiting room. It can carry information about surgery arrangements, health education notices and advice about other sources of help that are available to special groups such as expectant mothers, young mothers with children, the disabled and the elderly.

The secretary will have to lock the waiting room door at the end of each surgery otherwise she may find that a constant trickle of casual patients will prolong the work unnecessarily but she must, of course, unlock the door some minutes before the next surgery is due to begin.

THE CONSULTING ROOM

This is the point in the surgery where a quiet, private and unhurried discussion between doctor and patient can take place. The doctor will want the patient to feel able to discuss and explain his symptoms and to listen to the advice given in absolute privacy. There is no place for a secretary in the room and usually only the parents of children or the husband or wife of a patient are admitted during a consultation. The exception to this rule is where the consulting room contains the examination couch and the secretary may then be asked to chaperone or to assist with treatment.

Generally the consulting room contains a desk, two or three chairs, bookshelves and a wash-basin and it reflects the doctor's personality like a mirror. Most doctors do not like their own consulting room arrangements altered. The chairs and light are arranged to suit them and the books surrounding them are the ones that they need. Therefore, tidying-up must be done in a rather tactful way. The doctor's desk will usually carry one, two, or three trays for work, often 'In', 'Out' and 'Pending'. The 'Out' tray will be emptied frequently, preferably at the end of each surgery and the 'In' tray filled with letters, reports and notes needing his attention. A clock or calendar on his desk will be altered when necessary and the secretary will see that clean blotting paper, ink and stationery are always in the proper place. The doctor will keep in his consulting room a number of the forms that he constantly uses (the main stock being kept in stationery cupboards in the office) and these must be replenished when they are getting low. She will see that a clean towel and soap are by the wash-basin and that medical equipment kept in the consulting room is maintained. This might consist of cotton wool and spirit for injections, sterile syringes, torch, thermometer, throat spatulas, etc., but here again individual doctors will vary in their requirements.

If there is an appointment system the secretary will put the notes, in the order in which the patients are to be seen, on the doctor's desk before the surgery begins and will attend to the curtains, ventilation, light and heat at the same time.

During the surgery the doctor will be left alone in the consulting room with the patient. There will normally be an intercom system of lights, buzzers, bells or telephones and he will signal to the secretary by these when he needs another patient, wants to speak to her, etc. Each doctor develops a different technique that his secretary will soon learn and may even have a system whereby she can arrange an interruption of an over-long telephone call or consultation.

THE EXAMINATION ROOM

Some doctors prefer to have a couch in their consulting room on which the patient can be examined, and have a screen or curtains on runners to give the patient privacy whilst undressing. The doctor can talk to the patient or write notes or a prescription while the patient is dressing and consequently little time is wasted. Where there is adequate space, it is better to have a separate examination room. Old people and children often take a long time dressing or being dressed and another patient can be seen during this time. If a nurse is employed in the practice, as well as a secretary, the care of the examination room will be her prerogative, but where a secretary only is employed she will be expected to keep the room ready and on occasions to act as a chaperone.

The examination room should be kept particularly warm but also well ventilated. Fire precautions are important where dressing and undressing are done in a confined space. The couch should be covered with a clean sheet and another clean folded sheet should be put on the couch to cover the patient. The equipment used in the examination room will vary very much with the doctor, but will certainly include a thermometer, tongue depressors, torch, patella hammer, stethoscope and sphygmomanometer. Other equipment may be carried into the room when needed. The care of all the doctor's equipment is dealt with in Chapter 35. A small desk or flat surface for writing on is a useful feature and this may include a supply of certain forms which will need checking periodically.

The doctor will normally direct patients into the examination room after he has taken the history, but sometimes the secretary will know that a patient is to be examined and may show them straight in herself. She must then inform the doctor that there is a patient in the room otherwise he may either forget them or put another patient in, causing some embarrassment.

THE TREATMENT ROOM

Once again the possible variations are numerous. One doctor may consult, examine and treat all in one room, another may use separate rooms for each function, while a third may carry out very little physical treatment at all. Indeed some doctors may perform a wide range of minor operative procedures, dressings and injections, with or without the presence of a nurse whilst his colleague, round the corner, confines himself to examining and prescribing.

Care and maintenance of the equipment used are considered in the next chapter but every treatment room will contain a couch that needs clean sheets and a wash-basin that needs soap and towels. Once again, if a nurse is not employed the secretary will find herself doing a wide variety of tasks and here the doctor may teach her to help him with dressings and treatment.

Other rooms to be found in surgeries will include lavatories (sometimes separate ones for staff and patients) and the secretary may need to see that soap, towels and toilet paper are there, dark-rooms for examining fundi and transilluminating sinuses, laboratories, dispensaries, cleaner's room, and store rooms.

So much for the structure of the premises. The secretary may be responsible for supervising the cleaning. This will have to be done at some time when the surgery is not being used and thus it may be an early morning, midday or an evening cleaner that is required. She must find out what the pay is to be and see that the cleaner is paid for the correct amount at the same time each week and that any deduction for insurance stamps is made and recorded in the wages book. She will have to order fresh supplies of cleaning materials when the cleaner needs them and keep an observant eye on corners and dust-traps so that she can tactfully point out things that are being missed. Where a vacuum cleaner or electric polisher are used she should make arrangements to see that they are regularly serviced and may well keep a small card to record these dates. The doctor may leave her to appoint a new cleaner when required. If an advertisement is put in a local paper, it is better to give the doctor's name and address and not a box number, and when checking on references it is very important to remember that confidential papers may be left in trays and baskets and that a cleaner with a reputation for integrity is essential. Outside windows, paths and drives may be kept clean by a handyman and here again the secretary is responsible for paying the wages and keeping an overall eye on things.

This role as 'practice manager' will mean that other duties, including paying rent, rates, fuel bills and making arrangements for laundry and milk deliveries, are all part of the job and last but not least is the one of making tea. This is normally done at the end of the surgery and 'tea-time' is a very important part of the doctor's and the secretary's day. It is often the time when repeat prescriptions are done and it gives the doctor and the secretary the opportunity to discuss their problems and the patients. At this rather unguarded time the secretary should be careful not to take lighthearted remarks too seriously. Doctors cannot be serious all the time and their humour is a relief from responsibility and often a mark of their understanding.

GROUP SURGERIES AND HEALTH CENTRES

With the move towards working in larger groups premises have become larger and more complex. There may be more than one group practice operating from central premises and there may thus be more than one reception and waiting area. Similarly, space has to be found for other professionals; health visitors, social workers, clinical psychologists, physiotherapists and so on to work as part of the team. All this increases the complexity and sometimes for patients the confusion of finding their way around. Secretaries must be on the lookout for patients who are lost or bewildered in the general noise and bustle.

HALF DAYS

All doctors will require time off from their work. The idea that any one should be expected to be on call for long periods without the relief that a half-day would bring is completely outmoded. It is not only unfair on the doctor but is unfair on his patients, for a tired doctor is often an impatient or an uninterested doctor and neither of these go with good medical practice. The secretary must therefore guard his half-days and off-duty periods jealously. If patients attempt to put pressure on him at such times, the good secretary will politely absorb this pressure and she has every justification for being firm on this point. The annual holidays must be treated in the same way, but under his terms of contract the doctor is bound to notify the FPC of the deputizing arrangements he has made before he goes away. The secretary may remind him of this. This attitude to the half-day and holiday does not mean that the patient need be worried about being left untreated, for the secretary must find out what locum or deputizing arrangements have been made so that she is always in a position to advise the patient on this point.

The amount of time-off that the doctor can take will vary with circumstances. In the case of the unassisted country doctor it may be very limited, whereas in big group partnerships efficient systems can easily be worked out.

The secretary should be careful to arrange her own half-days and holidays with her employer when she first accepts the post. Generally they should be at times when the practice is reasonably quiet and if possible when a locum secretary can be obtained.

27

Office Work in General Practice

FILING IN GENERAL PRACTICE

Documents are filed to ensure accurate, quick and simple reference, and whatever method is adopted should satisfy these three criteria. The documents are of eleven types:

1 The medical record envelope (forms FP 5 and FP 6)
2 The medical record card of private patients
3 Medical records of temporary residents
4 Records of immunization and vaccination procedures
5 Antenatal records
6 X-rays
7 Advertising literature from drug firms
8 Private correspondence
9 Circulars from the FPC
10 Cards and registers for statistical and research purposes
11 Documents relating to bookkeeping
12 Special registers—'at risk', 'follow-up', etc.

The medical record envelope (forms FP 5 and FP 6)

The bulk of filing work in general practice is concerned with this envelope and its contents (Fig. 27.1). There will be one held for every patient on the doctor's list apart from the temporary residents and private patients. There will, therefore, be an average of over 2000 envelopes held by every GP. It is true to say that the following are two basic rules.

1 No patient should ever be seen by a doctor in the surgery or at home without the medical records being available.

2 No correspondence or report concerning a patient should be presented to the doctor without the medical records being available.

These envelopes are always filed in the vertical position, except in Scotland where they are filed in the horizontal position because of their special layout. There are three different storage methods available: (a) closed drawer (see Fig. 27.2), (b) open shelf, (c) rotating drum.

Drawers have the advantage of good security but the disadvantage of taking up more space because they take up a lot of room when they are fully opened. Shelving is the commonest method and is cheap. Security is poor unless a system of lockable shutters is provided but shelves are a very economical use of space and can be converted to A4 size, if this is needed. Drum filing is the most expensive, but it is very economical in the use of space and allows easy access.

226

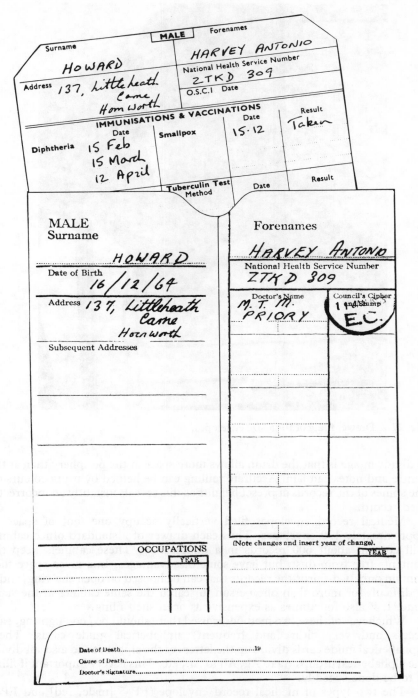

Fig. 27.1 The medical record envelope (forms FP 5 and FP 7a).

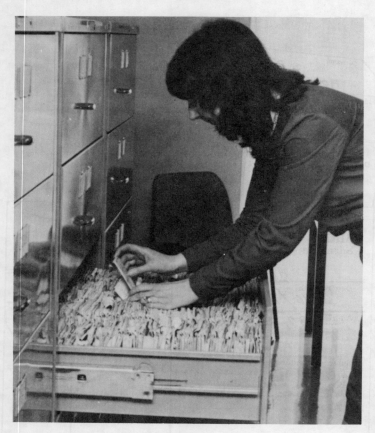

Fig. 27.2 Drawer filing of FP 5-size envelopes.

A disadvantage is that the drum allows more space at the periphery than at the centre and notes can jam. Accurate refiling can be helped by using colours on the spines of the records at preset heights as this reveals instantly an incorrectly filed record.

Medical record envelopes filed vertically occupy one foot of space to approximately 130 envelopes. Thus each drawer of a standard office cabinet will contain about 600 records in a double row. These cabinets keep the contents free from dust, but have some disadvantages. In a given space they contain only two-thirds the records that can be housed on open shelving, and it is difficult for more than one person to search the same cabinet at the same time. It is also four times as expensive as open-shelf filing.

Whichever of these two methods is used there should be good lighting, easy access and very clear (and frequent) alphabetical guide cards. These alphabetical guide cards divide up the letters of the alphabet and also subdivide the alphabetical groups Aa to Ag, Ah to An, etc. This is very important if filing is to be done speedily.

The two types of medical record envelope (FP 5 [male, red] and FP 6 [female, blue]) may be in one straight run, both types intermixed, or may be kept separately: either in two columns in one drawer, or in two separate drawers. The only advantage in storing them separately is that this may be of help in collecting statistics where the sex of the patient is a feature. An interesting development in the system of filing record cards that has been suggested by some doctors is to file in 'families'. Thus Leslie and Margaret Jones and their three children are all filed together. The advantages of this method are that the doctor never sees one member of the family without all the family's records and is therefore in a position to treat an illness as a family problem. This system makes searching for the cards more difficult, as reference has to be made to the name and address.

The record envelopes of patients attending the surgery with appointments should be removed from the file before the surgery begins and placed on the desk of the doctor in the correct order. The records of patients attending without appointment are extracted at the time and taken to the doctor before he sees the patient.

When removing an envelope from the file the use of a tracer card or marker to identify the position from which it has been withdrawn will greatly speed refiling. These tracer cards carry an identifying number and each one is accompanied by a slender marker card of the same colour and carrying the same number. The tracer card is inserted in the position in the file formerly occupied by the notes and the marker slip is put in the notes. When refiling it is only necessary to match marker and tracer to find the right place in the file. In some surgeries it is customary for the patient to take his own records in to the doctor. This is not a good principle and should only be done under circumstances which ensure that the patient is unable to read the records. The use of medical record envelopes with correspondence is dealt with later. It is important that these record envelopes are replaced in the files at the earliest opportunity, otherwise they can easily be lost. Before refiling them, they should be placed in an order corresponding to the filing system and then taken to the files. Thus record cards A–L are placed in that order near the appropriate shelf or drawer so that they can be put back into the files without the secretary having to do any more walking about than necessary. Gusseted envelopes can be obtained from the FP Committee to replace envelopes that become too full.

Keeping the contents of a medical record envelope in order has become recognized as a most important requirement for good medical care. In many practices staff will be involved in this work. Continuation card forms (FP 7) will have to be fixed in chronological order usually using a 'treasury tag'. They may be preceded by an FP 9A and 9B, used for summaries of patients' problems and for drug cards.

Letters about patients will also be fixed in chronological order and may be folded in special ways.

In some practices the medical records on either FP 7s or on A4 sheets will be typed. Here the doctor will use a dictating machine in his consulting room and transcription will be done later.

Numerical filing

Occasionally practices adopt numerical filing. This always entails setting up a central register cross-referencing the patient with their number. Systems can use sequential filing or terminal digit filing (see Chapter 17) but an alternative is to file by date of birth. The file then becomes an age–sex register itself (see page 233). This system becomes too bulky if more than 10 000 records are kept.

Whenever a numerical filing system is used it becomes important to ensure that any letter or reports about a patient bear the correct number as this greatly simplifies refiling.

A4 folders

The medical record envelope (FP 5 and 6) has been in existence since the first National Insurance Act of 1911. If it is well kept it is still an extremely useful tool for the storage and retrieval of medical data. Unfortunately, the amount of information that should be recorded grows year by year and it is now apparent that a different system of documentation is required. One possibility is to convert to A4 size (31 × 24 cm) folders. Many practices have made the change. There is a stout manila cover, sheets for personal data, clinical notes, laboratory and X-ray reports and so on and a pocket to take the old FP 5 or 6. (This will be required if the patient transfers to a practice that does not use A4 records systems.)

It is, however, possible that records may be computerized and thus the wholesale conversion to A4 records superseded. In the meanwhile we shall have to live with both systems. Other A4 records are described elsewhere.

The medical records of private patients

These are filed in a similar manner to the NHS medical record envelope. There is, however, no standardization of these records from one practice to another. They are usually in card form and not in envelopes. Consequently there may be a number of cards for each patient. These should be stapled together in the correct chronological order, and some system has to be devised for storing and filing letters and reports referring to these patients. If they are fastened to the record card they may easily become detached and lost. A better method is to make an entry on the record card referring to the report, e.g. 19.6.65—'see letter from Dr Smith', and file these letters in alphabetical order in a separate series of box or suspension files.

The medical records of temporary residents (forms FP 7 and FP 8)

These consist of a single card to which is attached an acceptance slip sent out by the FPC (see page 253). They should not be stored with the record envelopes, because (a) they are flimsy and can easily be pushed to the bottom of a file and lost, and (b) they have to be returned to the Committee after three months and must be filed somewhere where these dates can be checked periodically, for example a box file arranged in date order.

Medical record cards GP 7 and GP 8 are used in Scotland. A stock of these is held by the doctor, who automatically completes one when he sees a temporary resident. If the doctor feels he needs to communicate with the patient's own doctor he does this by letter. He claims his fee by completing form GP/19 (Scotland) and sending it to the Primary Care Administrator of the Health Board.

Records of immunization and vaccination procedures
See Chapter 33.

X-rays

In most cases X-ray films are retained within the radiology department of the hospital which the patient has been attending and a report is sent to the GP. Only occasionally, when X-ray examinations have been carried out privately, are the films sent to the doctor. These should be placed in jumbo-sized files.

The reports or X-rays are presented by the secretary to the doctor with the records of the patient. They are then either abstracted into the notes or, more usually, filed with them. Some A4 record systems contain special sheets on which X-ray reports can be gummed sequentially.

These X-rays, unlike medical records, will not be kept indefinitely, and sooner or later it will be necessary to throw out the older films. The doctor will decide how long they are to be kept and may decide to retain some films for an extra length of time. A method which makes this possible is to store these films in groups of one year together. Thus if it is decided to keep films for five years only, at the end of 1985 those films taken in 1980 will be removed and the drawer relabelled 1986. The films are not burnt but are sold to firms that reclaim silver from them.

Just as a patient should not be seen without his records, so should any X-rays taken since his last appointment be presented to the doctor at consultation. If a patient is being sent for X-ray the doctor should see that the word 'X-ray' is written in the appointments book by the secretary opposite the patient's next appointment.

Advertising literature from drug firms

Drug firms keep in contact with doctors in three ways: by advertising in medical journals, by sending representatives to visit doctors and by mailing advertising material directly to them.

The direct mailing is often glossy and attractive but bulky. Nevertheless certain mailed advertisements may be useful for the doctor and these he will wish to keep.

The most useful literature to keep is the data card. This has to be produced by the drug firm for every product marketed and contains all the essential information about the product. The cards should be filed in alphabetical order. A volume entitled the *Data Sheet Compendium* is produced annually by the organization representing the pharmaceutical industry and sent to most GPs. It contains the same information as the data sheets but these are listed under the manufacturer's name.

Private correspondence

Where this is non-recurrent and limited in scope it can best be put into a box file. This is a cardboard box with spring-clip and alphabetical index sheets and the letters are placed in it under the appropriate initial of the subject or name.

Where there is a larger quantity of correspondence it may be better to use an individual folder of the suspension file variety that is numbered. Here there is a separate small card-index file referring to the correspondence, e.g. BMA file no. 17 would contain, amongst other correspondence, letters to and from the Practice Organization Committee and to and from the local BMA secretary; cards would be made out for both of these, referring to file no. 17.

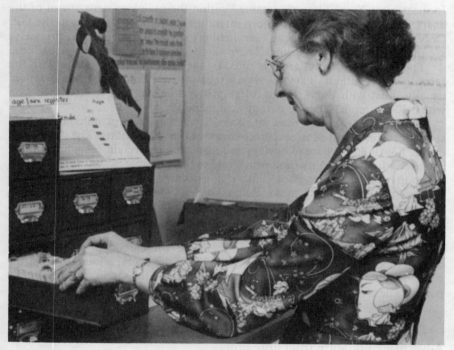

Fig. 27.3 Files for special records.

Circulars from the FPC

Every GP under contract with the NHS receives frequent circulars relating to fees, allowances and the conditions and terms of service. These arrive almost weekly, usually replacing a previous circular. They carry a paragraph number and are fitted into a ring file (the 'red book') entitled 'Statement of Fees and Allowances'. It is most essential that this is kept absolutely up-to-date and the secretary must ensure that each new arrival is accurately filed. For example, if a new scale of capitation fees is agreed, circulars numbered SFA para. 21.1 (Northern Ireland N1 para. 20) will arrive and replace the previous pages of that number.

Cards and registers for statistical purposes
(See below.)

Documents relating to bookkeeping
(See Chapter 11.)

Special registers ('at risk', 'follow-up', 'contraception', etc.)

There may be patients in the practice whom the doctor requires to see at intervals because he considers they are at risk of developing a disease or complication or need periodic reviews. There are a number of ways in which such a register may be kept—notebooks, loose-leaf ledgers or sometimes a special file.

In the latter system a convenient method is to divide the file into sections for each month of the year. An FP 7 or 8 for the patient is placed in the month or year in which they should be reviewed. At the appropriate time the patient should be sent for and the doctor notified if they fail to attend.

RESEARCH IN GENERAL PRACTICE

The Research Executive of the Royal College of General Practitioners has been concerned with the study of the incidence of disease, its causes and results. As well as individual methods of collecting data, such as punched card systems, standardized methods of data collection have been developed which can be used under many circumstances and which would enable the data collected from many different sources to be strictly comparable. A number of these systems are now being extensively used and many medical secretaries will be involved in their usage. They therefore need careful description.

Age and sex register

This is the basic tool in any practice doing research and it is also important in the clinical care of patients, particularly in preventive care, and in the administration of the practice. The NHS, by providing each doctor with a known population for which he is responsible, has enabled him to determine the incidence of events in the practice. That is, he can determine the rate per 100 or per 1000 patients that a disease, such as pneumonia, occurs, or the average number of consultations per patient per year, and so on. Countries where patients do not register with one doctor are unable to do this because a patient may sometimes attend one doctor and sometimes another in a different town; thus neither knows what the incidence of events is even though both can tell you the total number they have seen. A doctor can tell you, then, that he has seen 50 patients with pneumonia in a year, but he cannot tell you that the incidence of pneumonia that year was, say, one in a hundred. Furthermore, if the doctor has a register including the age and sex of each patient, he can tell you the incidence of occurrence in either sex and in different age groups.

The age–sex register is also valuable for the clinical care of groups of patients identified by either age or sex or both. For example, all small children require immunization against certain diseases at certain ages. All children in the appropriate age group can be identified and sent for. The cards can be tagged by clipping out a hole or by marking in some other way when this is done and this identifies the key members of the group, those who have *not* been immunized.

Common groups who need identifying include:
- all pre-school children for developmental assessment or immunization
- all girls under 12 for rubella immunization
- all women over 35 for cervical cancer screening
- all men and women between 35 and 65 for blood pressure screening
- all men and women over 65 for general health screening

Because GPs are paid some money for special groups of patients it is possible to use the register to check that these sums have been correctly calculated by the FPC. This might include extra payments received for the patients over 65 and over 75 years of age. Health visitors in particular find the register of the greatest value.

There are two methods by which an age–sex register can be set up:

1 *Loose-leaf method.* Here a loose-leaf folder is required and one page is used for each year. On this page will be put, on the left-hand side, all the males in the practice who were born in that year, and on the right-hand side, similarly, all the females. Every card in the practice is worked through and the details put on the appropriate page. Newcomers will be entered and those who die or leave the practice will be ruled through with the appropriate note made. The date and month of birth are recorded in figures.

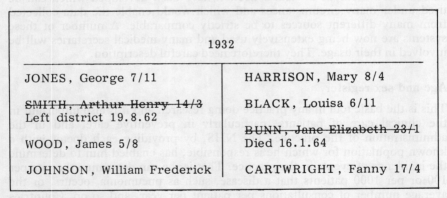

Fig. 27.4 The loose-leaf method of recording.

2 *Card index method.* This system uses cards designed by the records and statistics unit of the Royal College of General Practitioners. They are part of a series of data recording systems that are capable of central analytical or computer analysis. These systems are necessary when facts from a large number of doctors or practices are to be collected and in which strict comparability is required, or when a very large number of facts from a smaller number of sources need to be analysed.

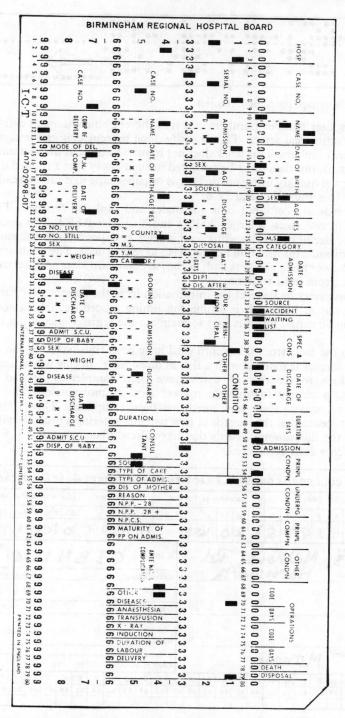

Fig. 27.5 A punch card for computer input.

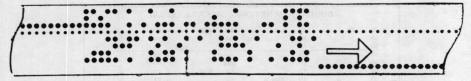

Fig. 27.6 Paper tape for computer input.

A computer handles numbers and it is therefore necessary to convert the facts into numerical series. This is easily done by replacing the letters of the alphabet by numbers. This work does not have to be done at the secretarial end of the system, but data must be collected in such a way that a trained operator can convert it quickly into punched cards or paper tape that can be read by the computer (see Figs 27.5 and 27.6).

The cards are coloured blue for males and pink for females. They are prepared in two sizes, a larger ASR2a and a smaller ASR2. The doctor will choose the size of card he is using for his register depending on the amount of future additional information he may wish to record on it. The cards are stored in small drawer filing cabinets and, as they are standard sizes, divider cards can be bought from local stationers.

It is necessary to abstract the information from the patient's record card in the same way as before. It is a time-consuming procedure, taking about one hour to do 50 cards, but it is easy to maintain the register once it has been set up.

When the facts from the record card have been transferred to the age–sex card, the former is marked with a tick in one corner. In this way a final check can be done to see that all cards have been completed. As the process continues, a clearly identifiable marker card is moved along the files of patients' records to show how much has been completed. This is important because it means that the records of new patients entering a practice will not be added to the files amongst cards that have already been abstracted. Fig. 27.7 shows such a card completed.

A.S.R.2a	COLLEGE OF GENERAL PRACTITIONERS RECORDS and STATISTICS UNIT																

Fig. 27.7 An ASR2a card.

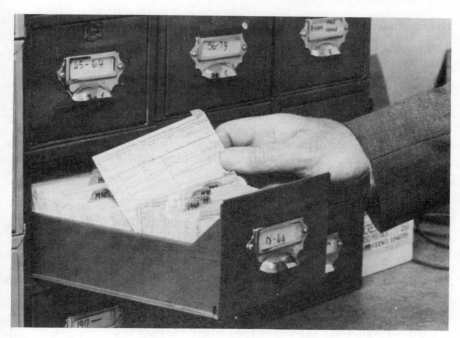

Fig. 27.8 The age–sex register.

The doctor's code is given to him by the FPC and can be found stamped with his name and address on each prescription form (FP 10). To doctors outside the NHS a number is allocated by the records unit.

The code used for the patient consists of the first three letters of the surname, the first letter of the first forename and the date of birth written numerically. A single figure date such as 1st January, 1908 is written 01 01 08 and 7th October, 1934 becomes 07 10 34. Thus, on the card the patient's identifying code has become BROH 010819.

Other boxes are filled in according to the standard instructions of the records and statistics unit. Many NHS record envelopes (FP 5 and 6) do not have the patient's date of birth—about 15% in most practices. If a marker card is placed inside these envelopes, they can often be completed when the patient attends surgery. But most FPCs will supply this information on request.

It is absolutely essential that the register is kept up-to-date. Otherwise it is soon useless. New entries must be made as every patient registers with the practice and entries deleted as soon as medical record envelopes are returned to the FPC.

The cards for new entries are filed in a separate drawer until the records are received from the FPC. This enables identification of patients who present but whose records cannot be found because they have not been received. Similarly the cards of patients who leave the list and whose records are sent for on form FP 22 are filed separately as these may still be required for research purposes.

In some practices age–sex indexes are computerized and the register is produced either as a total print-out or that part that is required at a given time is printed for the user.

Diagnostic index ('E' book)

This is used to record the numbers of particular types of illness that occur in the practice. The key is the diagnosis given to the patient's illness, the identifying details of the patient being entered under the appropriate diagnosis.

Each diagnosis is given a number obtained from a list prepared by the Royal College's record unit. It differs from the International Classification of Diseases, Injuries and Causes of Death in that it is shorter. This is because it contains only those diseases which occur reasonably frequently in general practice in Britain. Fig. 27.9 shows a page from the 'E' book; 282 is the number given to appendicitis.

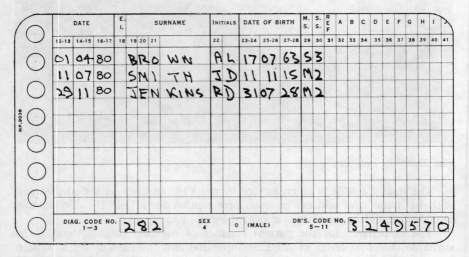

Fig. 27.9 The 'E' book.

There is one page for each diagnosis and this will contain the names of patients suffering from that condition. Males are written on one side and females on the other. Each page is clipped onto the 'E' book in such a way that it does not cover the last line of the underlying page. Each of these exposed lines lies opposite to the diagnosis and code number, and thus one can rapidly turn to the appropriate page to fill in the details.

The medical secretary may be expected to complete these each day from the diagnosis entered on the record card (FP 7 or 8).

Each year these pages are sent to the records unit for analysis. In this way, many practices are contributing to our knowledge of the incidence and causes of disease.

Summary cards ('S' cards)

In the 'E' book the diagnosis is the key factor, but in general practice it is usual to record information in relation to the patient rather than to the diagnosis. For this reason another system has been designed in the series. In this the routine notes about the patient are made on a card (S4A) which fits into the record envelope. After each episode of illness, the details are entered on a summary card (S4) made out for that patient, which, at the end of the year, will therefore carry particulars of all the illnesses from which the patient has suffered. This information is capable of being punched onto cards or tape.

To summarize the differences between 'E' book and 'S' cards, it will be seen that at the end of one year a page in an 'E' book will contain the names, addresses and ages of all patients who suffered from, say, pneumonia and may include, say, Mary Smith. At the same time, Mary Smith's 'S' card will list all the illnesses she had that year including the episode of pneumonia.

It may well be the medical secretary's responsibility to complete these cards, but the system used by a particular practice—'E' book, 'S' cards or a combination of both—will depend on the requirements of the doctor and will have to be worked out and practised by the doctor and his secretary.

Three other systems in the series deserve mention:

1 *The 'L' book*. This is a loose-leaf ledger with foolscap-size sheets. It is designed to measure workload at the same time as it records identification details about the patient and the diagnosis. It can be modified to suit the particular study or interest of the doctor but could, for example, record the number of visits or consultations, the type of pathological investigation, the hospitals to which patients are referred, and so on.

2 *The 'F' book*. This differs from previous methods of recording in that it is built around the family as a unit. It is a visible-edge indexing system like the 'E' book, but an entire household is recorded on one sheet. The facts recorded are partly administrative—date of leaving practice, relationship within household, etc.—and partly clinical—blood group, morbidity by code number, 'twins', illegitimacy, adoption, and so on. A method has been evolved by which, once the 'F' book has been built up, it can be maintained entirely by secretarial staff.

3 *The 'W' book*. This was originally called a practice index book, which gives the key to its use. It does not record morbidity as the 'E' book does but shows where the records with the information will be found. A very simplified classification of diseases with eight groups is used. There is one page for each, on which only the date, name and diagnosis are put. All other details can be extracted from the records if required.

CORRESPONDENCE

Incoming post

The amount of post arriving at a doctor's surgery each day is usually considerable. Amongst it are letters and reports of the highest medical importance, and some proper system of dealing with it must be developed. The secretary will find that the use of labelled letter trays will be of great help for sorting correspondence. A letter placed in an appropriate tray will rarely be mislaid, but those opened and left on the desk may be inadvertently swept into wastepaper baskets, into books or other envelopes. The number of trays she will need will depend upon the number of doctors that she serves. There are five types of incoming letter, thus she may use up to five letter trays. These are:

1 letters and reports from hospitals, doctors and patients, etc.

2 documents arriving from the FPC
3 bills, receipts and payments
4 personal letters
5 advertisements and medical journals

The post should be opened early in the day as there may be letters about patients who have to be seen that very day. It should be sorted into the appropriate tray and scanned quickly through. It can then be left until later in the day unless it requires immediate attention.

Most of the incoming material will require the attention of the doctor. It will, therefore, find its way into the 'In' tray on his desk, but before that occurs it has to be attended to by the secretary.

1 She must attach any letter or report about a patient to the medical record envelope of that patient and place it in the 'In' tray of the doctor to whom the letter was addressed. Similarly any letter from a patient or his relative should always be presented to the doctor attached to the appropriate medical record envelope.

If the letter requires an immediate reply, and particularly if it requests a visit, the doctor's attention must be drawn to this fact. It may be his habit to reply to letters the following day, and thus an urgent matter may be delayed. This is of particular importance where a notification of a patient's discharge from hospital is received. There is an increase in the number of patients discharged very early from hospital and many of these require visiting.

2 Any letter from the FPC to the doctor will need his personal attention. Other documents such as requests for the return of cards may not. The method of dealing with these is described in Chapter 29 under 'FPC forms'.

3 Bills, receipts and payments are dealt with in the section on bookkeeping (Chapter 11).

4 Personal letters, marked as such, or those in the recognized handwriting of friends or relatives should be left unopened unless the doctor has specifically authorized the secretary to open them.

5 Advertisements will be opened, removed from their envelopes and put into the doctor's 'In' tray, as will medical journals.

When the doctor has attended to the papers in his 'In' tray he will put those that require attention in his 'Out' tray. Letters and reports about patients that need to be placed in the medical record envelopes will either be dealt with by the doctor or he will return them to the secretary, having initialled them, for her to deal with. It is important that the contents of the medical record envelope are kept tidy, in the correct order, and limited to those that are really necessary. As a general rule all letters that must be kept will be folded with the headings on the outside so that they can be recognized immediately on withdrawal from the envelope. Where possible they will be stapled together in chronological order, the top letter being the most recent one.

The same treatment can be given to X-ray and pathological reports when the doctor has indicated that he wishes them to be included in the medical record envelope.

His 'Out' tray may also contain completed insurance reports for posting, advertisements that he wishes to be filed and papers relating to bookkeeping.

The doctor will take away with him those journals that he wishes to read. He may throw them away when he has finished them or he may keep them on his bookshelves. The secretary will only be involved if he does his own abstracting from journals, in which case she will file the article that has been removed in either a box file or a suspension file.

Outgoing post

This can be divided into five groups:
1 Letters to consultants (see page 67).
2 Reports on patients, e.g. insurance examinations (see page 263).
3 Letters to FPC (see page 252).
4 Private correspondence.
5 Bills and accounts (see page 77).

As these are described elsewhere it is only necessary to say here that where the consultant is seeing the patient at hospital the letter may be written on the doctor's headed notepaper or the hospital may provide a letter form on which the letter can be typed, folded once and sealed, and then details needed for the registration of the patient at the hospital can be filled in before folding again and sealing for post.

After dealing with the outgoing post the secretary should check that:
(a) all letters are correctly addressed
(b) all letters are correctly stamped, bearing in mind the different rates of postage
(c) envelopes are strong enough for the material they hold. It is possible to reinforce the sealing of flaps with Sellotape
(d) parcels are securely wrapped and tied, and where necessary sealed

---

Diploma Questions

1 You are secretary to a private doctor who deals extensively with medical examinations for a large number of organizations. Outline a possible filing system for patients' case notes and other related information. Give examples of the type of data, returns, and information that might be required by the doctor, and the system of retrieval you would use.
2 Describe the various methods of storage data in a large group practice.
3 Outline the ways in which a medical secretary can assist in clinical research in general practice.
4 A scientific paper reporting medical research usually has conventional sections. Briefly describe these and set out the various steps that have to be taken by the typist to ensure that a paper to be published is prepared in an acceptable form.
5 State the purpose of the age–sex register and state the matters to be considered when setting up such a register.
6 What procedure would you follow in dealing with the incoming and outgoing mail in general practice?

28
Practice Management

General practices, because of their small size, have considerable freedom to decide on and alter the way in which they work. The smallest unit would consist of one doctor and one receptionist, but as group practices have developed the management has become more complex and the task of keeping the administration running smoothly for the benefit of patients has begun to need more specialized skills.

The size of groups has steadily increased over the last 15 years. There are now less than 9000 GP 'units' accommodating more than 25 000 doctors and amongst these the number including five and more has increased most.

Such a group may include seven to ten receptionists, often working part-time, attached and employed nurses, health visitors and midwives, cleaning staff, sometimes a resident caretaker, telephonist, gardener and so on. Considerable management skills are required to organize such a group in terms of personnel, finance and the buildings and equipment.

The practice manager or administrator has certain defined skills:

1 Planning the services and making the best possible use of accommodation and equipment.

2 Financial control and preparing practice accounts for annual audit (Chapter 11).

3 Engagement and supervision of administrative and domestic staff.

4 Training of reception staff.

5 Responsibility for statutory and other returns.

6 Data collection and other statistics (Chapters 13 and 27).

7 Dealing with other health service agencies and visitors.

Some of these tasks are covered in other sections of this book. The remainder are dealt with here.

PLANNING THE SERVICES

There is a well recognized circle of action involved in administration (see Fig. 28.1).

Most decisions about administrative change take place after a process of consultation. This is often at the practice meeting and it is here that the practice manager will need to keep the minutes (Chapter 10) and initiate the action that is required of her. Once this decision has been taken it will be her responsibility to discuss the steps with other staff and ensure that they have all the necessary information to feel well motivated towards the change. Staff should be invited to comment and make decisions.

242

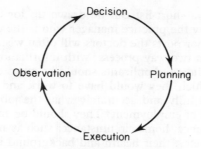

Fig. 28.1 Action involved in administration.

Execution requires all the steps to be detailed and the times fixed and may need further training, documentation or equipment set up before the activity begins.

The final step is almost the most important. It is necessary to observe and where possible measure and record the effect made by the changes. This will enable the practice administrator to report back at an appropriate time and complete the circle.

ENGAGING AND SUPERVISING STAFF

The steps in this involve:
1 drawing up a job specification
2 advertising and interviewing
3 providing a contract
4 staff training and occasionally dismissing staff

Getting the right person into the right job needs some skill. The first step is drawing up a job specification. This will include the skills required and the experience and attitude looked for in the applicant.

The job specification for a medical secretary might list the age range, educational attainments, typing and shorthand skills, knowledge of medical terminology, experience in dealing with confidential matters, ability to take decisions and work with other people, flexibility of approach to job, domestic commitments and so on.

Once the specification has been approved within the practice, an advertisement is drawn up. For junior staff the 'jobs vacant' column of a local newspaper is usually the right place, but for more senior staff it is often put into one of the medical weekly papers. The advertisement should be as specific as possible in order to avoid interviewing unsuitable staff. Under the Sex Discrimination Act of 1975 it is not permissible to specify the sex of an applicant but it should certainly specify all other essential requirements. Applications should be invited from both men and women. Applicants should be asked to write or telephone and then should be sent a standard application form to complete in their own handwriting. This should list name, address, date of birth, present occupation, schools attended, examinations and certificates obtained and previous experience (what were they doing and why did they leave?).

From the replies a short-list can be drawn up for interview. Interviews should be arranged by the practice manager who is the usual leader for more junior posts. For senior posts the doctors will often wish to be involved. The interview should be a two-way process, with information being given to and sought from the candidate. Applicants should be given the chance of looking round the area in which they would have to work and of asking questions. They should be told fully and accurately what the job consists of, and the terms and conditions of employment. They should be encouraged to describe their previous experience, home circumstances such as arrangements for child care, travelling time etc., their health and background information and their interests. If shorthand and typing skills to a good standard are required then a brief test of these, using a sample letter, can be a very helpful indication of suitability. References should always be asked for and should be taken up before an appointment is made. Sometimes applicants are told of the result of an interview at the time of the interview but it is more usual to inform them in writing.

Contract

A contract or Statement of Terms and Conditions of Employment must be given to any employee who works for more than 16 hours per week, and is not the husband or wife of the employer, not later than 13 weeks after starting work.

The law is stated in the Employment Protection (Consolidation) Act (1978), which lists the facts that a contract of statement must specify, these are:

1 the names of the parties to the contract
2 the date employment began
3 whether previous employment counts for purposes of continuous service
4 the rate of pay, the way it is calculated and the pay period (hourly, weekly, monthly)
5 the hours of work
6 holiday and sick pay entitlement
7 pension rights and whether the scheme is contracted out of the state scheme
8 the length of notice the employee is entitled to, and must give
9 the title of the job

Forms of contract can be drawn up or standard forms can be obtained from stationers. A standard contract will cover the following points in addition to the above: incremental date, overtime payments, maternity leave (Employment Act 1980), health and safety at work, and disciplinary procedures. (Further advice can be obtained from the Industrial Relations Officer, BMA House, Tavistock Square, London WC1H 9JP.) There must also be a complaints procedure laid down. The parties to the contract may include the senior partner or all partners. It does not matter which providing they have a partnership agreement. It is important to consider the status of previous employment as sometimes a partnership is dissolved on retirement of a senior partner and new contracts have to be drawn up for employees.

Holiday and sick pay entitlements are not mandatory but four weeks or twenty working days are customary for holidays with added days for length of

Table 28.1 Summary of employment law relating to employees of general practitioners. (Details to be found in leaflets relating to the appropriate act.)

Any *new applicant for a job* has the right
— not to be discriminated against because of sex or marriage[1], or because of colour, race, nationality or origin[2].

Any *employee* has the right
— to receive equal pay with a member of the opposite sex doing similar work[3]
— to have time off for certain trade union activities or to belong to a trade union[4]
— to receive an itemized pay statement[4]
— to have certain rights of sickness absence[5]
— to have paid time off for pre-natal care[6]

Any *employee who works more than 16 hours a week* has the right
— to be given a minimum period of notice based on length of service[4]

Any *employee with at least 13 weeks of service* has the right
— to receive a written statement of terms of employment[4]

Any *employee with at least 52 weeks of service* has the right
— not to be unfairly dismissed (unless they have worked for less than two years for an employer with 20 or less staff)[4,6]
— has the right not to be dismissed on the grounds of pregnancy[4]

Any *employee with at least 104 weeks service* has the right
— to receive maternity pay and return to work up to 29 weeks after giving birth[4]
— has rights if made redundant[4]

References: 1, Sex Discrimination Act 1975; 2, Race Relations Act 1976; 3, Equal Pay Act 1970; 4, Employment Protection Act 1978; 5, Social Security and Housing Benefits Act 1972; 6, Employment Act 1980.

service and most employees can expect their sick benefits to be made up to full pay for a few weeks and then to half pay for a few weeks. Maternity leave has to be offered if a staff member has worked for two years by the time she is 29 weeks pregnant and has to be offered her job back afterwards. The employer can claim a rebate to recover the statutory maternity pay in full through the Department of Employment.

The 1978 Employment Protection (Consolidation) Act lays down minimum lengths of notice required to be given by the employer. It is one week if the employee has worked for more than four weeks and less than two years, and thereafter one added week for each year up to a maximum of twelve. It may be necessary to stipulate longer notice to be given by the employee if replacement of the staff could be difficult. Any change in the written terms of employment must be notified to the employee within four weeks of the change.

Staff training

Every member of staff requires some training. Senior doctors are involved in continuing education inside and outside the practice. Trainee doctors have formal periods for education each week. Administrative staff require induction training when they join the practice and continuing education both inside and outside the practice. It is often the task of the practice manager to support and arrange such training and so it is dealt with in detail in this section. Although different categories of staff have different requirements there may be many occasions when it will be more profitable for, say, nurses and doctors or all the staff to attend a particular session. This requires special arrangements to be made.

Training and continuing education for doctors

About one-in-ten practices are designated as 'training practices' and will have a young doctor with them, usually for one year. These trainees have spent two years in approved hospital practice and are now completing their third year of vocational training in general practice.

Training consists of consulting and visiting patients, under close supervision initially and later accepting more responsibility. As well as this there are formal teaching sessions within the practice and regular attendance at a series of half-day courses outside the practice. The trainee is, of course, a fully registered doctor. To begin with they often work at a much slower speed than their more experienced colleagues but will gradually become more familiar with the task. They will not sign claim forms for money for the practice but otherwise, they function very much as a partner.

During the week there are sessions set aside with one of the senior doctors, designated as a 'trainer', where joint consultations are undertaken or 'topics' discussed. These are important times when the two doctors should remain undisturbed by outside telephone calls as far as possible.

Apart from formal training for trainees all the doctors will meet from time to time, often for a regular weekly lunchtime meeting. Some of these sessions will be devoted to audit or performance review, others to specific topics. Doctors also attend courses away from the practice. The secretary may need to make travel arrangements for this and for some of them a reimbursement of expenses is claimable under Section 63 and the appropriate form must be obtained at the course and then completed and returned to the appropriate FPC.

Training and continuing education for employed staff

Many employed staff will have had specific training before employment. They may possess appropriate qualifications in nursing, secretarial or reception work but even when relatively experienced they will need some induction training at the start of their job. Other people will not have had specific 'medical' training or 'general practice' training and will require considerable formal training.

Training is aimed at three areas: knowledge, skills and attitudes. *Knowledge* is acquired by listening to what you are told, by watching what is happening and by reading. *Skills* are, in the main, acquired by practising the tasks that have to be done after having been told or shown the desired way. *Attitudes* are more complex. They depend partly upon past experience but can be changed if a situation is set up where there is conflict between the present attitude of the learner and the change or effect that the learner desires. Learners will then find that altering their attitude leads to a more desirable effect.

For example, the trainee receptionist must learn that there are several different appointment systems that can be used and will learn the advantages and disadvantages of them. This knowledge is put to work by practising making new and old appointments and by being helped by the supervisor. The learner has then acquired the skill. She may however believe that people with minor symptoms should not present themselves to doctors and this attitude may lead her to be brusque or rude to patients. During the course of training she may discover a conflict between this attitude and the fact that some minor symptoms are the first warnings of serious disease or of great anxiety. A resolution of this conflict will lead her to change her attitude and thus alter the behaviour that stems from it.

This ability to accept criticism from within and without and to change appropriately is an important and surprisingly pleasant lesson to absorb.

Induction training

Every new member of staff needs time set aside at the start of the job to learn the 'local' rules. They will be told to whom they are responsible, introduced to all other members of staff and shown the layout of the building. If there are rules that are essential these should be given to the employee at the start of employment. There is usually a period of one week during which the new member 'sits in' with a more experienced member of staff and watches what goes on. After this a specific time (e.g. 30 minutes) should be set aside each day to deal with a specified topic.

For a new receptionist a list of suitable subjects will include:
1 confidentiality relating to documents and telephone calls and how to deal with doctors and other people making enquiries
2 the reception of patients at the desk and on the telephone
3 forms relating to reception work
4 the appointment system
5 medical records and related documents, how to file and retrieve
6 chaperoning
7 the prescription, prescription cards and repeat prescriptions
8 forms relating to sickness benefits, insurance, etc.
9 the hospital service, ambulance service, FPC and Social Services
10 the emergency situation

Continuing education

A senior member of staff, usually the practice manager or senior secretary, will have to develop skills as a teacher. To do this she has to help her colleagues to learn, to create suitable conditions for this to happen, and to be receptive to new ideas and change herself.

When new systems occur or old systems need reviewing she should be prepared to set aside time for these to be discussed in detail, so that all can become familiar with the objectives of the tasks and the methods required. Once again, the practice manager is faced with the triple task of encouraging change, acquiring new knowledge and skills, and facilitating change. It cannot be overemphasized how important a part 'feelings' play in all this. If the learner is encouraged to feel that he or she has an important role to play in the search for quality of performance, good practice will be reinforced or errors corrected, but if the learner feels threatened or criticized any change will be blocked. Both teacher and learner need to recognize these feelings, which are present in everyone and are a measure of immaturity. The degree of enthusiasm and sense of fun that the practice manager brings to this aspect of her work is critical.

As well as this 'on-the-job' learning, which should form a part of every person's activity, there is a limit to what can be done here. If the practice remains a closed unit, new ideas have difficulty in gaining entrance. 'Off-the-job' learning, particularly where the learner has the opportunity to meet colleagues doing similar jobs in different places, is very important and every member of staff should have the opportunity to attend courses outside the practice.

Courses are now regularly run and the practice manager should make herself aware of those in her neighbourhood, or may actually be the initiator of a course. The British Medical Association, the Royal College of General Practitioners and the organizations concerned with receptionist training have set up an organization to help in this work.

Courses arranged for staff (receptionists, secretaries, practice managers and practice nurses) attract financial support under paragraph 52 8–9 of the 'red book'. Seventy per cent of travelling expenses, subsistence, and course fees are reimbursed for courses organized by, or in association with, health authorities, the local Faculty of the Royal College of General Practitioners, or the education authority. The claims are made on form ANC 3.

Other forms used in employment

Seventy per cent of the salary of staff involved in the care of patients, up to a maximum of two full-time equivalent staff per doctor, is refunded by the FPC. Staff must work for a minimum of five hours per week and full-time means thirty-eight hours per week. Qualified staff must be employed for nursing and treatment, secretarial and clerical work, receiving patients, making appointments or, dispensing.

Private practice involving more than 10% of the gross receipts of the practice will result in a reducing scale of refund.

Form ANC 1 is made out for each new employee in duplicate. One copy is sent to the FPC and one copy retained to check that details on the quarterly claim form (ANC 3) are correct (see Chapter 29). An updated ANC 1 must be completed each time an employee's salary is varied. Claim forms must state correctly the weekly pay, and any variations due to overtime and so on must be included. The National Insurance contribution of the employer is set down, as this is completely refunded and the forms must be sent in before 10 days after the end of the quarter that they refer to.

Dismissing staff

Chapter 71 of the Employment Protection Act (1978) lays down the rules and regulations that must be followed when dismissing staff. Once a person has been employed continuously for 52 weeks they have the right to appeal to an industrial tribunal that they have been unfairly dismissed, and a tribunal may order compensation or recommend re-instatement. Dismissal on the grounds of pregnancy or trade union membership are unfair reasons for dismissal.

Employees who have been disciplined should have been warned verbally, and then in writing, of the required improvements. Advice on dismissal and related matters can be obtained from the Advisory, Conciliation and Arbitration Service (ACAS) who also publish pamphlets on Codes of Practice on employment matters. The Department of Employment also publishes helpful advice on such matters as maternity pay, contracts of employment, redundancy and so on.

FINANCE

The practice manager will be responsible for keeping the books herself or ensuring that they are kept up-to-date, and may be asked to produce a breakdown of income and expenditure for practice meetings, obtain competitive estimates when buying goods or services, present accounts to the practice accountant and try to maximize the practice profits.

Income

Most income is received from the FPC. A quarterly statement of account is sent to the practice in which the income is set out under a number of headings as described in the 'red book'—the Statement of Fees and Allowances.
   Headings will include:
1 basic practice allowance
2 seniority payments
3 vocational training
4 group practice payments
5 capitation fees and supplements
6 night visits
7 vaccination and immunization
8 cervical cytology
9 family planning
10 maternity payments
11 out-of-hours responsibilities
12 temporary residents
13 rural practice payments
14 capitation drugs and drug tariffs

It may be helpful for a statement to be drawn up for practice meetings setting out changes, particularly in earnings for item-for-service payments, as these show the activity in any particular area and can form the basis to make changes.
   Advances on payment due can consist either of half the estimated amount in the middle of a quarter or one third monthly. Advances may also be made for leave payments and the manager may indicate when these should be sent for.

Expenditure

Expenditure will either be constant: lighting, heat, staff salaries, telephones, etc., or variable. In any case the money required to meet the month's bills will have to be retained before the partners can draw a share of the profits. In some practices a tax reserve account will be built up to cover anticipated tax demands and this should be put to work to earn interest. The accountant will advise.

Estimates

When either goods or services are purchased it may pay to have several estimates to ensure the 'best buy'. These can be presented at partnership meetings for decisions to be taken.

Profits

The final financial role of the practice manager is that of maximizing profits. This can be done by seeing that all practice accounts are sent out promptly and that proper fees are charged (the BMA provides members with a list of appropriate fees).

The item-for-service payments offer the greatest opportunity for increasing practice earnings and as these are related to clinical work they increase the quality and quantity of care given. There is good evidence that practices employing the largest numbers of staff per doctor (up to two full-time per doctor) are the ones that earn the largest sums from item-for-service payments and the practice manager may need to consider carefully this relationship between staff numbers and profit.

The Statement of Fees and Allowances should be kept up-to-date by incorporating all the changes notified and the contents should be familiar to the practice manager.

Diploma Questions

*Denotes an incomplete question

1 As secretary to a group of GPs, describe four methods of payment through a bank which you might use for them. Give examples.

2 You are responsible for making up the weekly wages for two secretaries, one receptionist and one part-time cleaner. What deductions from salary are statutory and what information and documents do you require to enable you to calculate these deductions?

3 As secretary to a group of general practitioners describe how you would deal with:

(a) private patients' accounts

(b) remittances received in the morning post

(c) a bank statement which does not agree with a cash book balance.*

4 You are senior medical secretary in a large group practice and your employers are considering paying the staff monthly by credit transfer rather than by current weekly payment in cash. Write a report for them stating the advantages and disadvantages of this method of payment to both the practice and the employees.

5 Write about the following administrative procedure: rota systems for doctors and staff in group practices.*

6 In general practice the telephone represents one of the most important means of internal and external communication. It is essential, therefore, that this service is well-organized. Draw up a list of instructions for the guidance of staff in the use of this system.

7 Suggest, with reasons, six examples of published information which would be essential in the office of a health centre.

29

Forms in General Practice

The forms and certificates dealt with in this chapter will complete the rather formidable list that the GP has to handle. When one has been described in detail already only a brief reference to it will be made. The secretary will be expected to keep stocks of these forms available so that they can be produced whenever they are needed. They should be kept neatly in cupboards or drawers that are readily accessible. (Stocks of prescription forms should be kept in a securely locked cupboard or drawer.) Where possible they should be grouped together logically so that the minimum of walking about is done when a variety of forms are needed at one time, for example, all forms relating to antenatal work or immunization procedures will be kept together. They should also be kept in that part of the office where they are most frequently needed, for example forms relating to the registration of patients may be kept in the reception area. The secretary must not only be familiar with the uses of the forms but must also know how to order further supplies when necessary.

FPC FORMS

The list below includes all those forms that are commonly met with in general practice.

1 *FP 1 (Scotland GP 1, Northern Ireland HS 22X)*—registration form for patients who have lost their medical cards or for immigrants (see Chapter 30).

2 *FP 1C (Scotland GP 1C, or local FPC form)*—notification to FPC of change of address or name of patient.

3 *FP 3 (Scotland GP 3)*. This is the large envelope provided by the FPC and already addressed to the administrator. It is used for sending medical record envelopes, medical cards, etc., backwards and forwards between the Committee and the doctor. Care should be taken when putting medical cards and small forms into the large envelope to see that they do not slip inside medical record envelopes that are being sent back.

4 *FP 4 (Scotland GP 4, Northern Ireland HS 23)*—patient's medical card. This is retained by the patient. It bears the name, address and date of birth, the NHS number and the name of the doctor with whom the patient is registered. It contains some general information and two parts which can be completed when the patient changes doctor (see Chapter 30).

5 *FP 4B (Scotland GP 4B)*—transfer authority slip. This is attached to form FP 4 by the FPC when the patient wishes to transfer to another doctor without changing address and has sent his card and notification to the Committee.

6 *FP 5 (Scotland GP 5)*—male record envelope (see Chapter 27).

7 *FP 6 (Scotland GP 6)*—female record envelope (see Chapter 27).
8 *FP 7 (Scotland GP 7)*—male continuation card.
9 *FP 8 (Scotland GP 8)*—female continuation card.
10 *FP 5B and 6B (Scotland GP 5B and 6B)*. When the record envelope has become damaged, or too small for its contents, it can be returned to the FPC who will then issue a gusseted envelope FP 5B or 6B (Scotland GP 5B and 6B) (male or female).
11 *FP 7A and 8A (Northern Ireland HS 26A and 27A)*—male and female inoculation record cards (see section on 'Documentation' in Chapter 33). (In Scotland the immunization record is on the back of the medical record envelope.)
12 *FP 7B and 8B (Scotland GP7B and 8B)*—continuation cards (male and female) pending receipt of medical records.
13 *FP 9A and 9B (Scotland GP 9A and 9B)*—summary of treatment cards, coloured blue (female) and red (male) for insertion in medical record envelopes.
14 *FP 10 (Scotland GP 10, Northern Ireland HS 21)*—prescription pads. These will be dealt with in more detail later (see Chapter 34). They are stamped with the doctor's name and address and an identifying number. They are important documents and care should be taken to see that they are not lost or stolen.
15 *GP 10A*. This prescription form is used only in Scotland. It is used by the doctor to replace drugs which he has supplied to a patient from his surgery in circumstances when the patient is unable to get them from the chemist in time. Doctors in England and Wales cannot issue this form because they are paid, unlike doctors in Scotland, 25 pence per hundred patients in respect of their liability to supply such drugs.
16 *FP 10D*—prescription form for dispensing doctor.
17 *FP 10HP*—prescription form for hospital.
18 *FP 10S*—prescription form for HM Services.
19 *FP 13*. This is the form issued to persons who have completed service with HM Forces. It is handed by them to the civilian doctor with whom they wish to register.
20 *FP 19 (Northern Ireland HS 15, Scotland GP 19 [where it is used differently])*—notification of treatment given to a temporary resident (see Chapter 30).
21 *FP 22A–E*—application for return of medical records and notification of removal from doctor's list. This is sent out by the FPC in their weekly postal packet. It contains the names and addresses of patients removed, the reason for their removal and their new FPC. The records listed should be returned immediately as they are required for onward transmission to the patient's new doctor. The form should be shown to the doctor by the secretary, together with the cards, listed so that he can check and add any notes that are necessary. Form and cards should be returned to the council together.
22 *FP 24 and 24A (Northern Ireland MMS1, Scotland GP 24 and 24A)*—forms for application and claims for payment for maternity medical services (see Chapter 32).
23 *GP 24 (Scotland) (England and Wales MCW 01 and 01A, Northern Ireland MMS2)*—maternity services record card and envelope. Maternity claim form as used in Scotland.

24 *FP 27 (Scotland GP 27, Northern Ireland HS 13).* Where a patient claims to be on a doctor's list, and cannot produce evidence of the fact by showing his medical card, the doctor may claim a deposit and must give a receipt on this form. If the patient is on the doctor's list he can then claim back the deposit from the FPC, who make the appropriate adjustment with the doctor.

25 *FP 30 (Scotland GP 30)* (Fig. 29.1)—requisition card for a further supply of FP forms. It is usually completed by the secretary and can be included in the weekly envelope sent to the FPC.

26 *FP 31 (Scotland GP 31, Northern Ireland HS 13)*—claim form for a fee to be paid in the case of an emergency where a colleague has to administer a general anaesthetic.

27 *FP 32 (Scotland GP 32, Northern Ireland HS 14)*—claim form for special payment for an emergency attendance on a patient not on the doctor's list. It is used for visitors staying in the practice area for less than 24 hours, but for treatment given on the last day of a holiday form FP 19 should be used.

Form FP30/EC30

DOCTOR'S NAME.. No.........................

ADDRESS..

No. Required	Please supply the following:—				Form No.	No. in hand
	Books of Prescription Forms	....	....	....	FP 10/E.C. 10	
	ditto (Dispensing Doctors)		....	....	FP 10D/E.C. 10(D)	
	Books of Certificate Forms:—	....	....	....	Med. 3	
	ditto Supplementary		....	....	Med. 5	
	Application for Welfare Foods	....		....	F.W. 8	
	Acceptance Forms	....	....	....	FP 1/E.C. 1	
	Medical Record Envelope	....	....	....	FP 3/E.C. 3	
	Continuation Cards (Men)	....	....	....	FP 7/E.C. 7	
	Continuation Cards (Women)	....	....	....	FP 8/E.C. 8	
	Summary of Treatment Cards (Male)	....		....	FP 9A/E.C. 9A	
	Summary of Treatment Cards (Female)	....		....	FP 9B/E.C. 9B	
	Claim for Temporary Resident Fees	....		....	FP 19/E.C. 19	
	Books of Maternity Medical Service Forms (General Practitioners Obstetricians)			....	FP 24/E.C. 24	
	Books of Maternity Medical Service Forms (Doctors not on obstetric list)		....		FP 24A/E.C. 24A	
	Receipt or notice of account	....	....	....	FP 27/E.C. 27	
	Requisition for forms	....	....	....	FP 30/E.C. 30	
	Books of Medical Recommendations for sight testing	....	....	....	O.S.C. 1	
	Books of Expected Confinement/Confinement Forms	....	....	....	Mat. B1 & 2	
	Steroid treatment Cards	....	....	....		
	*Certificate A	....	....	....	H.S.A. 1	
	*Certificate B	....	....	....	H.S.A. 2	
	*Notification to Chief Medical Officer	....	....	H.S.A. 3	
	Request, Fitness for Work		....	....	R.M. 7	

*Abortion Act. 1967.   11098 352246 320m (5) 9.74 WPLtd Gp709

Fig. 29.1 Form FP 30.

Road-traffic accidents are not included and should be claimed for on the special BMA form.

28 *FP 33*—claim form for a service to a patient requiring special skills. This application must be supported by the local Medical Committee.

29 *FP 53 (Scotland GP 53)*. When a patient, who has recently been invalided from the Forces, is taken ill, it may be desirable to have a copy of his medical history while in the Forces. In these circumstances this can be obtained by submitting this form to the FPC.

30 *FP 58 (Scotland GP 58, Northern Ireland HS 123)*—registration form for an infant (see Chapter 30). If the birth has not been registered or the card has been lost, FP 1 (Northern Ireland HS 22X) should be used.

31 *FP 58B and C*—registration forms for adopted children (see Chapter 30).

32 *FP 69 (Northern Ireland HS 8, Scotland GP 69)*—warning that the patient may be removed from the list unless he or she can be traced.

33 *FP 73 (Northern Ireland VAC, Scotland FP 73)*—claim for payment for vaccinations and immunizations (see Chapter 33).

34 *FP 74 (Northern Ireland CYT/1, Scotland FP 74)*—claim for payment for cervical cytology test (see Chapter 33).

35 *FP 81 (Northern Ireland NV/1, Scotland FP 81)*—application for night visit fee (see Chapter 31).

36 *FP 106 (Scotland CP 105, Northern Ireland HS 14T)*. This form is used for immediately necessary treatment when refusal has been made to treat a patient as a temporary resident or take them on the permanent list. The form must be signed by the patient.

37 *Forms FP 111*. These are all record sheets for A4 folders:
  (a) FP 111F—clinical notes
  (b) FP 111G—summary of important problems
  (c) FP 111H—immunizations and screening procedures
  (d) FP 111J—maternity record
  (e) FP 111K—paediatric development sheet and card
  (f) FP 111L—mount page for laboratory and X-ray reports
  (g) FP 111M—nurse and health visitor's records
  (In Scotland these forms are prefixed GP and there is also a form GP 111N for contraceptive record.)

38 *FP 1001 and 1002 (Scotland GP 102–104)*—registration forms for contraceptive advice.

NATIONAL INSURANCE FORMS (DHSS)

(see DHSS leaflet NI 16, NI 16A)

Sickness benefit

This is a contributory benefit paid to people who are unable to work because of illness. It is paid for the first 28 weeks of illness (except for the first three days) when, for those still incapable of work it is replaced by invalidity benefit. Sickness benefit claim forms are commonly dealt with by the medical secretary, especially those working in general practice.

Sickness Benefit
claim form And Invalidity benefit

Statutory sick pay

- If you are an employee you can use this form for Statutory Sick Pay (SSP) if your employer wishes
- To get Statutory Sick Pay, you must be sick for at least 4 days in a row counting Saturdays and Sundays
- For Statutory Sick Pay you only need to fill in sections 1-5

Sickness benefit and Invalidity benefit

- You can only get benefit if you are sick for at least 4 days in a row counting Saturdays but not Sundays
  (Patients getting dialysis, radiotherapy or chemotherapy treatment should look at Leaflet NI16, as different rules can apply to them)
- If you are sick for 4, 5 or 6 days in a row counting Saturdays but not Sundays, wait until your last day of sickness and then fill in this form
- If you know you will be sick for more than 6 days counting Saturdays but not Sundays, fill in this form immediately

---

- Doctors do not have to issue sick notes for the first week of sickness, but don't delay seeing your doctor if you need medical advice
- Further details for Statutory Sick Pay are in leaflet NI244
- Further details for Sickness benefit are in leaflet NI16

---

1 Yourself

PLEASE USE BLOCK LETTERS
If you cannot fill this form in yourself, ask someone else to do so and to sign it for you

| Surname: Mr/Mrs/Miss/Ms |
| First names |
| Present address |
| Postcode |
| Date of birth |
| National Insurance number |

SC1(Rev)   Now turn over the page

Fig. 29.2 Sickness benefit claim form.

A patient does not need a statement from his doctor for the first week of sickness. He completes a 'self-certificate' form, SCI(Rev) (Fig. 29.2), and sends that to the social security office. These forms are obtained from the doctor's surgery, the local hospital or the social security office. A patient has to be ill for four consecutive days (excluding a Sunday) to qualify for benefit. If they are ill for four to six days they complete SCI(Rev) and send it off on the last day; the time limit for claiming may be extended for up to one month by the DHSS if there is good reason.

After the first week of illness the patient needs a doctor's certificate (form Med 3) to carry on claiming benefit (see page 259).

2 Details of sickness/injury

Give details of your sickness. Words like 'illness' or 'unwell' are not enough

Please say briefly why you are unfit for work

3 Period of sickness

date month year

Date you became unfit for work | day | | | 19

Date you last worked | day | | | 19

Time you finished work | time | am/pm

date month year

Night shift workers only

When did your last shift begin? | time | am/pm | day | | | 19

Tick one box

Do you expect to be unfit for work for more than 7 days? yes □ no □
If you ticked yes, go to part 5

4 Returning to work

date month year

Last day of sickness before starting or seeking work | day | | | 19

Date you intend to start or seek work | day | | | 19

Night shift workers only

Shift will begin at | time | am/pm | and end next day at | time | am/pm

5 If you are claiming Sickness or Invalidity benefit

Carry on from part 6 'Your work' — do not sign below

If you are using this form for Statutory Sick Pay

Stop here. Sign below, and send this form to your employer

Signature | Date

Remember, if you are sick for a second week, your employer may want a doctor's sick note

Fig. 29.2 Continued

If the patient is ill again within eight weeks the sickness benefit for the next period is paid immediately, that is without the three waiting days, so it may be advisable for a patient to complete an SCI(Rev) form for a short period of illness.

If the patient is ill for longer than 28 weeks he will require regular certificates from the doctor in order to claim invalidity benefit (leaflet NI 16A).

There are several important points about form Med 3 that the secretary should understand:

(a) The doctor must always see the patient when issuing a form Med 3 or a certificate of expected confinement (form Mat B1) and the statement

6 | **Your work**

	Are you?	Self-		
Tick one box	Employed ☐	employed ☐	Unemployed ☐	Other ☐

Tick one box   Has any employer paid you SSP in the last 8 weeks?   yes ☐   no ☐
If you ticked <u>yes</u>, please state the employer's name and address

```
[                                                            ]
[                                                            ]
```

7 | **Your doctor**

```
Doctor's name and address
[                                                            ]
```

8 | **In hospital**

Tick one box   Have you been a hospital in-patient since you became
unfit for work?   yes ☐   no ☐
If you ticked <u>yes</u>, please state the name and address of the hospital

```
[                                                            ]
[                                                            ]
```

9 | **Industrial injury or prescribed disease**

If you think that your sickness is due to an accident at work or to a
prescribed industrial disease caused by conditions at work, tick one box
accident at work ☐   prescribed industrial disease ☐

10 | **Your family**

Tick one box   Are you?   single ☐   married ☐   widowed ☐   divorced ☐
You can claim extra benefit for one adult dependant and for a child
or children
If you want a claim form sent to you, tick the box or boxes below:
Tick one or   woman (not wife)
more boxes   Wife ☐   husband ☐   children ☐   caring for children ☐

Now turn over the page

Fig. 29.2 Continued

on form Med 3 must be based on an examination which took place not
more than one day earlier.
(b) The certificate must not be signed by the doctor until the patient's
name and diagnosis have been entered.
(c) Form Med 5 should be issued in all circumstances when form Med 3
cannot be issued.
(d) Each certificate must be stamped with the doctor's name and address
(this is normally done by the FPC). Payment is usually made by means
of a postal draft which can be cashed at a post office.
(e) Certificates are not issued for illnesses lasting less than seven days.

11 | Other benefits

**Tick one or
more boxes**

Tick any of these benefits that you are getting or claiming
Supplementary benefit □
War pension (including war widow's pension) □
Youth training scheme allowance □
Enterprise allowance □
Unemployability supplement □
Job release allowance □

Tick one box

Are you getting or claiming any other social security benefit, pension or
allowance?   yes □   no □

If yes, state which

Tick one box

Is anyone getting or claiming extra benefit for you as a
dependant?   yes □   no □   If yes please state:

His/her name
Address
Postcode
Name of benefit

Tick one box

Have you received any money for training or rehabilitation in the past
8 weeks?   yes □   no □

If yes, where was it from?

12 | Declaration   Remem · if you knowingly give wrong or false info ..ation you may be prosecuted

I declare that I have not worked during the period of sickness which I have
stated and that the information given is complete and correct
I claim benefit
I agree to my doctor giving medical information relevant to my claim to a
doctor in the Regional Medical Service

Signature	Date

If you have signed on behalf of the person claiming, tick the box □

Send the form immediately to your local Social Security office to avoid losing any benefit

Fig. 29.2 Continued

All the above forms are obtained from the FPC and requisitioned on form
FP 30.

1 *Form Med 3*. These are the forms on which a patient claims sickness benefit.
They are issued to him by the doctor, who obtains them in books from the
FPC. The forms are stamped with the name and address of the doctor (or
partnership).

When a person is ill he will normally have completed a self-certificate to
cover the first six days. If the illness lasts longer a form Med 3 (Fig. 29.3) will
be issued by the doctor to follow or replace the self-certificate. If the doctor
believes that the patient will be fit for work within 14 days he issues a 'closed'

FOR SOCIAL SECURITY AND STATUTORY SICK PAY PURPOSES ONLY

<u>NOTES TO PATIENT ABOUT USING THIS FORM</u>

You can use this form either:

    1. For Statutory Sick Pay (SSP) purposes – fill in Part A overleaf. Also fill in Part B if the doctor has given you a date to resume work. Give or send the completed form to your employer.

    2. For Social Security purposes –
To continue a claim for State benefit fill in Parts A and C of the form overleaf. Also fill in Part B if the doctor has given you a date to resume work. **Sign and date the form** and give or send it to your local social security office QUICKLY to avoid losing benefit.

NOTE: To start your claim for State benefit you must use form SCI(Rev) if you are self-employed, unemployed or non-employed OR form SSPI(E) or SSPI(T) if you are an employee. For further details get leaflet NI16 (from DHSS local offices).

                        Doctor's Statement

In confidence to

Mr/~~Mrs/Miss/Ms~~ .... *John Williams* ....

I examined you today/yesterday and advised you that

(a) You ~~need not refrain from work~~   (b) you should refrain from work

                             for* .... *14 days* ....

            OR until† ....

Diagnosis of your disorder
causing absence from work ...... *Acute Lumbago* ....

Doctor's remarks

Doctor's signature   *M Drury*   Date of signing *5.8.85*

                                              Form Med 3

NOTE TO DOCTOR *†See inside front cover for notes on completion.*

Fig. 29.3 Form Med 3.

FOR SOCIAL SECURITY AND STATUTORY SICK PAY PURPOSES ONLY

Special Statement by the Doctor

In confidence to Mr/Mrs/Miss/Ms...... *Julie Donaldson*

(A) I examined you on the following dates

3.8.85
31.8.85

and advised you that you should refrain from work

from *3.8.85* to *2.9.85*

(B) I have not examined you but, on the basis of a recent written report from —

Doctor ...... (Name if known)

of ......

...... (Address)

I have advised you that you should refrain from work for/until ......

Diagnosis of your disorder causing absence from work ...... *Thyrotoxicosis*

Doctor's remarks

Doctor's signature *M. Drury*   Date of signing *31.8.85*

The special circumstances in which this form may be used are described in the handbook "Medical Evidence for Social Security and Statutory Sick Pay Purposes".

Hereford & Worcester F.P.C.
DRS. DRURY, COWAN, BLACKER, WYNNE & DYKES,
27 New Road, Bromsgrove, Worcs.

Form Med 5
3/83

PATIENT TO COMPLETE PARTICULARS ON REVERSE

Fig. 29.4 Form Med 5.

certificate, that is one in which the date when he considers the patient will be fit for work is entered after 'until' on the form. If he considers the illness will last more than two weeks he issues an open certificate by entering a period of up to six months in the space after 'for'. Each open certificate has to be followed either by another open certificate or a closed certificate when the date of return to work is not more than 14 days away.

Once the patient has been off work for six months it is possible to enter the words 'further notice' after 'until'.

2 *Form med 5* (Fig. 29.4). This form is used when the circumstances are not covered by the rules relating to form Med 3; for example where a doctor needs

to issue a certificate more than one day after examination, where a patient starts work without a 'closed' certificate, or where the doctor is satisfied, on the basis of a hospital report issued not more than one month previously, and relates the note only to one month ahead, that the patient is unfit to work.

3 *Form Med 6.* When the doctor does not wish the patient to know the true diagnosis he may issue a form Med 3 to the patient containing a vague diagnosis and simultaneously send this form with the true diagnosis to the Divisional Medical Officer (in Scotland, the Regional Medical Officer).

The three maternity benefits are explained in leaflet NI 17A.

4 *Form Mat B1.* This is a certificate of expected confinement (see Chapter 32).

5 *Form Mat B2.* This is a certificate of confinement. Both forms can be signed by the doctor or the midwife and should be accompanied by a completed form BM 4 (see Chapter 32) when making the claim.

6 *Form FW 8* (see Chapter 32). This claim for welfare milk tokens is sent to the local DHSS office. Part of the form constitutes a claim for a certificate of exemption from paying prescription charges.

Regional medical service forms

1 *Form RM 1 and 2.* If a patient has been off work an unduly long time for the diagnosis made, the Regional Medical Officer may send the patient a form RM 1 stating that he may be required to attend for examination. The doctor will then receive form RM 2 on which he can either give a history of the illness or state that he has issued a final medical certificate.

2 *Form RM 7.* Doctors who want a second opinion on whether the patient is fit to work may complete form RM 7, one of which is in each pad of forms Med 3, and send it to the Divisional Medical Officer (Regional Medical Officer in Scotland) who will then arrange for the patient to attend for an examination.

3 *Form RM 95L.* This is a certificate for a patient on the Disabled Persons Register.

Other services available for the sick or disabled

Whilst the secretary will not normally have to deal with forms relating to attendance allowances, invalid care allowances and mobility allowances she should understand in general terms what they entail.

Attendance allowances (leaflet NI 205) are tax-free payments made to severely physically or mentally handicapped people over the age of two. It is paid to the handicapped person and not to the carer. People may qualify for a lower rate if they need frequent attention or continual supervision during the day, and a higher rate if they also require help at night. A doctor, often a neighbouring GP, will examine the patient but the decision is made by a separate Board.

Invalid care allowance (leaflet NI 212) is a benefit for people of working age who are unable to work because they have to spend at least 35 hours a week caring for a person who needs an attendance allowance.

Mobility allowance (leaflet NI 211) is a benefit designed to help severely disabled people to become more mobile. It is for people who are unable or virtually unable to walk.

The *Disability Rights Handbook* is published annually by the Disability Alliance, 25 Denmark Street, London and should be available to the secretary who has to deal with enquiries, particularly in relation to health care.

BIRTH REGISTRATION

Every live and stillbirth must be registered within 42 days. The duty to give details rests on either of the parents, or in the case of an illegitimate child, on the mother. Where the doctor was present at the delivery or examined the body of a stillborn child he must sign a Certificate of Stillbirth and give this to the person who is informing the registrar.

DEATH CERTIFICATES

These books of certificates are issued to registered practitioners only. They may be obtained from the registrar for the subdistrict in which the doctor lives. Their issue is a statutory duty and no fee is chargeable. The certificate is only given by a doctor who was actually attending the patient in his last illness. The death must be registered within five days in the subdistrict of its occurrence. The duty of registration falls primarily on the nearest relatives who will obtain the certificate from the doctor and he will also give them a formal notice which will give guidance about registration. The patient's relative will often attend at the surgery for the certificate and the secretary should appreciate the situation and not keep him waiting in the waiting room, in fact it is usually kinder to sit him down somewhere else. She will frequently be asked the times at which the registrar's office is open, and should keep a note of the times for any enquiries.

CREMATION CERTIFICATES

A doctor may be requested to sign cremation certificates for patients he has attended during their last illnesses. These certificates need to be confirmed by another doctor and he may from time to time be asked to sign in either capacity, e.g. Part A or Part B certificates are usually obtained from the undertaker and a fee is payable to both doctors.

INSURANCE CERTIFICATES

These are of two varieties. 'Short certificates' are reports on patients who are on the medical list of the doctor. They do not call for any examination, but the doctor will require to see the patient's medical records. The secretary will present the form and records to the doctor together for him to complete. A fee is payable. 'Long certificates' are reports on patients who are not on the doctor's list. These patients require a full medical examination followed by the completion of a detailed form which takes anything up to half an hour or longer to complete. The insurance company will usually telephone the doctor and arrange an appointment and they will send the necessary papers through to the doctor by post. The secretary should check the time of the appointment with the doctor and make sure that the papers are ready before the patient attends. The report consists of two parts. In one the doctor will note the patient's answers to a number of questions and in the other he will note the results of a full examination. For this the doctor will need to measure the height and weight of the patient and to test the urine, which must have been passed at the time of examination (a diabetic might try to escape attention by bringing a specimen belonging to someone else!). A fee is payable.

SIGHT TESTING

1 *Form OSC 1.* The ophthalmic service is in two parts—the hospital eye service, where patients attend for diseases of the eye and are treated, and the supplementary ophthalmic service. There are three types of person providing this latter service:
  (a) Ophthalmic medical practitioners. These may also be specialists under the hospital eye service and they test sight only and prescribe glasses.
  (b) Ophthalmic opticians. These test sight and supply and repair glasses.
  (c) Dispensing opticians. Supply and repair glasses only.

The supplementary ophthalmic service is administered by the FPC through the Ophthalmic Services Committee and holds the three types of person above under contract. The sight test is free and if the person examining the patient decides glasses are necessary he will prescribe them. The adult must pay a certain sum per lens and prices according to quality for the frames. Bifocal lenses cost more but any lens can be fitted to suitable private frames. Patients cannot have a spare pair of glasses under the NHS even if they bought a pair of glasses privately. Glasses are free to children, patients in hospital and in cases of hardship.

PRIVATE CERTIFICATES

These are required by a patient as proof of illness and are sent to employers, sick clubs and occasionally to schools. The doctor usually has them privately printed, although one of the large drug firms supply books of them free to doctors. The doctor is under no obligation to issue them and may charge a fee for doing so. He generally resists issuing them as much as possible because of the burden of work and this particularly applies to the certificates that schools often demand. However they are often a necessity for the patient and it is certainly not their fault that they have to ask for them. It is not necessary for the doctor to visit a patient solely to issue a note for work and he will certainly refuse abuse of this sort.

Medical Certificate

This is to certify that in my opinion ....

of ....

$\dfrac{is}{was}$ suffering from ....

and is $\dfrac{unable}{able}$ to attend $\dfrac{work}{school}$

signed ....

date ....

Fig. 29.5 A 'private' medical certificate.

HOSPITAL FORMS

There are three types of form under this heading and the lay-out of them may vary from hospital to hospital. Some details such as name, age, address etc., can be completed by the secretary.

1 *Appointment form.* This is a form requesting an appointment for a patient to see a Consultant in a hospital. It usually contains details of the patient's name, address and date of birth, the doctor's name and address, and the Consultant with whom the appointment is to be made. There may be a space requesting details of previous attendances at the hospital and very often the form contains a space for the letter from the doctor to the hospital. Where this is done the form is folded and gummed in such a way that the clinical notes are only opened by the clinician. The appointment is usually sent directly to the patient, but the doctor may indicate on the form that the appointment should be sent to him. Full and accurate completion of the form is necessary so that pre-registration can be done at the hospital (see section on Pre-registration in Chapter 18).

2 *X-ray request form.* This form is given to the patient to take to the X-ray department. It should contain details and dates of previous X-rays, and for women of childbearing age the date of the last menstrual period. This latter is required because of the danger of X-rays to the unborn baby in the early months of pregnancy. Radiologists will then only X-ray these patients when it is safe to do so.

3 *Request for pathological investigation.* This is treated in much the same way as the X-ray request form. Where a specimen container is given to the patient the name should be written on it by the secretary.

MISCELLANEOUS FORMS IN COMMON USE

1 *Notification of infectious disease* (see Chapter 33).

2 *International certificates of vaccination and immunization* (see Chapter 33). These forms are included under this heading as they have to be countersigned by the local District Community Physician.

3 *Request for transport.* This is used in certain areas to request ambulance or car transport for patients when 24 hours' notice can be given. It usually contains details of the journey and time and whether it is a stretcher or sitting case.

4 *Request for supply of vaccines* (see Chapter 33).

5 *Form Med 133.* This is the summary of the medical history of a patient who has been invalided from HM Forces. It may be sent automatically or on request by means of form FP 53 (Scotland GP 53).

6 *Form Med 136A.* The request form sent by a civilian doctor for the service medical history. It is submitted to the ex-service person's last unit.

7 *Request for supply of Red Cross equipment.* The Red Cross may be able to lend equipment to patients for use at home, e.g. bedpans, urinals, rubber sheets, crutches, wheelchairs, etc., and some areas have a request form.

8 *DP 32.* Under the Disabled Persons Acts, 1944 and 1958, the Department of Employment and Productivity may make provision for disabled persons to secure employment. When the doctor thinks that it is in the patient's interest to be included on the register, he will ask the patient to obtain this form from the Department's local office, and he will complete part of it. The services provided are industrial rehabilitation and training, sheltered employment, and transfer expenses. Under the quota scheme any factory employing more than 20 people must employ 3% of registered disabled persons.

9 *Steroid therapy.*

10 *Anticoagulant therapy.*

11 *Tetanus immunization.* Small cards indicating that patients have been or are being treated along these lines may be issued to the patients. They are often supplied by the FPCs.

12 *Notification of unusual reactions to drugs.* A letter card has been produced by the Committee on Safety of Medicines for the notification of unusual reactions.

Form ANC 1, 2 and 3

GPs are entitled to a reimbursement of the salary paid by them to staff engaged on nursing or administrative duties for NHS patients. If the doctor has 1000 or more NHS patients, the allowance is paid in full, if less he gets that proportion. If more than 10% of his practice is private the repayments are also reduced proportionately. Each doctor can employ two full-time (or the equivalent number of part-time) staff and secure a repayment of 70% of their gross salaries, before deductions for income tax, National Insurance, etc. Form ANC 1 notifies changes in salaries and must be completed for each member of staff when first employed. Form ANC 2 must be signed by the doctor certifying that the sums claimed each quarter and set out on form ANC 3 are proper entitlements and conform to current regulations. These must be submitted to the FPC at the end of each quarter.

Forms Prem 1 and 2

Where practice premises are being used for the care of NHS patients the rates, and either the actual rent or an estimated amount of what a fair rent would have been, are repaid through the FPC. The original claim for rent to be determined is made on form Prem 1. Afterwards form Prem 2 with the receipted rate demands must be submitted to the FPC at the end of the quarter in which they have been met.

Diploma Questions

*Denotes an incomplete question

1 In addition to capitation fees, what other form of remuneration does the General Practitioner receive? Describe the documents which the medical secretary may have to complete on behalf of the practitioner.

2 The correct completion of FPC forms is a very important part of the medical secretary's job in general practice. Describe the most important of these documents and explain their uses.

3 Describe the various forms used in general practice for the registration of patients.

4 State documentation, office and general procedures necessary when patients attend general practice for medical treatment as temporary residents.*

30

Reception and Appointments

In this chapter we shall consider the work entailed in the reception of patients. Although it is described in relation to general practice the broad principles are common throughout the medical scene.

The work that faces the individual secretary in general practice is of a more varied nature. Her responsibility is often greater because she works alone, and, at times, has no other person to rely on when decisions have to be taken. This variation itself lends interest to her job, because, while planning and organization are part of the essence of general practice, they cannot be carried to the same lengths as they are in ordinary commercial practice or in the work of the hospital medical secretary. The unexpected will always turn up: one day is never the same as another and the dull, routine day is sure to be followed by one packed with interest.

In general practice the secretary will come into very close personal contact, not only with the doctor for whom she works, but with his patients. Thus the job calls for very special qualifications, many of which cannot be learnt from books. A sense of sympathy, a capacity for liking people just as they are, a pleasant and polite manner to patients, and an ability to remain calm are all golden qualities. They are nowhere more essential than in this job.

The work of the secretary in general practice falls under two headings:
1 the receptionist
2 the secretary

Such a clear-cut distinction is easier to make in theory than in practice.

The large group practice, with several employees, may attempt to divide the work along these lines, but in the great majority of practices the work overlaps into both types, and where only one person is employed she is more accurately described as a medical secretary/receptionist. For this reason no attempt has been made to divide these tasks in the succeeding chapters. Obviously where work of this latter nature is being done it is a more responsible post than when work as either a receptionist, or a secretary only is undertaken, but for the sake of convenience she is referred to throughout as a secretary.

THE RECEPTION OF THE PATIENT

The first contact that a patient makes with his doctor will usually be through the secretary. The tone set at this enquiry can colour every aspect of the consultation and treatment that follows, particularly when a sharp or unsympathetic reply is given to a nervous questioner.

268

Nearly every patient who attends the surgery has a high level of anxiety. They may be worried about their illness, worried that they may not present themselves accurately with their problems to the doctor, worried that they may be thought silly, or inconsiderate, or they may even be frightened of you—the receptionist. This anxiety may show itself in a variety of ways. Patients may appear brusque or aggressive, confused or stupid, over-casual or may exaggerate their symptoms. Some may not hear well, see well or understand the system that is being operated. Some may have an inadequate command of language or be unable to understand the words that you use. Whichever factor is operating the patient's anxiety can be increased or decreased by the behaviour of the receptionist and regrettably this is the area of practice about which most complaints are made and most unhappiness expressed.

Health care professionals are now increasingly aware of the problems that poor communication with patients cause. In their educational programmes time is devoted to this topic and methods such as using video recording of consultations and reception of patients, which can later be analysed by the health worker, are used in basic and continuing education. All this shows what a difficult area of activity it is and how much we must work at it.

Certain key elements of reception work can be identified:

1 Attend to the patient at the reception desk as quickly as possible. If you are busy then a word to the waiting patient such as 'I shan't keep you a minute' or 'Sorry to keep you waiting' helps to make them feel 'noticed'.

2 Welcome the patients by look, posture and words. Look at them, smile where appropriate and face them directly. Start with a phrase such as 'Can I help you?' or, if you know them, 'Good morning, Mrs Jones'.

3 Be aware of confidentiality. The patient may need to state their requirements and this may contain confidential matter, so try to deal with each patient by himself (or herself) and if in doubt move them to a quieter corner where a degree of privacy can be assured.

4 Try to say 'yes' to patients' requests even if you then qualify it to 'yes but...'. They may be asking for an appointment when none is available or a prescription which will have to be prepared later but even if they have to wait for this, or return at another time, they should be made to feel that you are trying to be helpful and that the systems that you operate are reasonably flexible.

5 Be ready to record the reason for their appearance at the reception desk in writing so that they are not forgotten and so that they can be properly addressed by name and title.

When the patient first comes into the waiting room, whether he has an appointment or not, he will have to register his attendance with the secretary. Christian name as well as surname should be taken and recorded on a list. A mental note should be kept of whether the lady said Mrs or Miss. Where the name is a common one it is often helpful to make a note of the address.

The value of this list is:

1 The records of patients who have not made a previous appointment can be removed from the file.

2 The order in which patients without appointments attend is recorded so that they can be called in turn. Nothing causes more trouble in a waiting room than calling patients in in the wrong order.

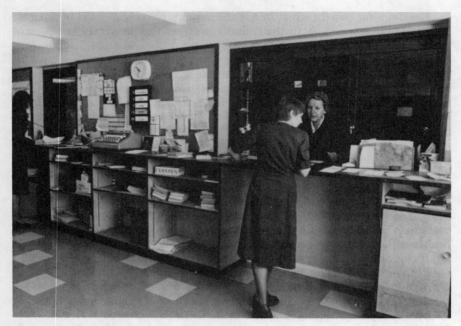

Fig. 30.1 Reception—the receptionist's view.

3 This list serves as an added record of patients who have attended. These lists will be retained for some weeks afterwards for reference as they may be of importance in the collection of statistics.

The reception desk is a place to which patients often come with requests for repeat prescriptions, appointments for later surgeries and a hundred-and-one other messages. It is often unfair to patients to ask them questions in such a public place. Where possible details of illnesses, ages or other points should be taken somewhere where they can be recorded with a degree of privacy. It is not possible to overestimate the importance of recording accurately all messages that are received. They should not be written down on loose scraps of paper, which have a habit of getting lost, but all should be recorded in a book kept for that purpose.

When the patient is called from the waiting room by the secretary she should use his name and title. 'Mr Jones' is correct. 'Next please' is not.

In most surgeries there is a system of internal communication between the doctor and his secretary which enables the doctor to signify his readiness to see another patient. This is usually done by means of a 'buzzer', light or internal telephone (see Chapter 12) and this enables the secretary to know when she should call the next patient in. In some surgeries patients are given a disc with a number on to indicate the order in which they will be seen. In others this is indicated by coloured lights or buzzers directly into the waiting room. Whichever system is used the supervision of the waiting room to see that patients are politely informed when it is their turn is important and stress upon patients can be much reduced if they are kept informed of delays when the doctor is getting behind with his appointments. It will calm some patients and give others the opportunity to make other appointments or fit other tasks in.

THE APPOINTMENT SYSTEM IN GENERAL PRACTICE

Nearly all general practices in Britain now see their patients by appointment. What was at first thought to be an introduction that would benefit all patients has now proved to have certain inherent problems and has become a potential source of irritation for patients, doctors and their staff. The advantages for the doctor of appointment systems are listed below.

1 He can plan his week so that the distribution of the work is much more even.
2 He can arrange his time off more easily.
3 By making further appointments he can follow-up patients better.
4 There is less rush and stress upon the doctor who knows that there is not a long queue waiting to see him.
5 He can arrange longer appointments for patients that need them.

The advantages for the patient are as follows.
1 The amount of time wasted in waiting rooms is enormously reduced.
2 He can arrange to see the doctor of his choosing.
3 The risk of cross-infection in crowded waiting rooms is cut down.

A badly functioning appointment system is a source of worry and frustration for patients and needs tact, skill and energy to correct.

It is essential that patients who believe they need to consult a doctor should have no barrier put between them and medical advice. If this occurs a major function of good family doctoring can be destroyed. About two-thirds of all appointments are made by patients before they leave the surgery. They are therefore predictable and can be fitted in conveniently. One-third are new appointments. Some are not urgent and the patient is anxious to wait for a convenient time and see a particular doctor. Others are believed by the patient to be urgent. These patients must be fitted in to the first surgery whether or not space is available. It is never the place of the secretary to act as a filter or dissuader. It is her place to facilitate the appointment, and this requires demonstrable sympathy and concern. No firm rules can be laid down for this as the essence of the exercise is flexibility. A good secretary will be highly sensitive to this point and will be very ready to consult her employer as soon as problems or the number on waiting lists begin to build up. She will be observant of the different speeds at which doctors work and will soon learn which consultations require time and which ones are 'quickies'.

Running an appointment system

1 The appointment system operates for the benefit of the patient.
2 Patients should be offered an appointment within 24 hours of requesting one.
3 Deferred appointments should only be made if the patient is willing.
4 If the patient insists on an appointment when no vacancies occur they should be marked as 'urgent' and the doctor informed. The doctor can then decide whether to discuss this with the patient.

5 Receptionists should try to ascertain which patients require a double booking.
6 A practice policy should be adopted about patients wishing to speak to the doctor by telephone during appointments.
7 A senior receptionist should monitor the system and inform the doctor if it is not running smoothly.

There are three main methods of booking appointments. The usual rate is about one every 10 minutes with other more urgent cases booked as 'extras'. This results in one person being seen about every seven minutes.

1 Sequential booking

There are two columns. Patients are booked in the left-hand column until this is full and then the right-hand column as required.

	Left		*Right*
9.00	Mary Jones	9.05	
10	Jane Smith	15	Samuel Baker
20	Henry Davies	25	
30	Albert Williams	35	
40	Elizabeth Waldron	45	Derek Thomas
50	Linda Reed	55	

2 Limited block booking

Patients are booked in at three every 15 minutes and blanks are left as required.

9.00	Mary Smith	Henry Davies	Sandra Jones
9.15	Edward Jones	John Bishop	LEFT BLANK
9.30	Samuel Kella	Brenda Waldron	LEFT BLANK

3 Block release booking

The appointment sheet is divided into three blocks of different priority. Block 1 can be booked at any time in advance. Block 2 can be booked 24 hours or less before the surgery. Block 3 can be booked only after the last surgery ends. Blanks are also left for urgent cases. This system allows the number of patients to be spread more easily during the week.

Left		Right	
9.00		9.05	
10		15	
20	can be booked	25	can only be booked
	any time in		24 hours or less
30	advance	35	before surgery
	(block 1)		(block 2)
40		45	
50		55	
10.00		10.05	can only be
			booked after
10		15	previous surgery
			(block 3)
20		25	

Where a patient has a common surname some other means of identifying him may be necessary. There may be three 'Leslie Jones' in the practice and so '2 KR' after his name will show that this one lives at number 2 Kings Road. There should also be a space to note any other important details, such as 'antenatal', etc. Another method of differentiating between appointments in the book is by the use of coloured inks, for example antenatal appointments may be marked in red.

There is a natural tendency for patients who have seen the doctor to walk out without making a necessary further appointment. They are often so preoccupied with what has been said to them that they will walk past the secretary lost in thought. It is the job of the secretary to try to ensure that those who need further appointments do not leave without making them.

Two problems calling for tact are (a) the patient who has not made an appointment, and (b) the patient who requests an appointment on a day when the list of the doctor is already filled.

As regards the former it should be possible to fit the patient in during the surgery if it is not a crowded one. If it is heavily booked then the patient should either be advised of the time he may have to wait or encouraged to make an appointment for a later surgery. If the appointment list is fully booked it may be possible to persuade the patient to come at another time or to see a partner. At such times it is useful to find out if the patient thinks his appointment is urgent. If he does, then the secretary must find room for him. It is not her job to decide on the degree of urgency, and if 'disciplining' is required then it is up to the doctor to do it.

The appointment card

In some practices it is the policy to give the patient requiring a further appointment a small printed card as a reminder. These cards bear the patient's and the doctor's name, and the date and time of the appointment (Fig. 30.3). They should be brought back by the patient when attending as they identify the patient and are a useful method of checking if there has been a mistake.

		30				
		40				
		50	Mr Special 29 Ab	✓	Mrs Byrne 20 Gl	✓
9		00	Mrs Jessop 17 Po	✓	Mrs Jones 1 Tl	✓
		10	Mrs King 3 So	✓		
		20	Julian Day 70 Gl	✓	Mrs Oval 1 OT	✓
		30	Iain McDougall	✓	Mrs Hendry 232 OM	✓
		40	Mrs Peters 4 Ma	✓	———	
		50			Mrs Flattery 22 Lo	✓
10		00	Mrs Ovary	✓		
		10	Mr Bottle 2 St	✓	Mrs Joker 106 Bl	✓
		20	COFFEE		COFFEE	
		30	Mr. J Chandler 17 Ja	✓	Joan Hammond 16 To	✓
		40	Mrs. Sink 467 So	✓	Mrs Drain TA Bl	✓
		50	Robert Jules 6 Po	✓		
11		00				
		10				
		20	ANTE-NATAL 2-30		Mrs Suza	✓
			Clinic 2-45		Mrs Tern 82 SA	✓
			3-00		Mrs Broughton	✓
			3-15		Mrs Bull 13 Ap	✓
		40				
		50	Mr Dodds 61 B Cl	✓	Mrs O. Time 10 thr	✓
6		00	Alan Horn 90 St	✓	Mrs Horn	✓
		10			Mrs Apple 109 Gr	✓
		20	Mr. Sinclair 13 Ob	✓	———	
		30	Mr. Hudson 35 Ma	✓	Mr. Sinclair 2 Son	✓
		40	Mr. Powers	✓	Eine Kliner	✓
		50	April May 42 Sot	✓	Mr. Rule 13 Fl	⟍⟍
7		00	Arthur Stevens 14 Ba	✓		
		10	Mrs Blake 206 Za	·	Bill Blake	✓
		20	———			
		30	Mr. Lowe 21 Ro	✓	David Lowe	✓
		40	Brenda Potts	✓		
		50	Mr. Sandys 43 Ce	✓	———	
8		00	Mr. A. Jones 4 The Bl	✓		
		10				
		20				

⟍ Failed to attend

Fig. 30.2 Practice appointments book.

DR. J. SMITH
23, HIGH STREET, JOHNTOWN
TELEPHONE: JOH 9999

M ....

Your appointment is

on ....

at ....

Please bring this card with you

Fig. 30.3 An appointment card.

THE REGISTRATION OF PATIENTS

As we have already seen one of the important functions of the FPC is to ensure that the medical records of every patient are in the possession of his doctor. The correct registration of the patient enables this to be done and also enables the FPC to keep the total number of patients on the doctor's list up to date. In order to ensure that the maximum payment for patients is credited to the practice it is important to remember that the closing dates for receipt of cards by the FPC are the first of January, April, July and October. Many practices like to make an appointment for the patient to be seen by the doctor when they first register. These introductory consultations are important. They enable patients to meet and identify their doctor. They enable a doctor to find out important data about the patient's medical and social history and the patient to explain his special needs. They enable information to be given about the systems that the practice operates, such as appointments, contacting a doctor 'out of hours' or in emergency, obtaining a prescription and so on. Finally, they are a time when basic preventive medicine can be practised, such as recording blood pressure or checking on immunization or cervical status. In some practices a form has been designed that can be completed by the patient whilst waiting for this first contact, which enables basic data on records to be completed. Registration is effected by one of four methods.

1 First registration

The first registration on a doctor's list is usually done by means of a card given to the parents by the registrar of births. This form (FP 58 or Northern Ireland HS 123) is partly completed by the registrar who allocates the child a number from his register, which afterwards becomes his NHS number. The parents then take the form to the doctor of their choice, who will, if he is prepared to accept the child on his list, sign it, and it is then sent to the FPC by the doctor. The FPC then issues the child with the medical card, enters him on their register and sends the doctor a medical record envelope. Adopted children may be issued with form FP 84B which maintains confidentiality by removing details of previous name etc. If it is a dispensing practice 'D' has to be entered in the box if drugs are to be supplied and the parent must sign the consent form. If it is a rural practice the distance from the main surgery is entered.

2 Transfer of patient on change of address

Where a patient transfers to a different address from the one given on the front of his medical card he can then change his doctor. This is done by entering his new address in Part A of his medical card (FP 4, Northern Ireland HS 23). He then hands this card to his new doctor who signs and sends it on to the FPC. On receipt they record the transfer, arrange for the patient to be removed from his previous doctor's list, and recover the medical record from his previous doctor for onward transmission to the new doctor.

3 Transfer of patient without change of address

Every patient has the right to transfer to a new doctor if he wishes and if the new doctor is willing to accept him. This can be done in one of two ways:
(a) The patient completes Part B of his medical card (FP 4, Northern Ireland HS 23) and takes it to his present doctor. If the doctor is agreeable to the transfer he will sign the card which is then taken by the patient to his new doctor. The card is signed by the new doctor and sent by him to the FPC, who then proceed as in 2.
(b) If the patient does not wish to approach his present doctor about the transfer, the card can be sent to the FPC with a letter from the patient stating that he wishes to transfer. The Committee will then return the medical card to the patient with a transfer authority attached. This states that he can register with a new doctor after 14 days have elapsed. If the card is not signed by a new doctor within one month the transfer authority will lapse and fresh application must be made. When registering patients record the new patient's telephone number and enquire if regular medication is required. Registration forms should be sent to the FPC without delay.

4 Temporary residents

Where a patient does not intend to stay in an area for more than three months he should not re-transfer with his medical record card, but should ask to be registered as a temporary resident. This of course, is only done if he requires treatment and in these circumstances form FP 19 (Northern Ireland HS 15) (Fig. 30.4) is used, and the doctor signs to certify that he has given treatment. These forms are in duplicate. The carbonized top copy is filled in by the secretary, signed by the doctor and patient, and returned immediately to the FPC. The card bottom copy has the clinical notes on the reverse and is sent back to the FPC either when treatment is completed or at the end of three months, so that the record of the illness and treatment provided can be forwarded to the patient's regular doctor for inclusion in the medical record

---

NATIONAL HEALTH SERVICE
RECORD OF TREATMENT OF
TEMPORARY RESIDENT

Cipher of Home FPC

Surname	Mr Mrs Miss	NHS Number	Date of Birth

Forenames

Temporary
Address

Home
Address

Name of doctor at home

To be completed by patient

I am temporarily resident at the address shown above and I expect to remain in the district for (tick whichever is appropriate)

not more than 15 days from today ☐

more than 15 days from today ☐

but not more than 3 months from the date of my arrival.

I have received treatment from the doctor whose signature appears below.

Patient's signature..Date................................

A person signing for the patient should state the relationship.

To be completed by doctor

I have accepted the person named above as a Temporary Resident and have given treatment which is not one of the exceptions listed in paragraph 32.6 of the Statement of Fees and Allowances.

*I also claim a Rural Practice Payment. The distance from my main surgery to

the patient's temporary residence is................miles.

Doctor's signature...

Date...Code No............................

*Delete if not applicable
Dd. 8011074. 4000M. 6.79 FM(P)Ltd.   Form FP 19 (Rev. 1977)

Fig. 30.4 Form FP 19.

envelope. When a patient stays on in an area for a further temporary period a new FP 19 form should be used. Each FP 19 must state whether the patient intends to remain for more or less than 15 days in the area. Where a visitor is in the area for less than 24 hours and requires treatment (or for emergency treatment of patients outside the practice area), form FP 106 (Northern Ireland HS 14T) must be used.

New patients who have just left the Forces register with form FP 13, which is given to the patient when he leaves the service.

5 Immigrants' registration

Immigrants register with a doctor by means of form FP 1 (Northern Ireland HS 22X) (Fig. 30.5), which they obtain from the doctor.

TO BE COMPLETED IN INK

Mr. /Mrs. /Miss: MR
SURNAME (*Block Letters*): RAYMOND
FOR OFFICE USE

Forenames (*Block Letters*): DAVID JOHN
National Health Service No.: QJBM 12/6

Former or any other Surname: —
Date of Birth — Day: 23 | Month: 12 | Year: 33
Town and Country of Birth: LONDON ENGLAND

Address: 17 DRAYTON CLOSE. HORNWORTH

Previous Address: 23. THE ELMS. CHATSTONE
(*insert date*)
If recently arrived from abroad: —
If recently returned from H.M. Forces ....

Application to be included in List of Dr. M.T.M. PRIORY

TO BE COMPLETED BY DOCTOR: Dr's CODE No. 1148
FOR OFFICE USE
I accept this person for inclusion in my list
Signed: M. Priory
Date: 17.12.86

IF SUPPLYING DRUGS enter 'D' here: D
IF CLAIMING A RURAL PRACTICE PAYMENT enter distance from main surgery to patient's residence and inform F.P.C. if claiming for other than ordinary distance
miles: —

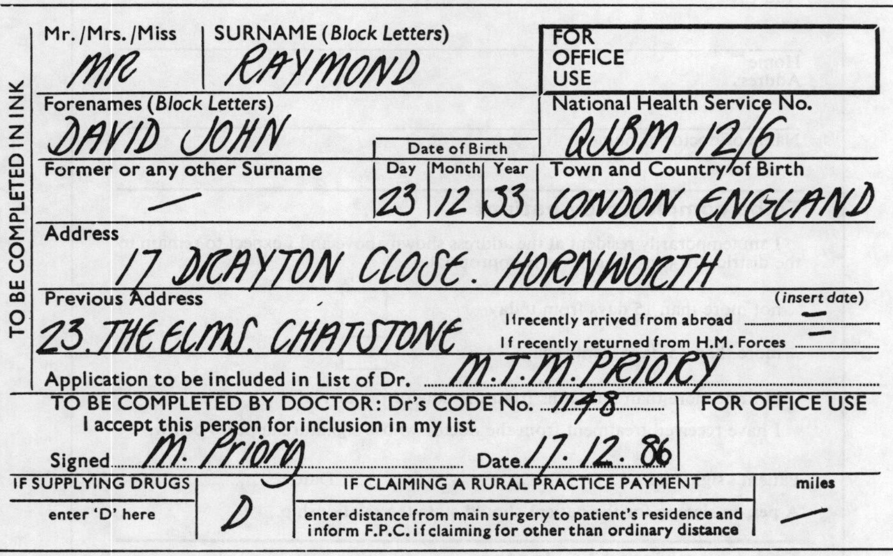

Fig. 30.5 Form FP 1.

6 Transfer when medical card is lost

Form FP 1 is used again, but here it is very important that the previous doctor's name and address are included.

Once a medical record envelope is issued it is important that the patient's name on it should not be altered without notification to the FPC, as otherwise it may not be possible for the Committee to trace the records at a later date; this can be done on Form FP 1C. It is also helpful if the patient notifies the Committee of a change in address. It is important that the secretary has a clear understanding of the methods of registration. Muddles and errors in this work lead to delays in the arrival of the patient's record envelope. This often hampers effective treatment. The necessary forms will be filled in by the patient and secretary and given to the doctor for him to sign. The secretary will then see that they are sent off in the first envelope leaving for the FPC.

To sum up, the types of acceptance with which a doctor's secretary may have to deal are:

(a) Infants—form FP 58 (Northern Ireland HS 123) issued to the parents by the registrar.
(b) Adopted children—form FP 58B issued by the Court.
(c) Other children and adults—form FP 4 (Northern Ireland HS 23) or if without medical card form FP 1 (Northern Ireland HS 22X).
(d) People discharged from HM Forces—form FP 13 issued on discharge.
(e) Temporary residents—form FP 19 (Northern Ireland HS 15).
(f) Emergency treatment (staying less than 24 hours)—form FP 106 (Northern Ireland HS 14T).
(g) Immigrants—form FP 1 (Northern Ireland HS 22X).

The secretary's part in all this is an important one. She should ensure that registration is quickly and correctly done and she should take the following steps:

(a) Select the proper form and see that all the spaces are correctly filled in.
(b) Ensure that every entry is in block capitals except the signature.
(c) Ensure that the patient's date of birth is recorded and, if known, the NHS number.
(d) Record the telephone number when possible.

FPCs issue a temporary medical record card FP 7B (male) or FP 8B (female) acknowledging acceptance of the patient on the doctor's list and allowing a record to be kept whilst awaiting notes from the previous doctor. It is essential that all registrations of patients should be received by FPCs before the first day of a new quarter so that payments can be made to the practice.

Diploma Questions

1 Outline the procedures necessary for introducing a patient appointment system in general practice, mentioning the advantages and disadvantages of this system to doctors and patients.
2 State clearly the disadvantages to patients in:
   (a) attending a surgery where there is an appointments system, and
   (b) attending a surgery where there is *no* appointments system.

31

The Doctor's Visit

VISITS AND ROUNDS

There is perhaps no aspect of the doctor's work on which the stamp of his individuality is laid more firmly than on the way in which he does his visits. For not only does the method of each doctor vary but the geography of his practice, the time of the year and the patient himself all have their effects. The country doctor may spend half a day on one or two visits, involving many miles of motoring and the opening and closing of innumerable gates. During this same time the city doctor may have seen a dozen patients and been able to walk to several of them. The summer months may give the doctor time to choose a favourite route, or leisure to take the family with him. Whereas a measles epidemic will hardly give him time to eat his meals.

In many houses the doctor's visit is looked upon as an important event. Bedrooms are tidied and relatives wait in all day to see the doctor. In others it is only at the third request that the television is turned down low enough to let him even use his stethoscope. One thing is certain—he must go straight to the point. The social niceties belong to a bygone era. Today they usually waste time and distract him from his job and as such they must often be firmly set aside.

With all these variations it is difficult to find a point on which to start to generalize. There are in fact, only two points on which everyone would agree. These are, firstly, that at the most only half as many patients can be visited at home at a given time as could be seen in the surgery in the same time, and secondly, that the medical records should be in the doctor's hand when he visits a patient. These two points will affect all the discussion that follows.

It is true to say that nearly all emergencies seen by a doctor are a result of a request for a visit. The 'sorting' of telephone requests thus has obvious risks and is a matter that calls for considerable experience. For if the doctor decides not to visit the patient at this time, he must know that the patient is sensible and responsible enough to call again if the circumstances change. The doctor not only visits the patient who *is* ill, but he visits the patient who *thinks* he is *ill*. He does not expect the patient to make a diagnosis, for fear or worry may be a sufficient reason to request a visit. He does, however, expect the patient to be considerate and polite. Just because a doctor is on call for 24 hours in a day it does not mean that he is expected to continue on unimportant work throughout this period. All these things must be clearly understood by the secretary for it is in this part of her duties that her most responsible tasks will lie.

REQUESTS FOR VISITS

The majority of these calls should come before the end of the morning surgery, and one of the most helpful ways in which a patient can be trained is to observe this simple rule. Many doctors arrange for notices to be displayed in their waiting rooms to this effect. Page two of the patient's medical card states:

'*Day Visits*. Please do not ask the doctor to call unless the patient is too ill to attend his surgery. Attendance at the surgery should be during surgery hours unless otherwise arranged by the doctor. When the condition of the patient does require a home visit, please try to give notice, if at all possible, *before 10.00 a.m. on the day on which the visit is required*.' It does no harm to point this out courteously to the patient, but understanding of the patient's problems is necessary also. Sometimes the patient has been hoping that he would recover and would not need a visit; at other times he has been sent home ill from work or school later in the day. As the prospect of a long night approaches the patient's fear may increase and his pain grow worse. All these points must be taken into consideration. *The secretary should never take it upon herself to refuse a visit.*

Every request for a visit must be written down at once, and this means that pen and book must always be kept by the telephone. The request must be written in the book by the telephone and not on a 'scrap' of paper. Requests that come in by post or on a note brought by hand should be stapled to the page in the book until they have been dealt with. This practice must be followed rigidly. Even if the visit is not urgent the note should be made, for, in the event of litigation against a doctor, who fails to visit, his case will be much weaker if these notes are not kept in this way. The record of the request for a visit should contain the following details.

1 *The time at which the request was received*. This will help the doctor when he comes to assess the urgency of the call. For instance, if a call to see a child with abdominal pain was received at the beginning of a surgery he may wish to visit him immediately the surgery is over, but if it came in just as the surgery ended he may feel this gives him time to do another urgent call first.

2 *The surname and Christian names of the patient, and, in the case of a child, the age*. Very often children have the same initials as a parent. What is urgent in a child may not be so in an adult, and *vice versa*. As the records will be taken when the doctor goes out to see the patient, the secretary will need these names herself.

3 *The address*. It is never sufficient to rely on the address on the card. There will be many occasions when a patient has moved house without notifying the doctor and nothing is more irritating than a two-mile journey to visit a patient, who now lives somewhere else. It is important to ensure that it is correct in every detail. Most towns have a Laburnum Street, Laburnum Crescent, Laburnum Close and so on, and they may be miles apart.

4 *The patient's symptoms*. Here the point must be made that the secretary is not asked to record a diagnosis but the symptoms of an illness. The diagnosis may be offered by the patient, but it is much more useful to have a note saying 'abdominal pain and sickness' than 'the patient says he has a chill'. These symptoms will help the doctor to arrange the priorities of visiting. He may know that Mrs Brown never sends unless she is really ill, but if 'she can't move her left leg' it may be urgent. Another helpful point is to mark the day book

(Fig. 31.1) by the telephone to indicate the messages that are requests for visits and to distinguish them from requests for prescriptions or other matters. This can be done by underlining or marking the call with the letter 'V'. Occasionally a call will come that requires attention immediately and will not wait until the end of the surgery. If the secretary thinks that this may be the case she should speak to the doctor before the caller rings off. In this way further information may be obtained by the doctor or advice given

There remain two other varieties of call that come in:
(a) the night call.
(b) the call that is made to the doctor's private residence.

TIME	TYPE OF MESSAGE			NAME AND ADDRESS	MESSAGE	DOCTOR
	PRESCRIP- TION	VISIT	CERTIFICATE			
9.0		✓		Mr. Thomas, 24 The Close Clean	Pain in stomach & vomiting	Dr. M.
9.5		✓		Janet Powell, The Firs, 21, Drayton Lane	Cold and cough	Dr. C.
9.8	✓			Mrs. Deacon, 16 Coal Lane	Repeat cough linctus	Dr. C.
9.30			✓	Mr. R. James, 39 Elm Way	Private note date for 30th Aug.	Dr. A.
9.45		✓		Ronald Jay, 1 Moss Way	? Measles	Dr M
9.47		✓		Mrs. Mary Brown, 5, King Edward Close	Diarrhoea and Vomiting for two days - go in through back door.	Dr. C.

DAY Monday   DATE 1st July

Fig. 31.1 The day book.

The secretary will not be directly involved with either of these but there is an important point of principle involved. The doctor will wish to record the symptoms, diagnosis and treatment on the record-card, and the secretary should enquire each day whether any other visits have been made that are not on the doctor's visiting list of the previous day. If so, she must present the card and fill in the register of visits. A fee is paid by the FPC to the doctor for a visit requested and made between the hours of 11.00 p.m. and 7.00 a.m. This is claimed for on form FP 81 (Northern Ireland NV/1) (Fig. 31.2). It needs to be signed by the patient (or other responsible person) as well as the doctor. When the patient dies or is very seriously ill, the doctor may put a note on the form explaining the circumstances in place of the patient's signature.

Where a patient is not a patient of the practice and is resident in the area for less than 24 hours a claim for emergency treatment is made on form FP 32 (Scotland GP 32, Northern Ireland HS 14). (A fee for immediate necessary treatment can be claimed on form FP 106 (Northern Ireland HS 14T) if care has to be given to a patient whom the doctor has declined to take on his list or is a temporary resident.

FP 81

National Health Service

HEREFORD AND WORCESTER
FAMILY PRACTITIONER COMMITTEE

CLAIM FOR NIGHT VISIT FEE

1   Between the hours of 11 pm on ___1 July 86___ and 7 am the
following morning I both received a request to visit and attended.

Surname of Patient ∅   *Richards*

Christian or Forenames   *Kevin*

Address   *207 Bransgore Road,*
Birmingham

2   The attendance took place

*   at the patient's home

*   ~~at the surgery~~

*   ~~at a local general practitioner hospital~~

*   ~~at a general practitioner maternity unit~~

and was in accordance with 1(a)-(c) overleaf.

3   Signature of visiting doctor

I hereby claim a night visit fee

Signature of claiming doctor   *M Bourne*

Doctor's FPC Code No   *1748*   Date   *1/7/86*

Name and Address   *Dr M Bourne*
8, Scotts Way
Birmingham

∅   If more than one patient was attended on the same visit to the same
location, this should be indicated and the name of each patient shown
overleaf.

*   Delete as appropriate

SEE OVER/.......

Fig. 31.2 Form FP 81.

THE VISITING LIST

This is the list of visits that is made out each day for the doctor. It will contain the names and addresses of all patients that are to be visited that day (Fig. 31.3). It can also usefully contain any other appointments and commitments that have to be kept, e.g. visits to hospitals, schools or factories, domiciliary visits with Consultants, meetings, and trains that have to be met. There should be space left next to the name for the doctor to indicate when he wishes to see the patient again. It is also helpful to have a column in which he can record charges for private patients or arrangements concerning, for instance, district nurses or ambulance transport that have to be made.

DAY FRIDAY	DATE 3rd January	DOCTOR	
	NAME AND ADDRESS	REMARKS	NEXT VISIT
1	A. Jones, 19 Forth St. Homworth ✓		7
2	T. Nelson, The Cottage Fir Way ✓	Take ear syringe	14
3	J. C. Bolyis, Raymond House Homworth ✓	Fix X-Ray and Ambulance Time	1
4	B. White, 72 Grey Road, Sealeigh ✓		off
5	J. Jones, 64 New Rd.	—	.
6	K. Benson, 28 Copton Close		
7	L. Harper 44 High Street		
8	S. Davidson 'The Beeches' ✓	£1.05	1
9	John Sunley 14 Crossfields ✓	Notify measles	1
10			
11			
12			
13			
14			
15	Local Medical Committee — 4.30 p.m.		
16			
17			

Fig. 31.3 The visiting list.

Some doctors have their lists made out in a book, which is taken around with them, but this is not a good idea because the secretary will want to prepare the next day's list as far as she can and unless she has the book this cannot be done. The importance of preparing the list early cannot be overemphasized. At the end of a busy surgery the doctor will wish to get on with the visits, and if all the re-visits are already down on a list made out the day before, he can make a quick start. Similarly the doctor should be encouraged to return these lists as soon as the visits are finished so that preparation of the next day's list can start at once.

It is sometimes the custom in a group practice for one of the doctors to start visits at 9.30 a.m. while his partners do the morning surgery. In such cases patients have to be trained to request visits early in the morning.

The visiting list must always be 'married' to the record cards of the patients who are to be visited. This entails removing them from the files at the earliest opportunity, checking surname, Christian names and age, and making a special note when the address on the record envelope differs from that in the day book. The system by which the cards and lists are carried by the doctor is mentioned later.

At the end of the surgery all new calls are added to the visiting list. It is often helpful to mark in some agreed way the new calls because the doctor may have a system whereby he tries to get these calls attended to early. Where there is more than one doctor doing the visits, these have to be shared out. This is usually done at the end of the surgery, over a cup of tea. The principles by which this sharing is done vary. The patient may express a preference for one doctor. Here the secretary should be careful not to leave the impression of giving a guarantee that any particular doctor will call as there may be other circumstances that she does not know about. If the patient is usually treated by a doctor or is suffering from a condition that he started to treat him for, then again this doctor will probably take the call. The remaining visits will be shared out on the basis of equality of work or geographical distribution. Geography is an important factor. There are doctors who dash here and there like ill-organized bees, but usually a visiting list is planned to cover the greatest number of patients in the shortest distance. It is here that intelligent anticipation by the secretary can save a great deal of time and energy. If the visiting book is made out properly she should be able to note where the visits are for the next few days. A call may come in for the doctor to visit a house which is close to one that is on his list to be visited within the next day or two. She may then suggest that this latter visit is advanced a little to save an extra journey.

One final point about the visiting list. The secretary will receive many calls that will sound to her as if a visit is not really necessary. A request for a visit by a patient who only needs a 'note', and one to visit someone with a cold are typical examples. Her she can genuinely justify her position as the doctor's first assistant. She may be able to speak to the doctor before the caller rings off, and a few words from him may save a visit. On the other hand she will know that a patient does not need to send in a first certificate (form Med 3) for six days, and thus the patient will be able to collect his own note from the surgery in a day or two. In this sort of way she can save the time, energy and enthusiasm of the doctor for patients who need his attention.

THE DOCTOR'S ROUND

When the list is prepared and the cards are ready the doctor can set off on his round. Many patients ask when the doctor will call. It is often a great nuisance to them not to know when he will be coming. They may have shopping to do or children that must be fetched from school. Unfortunately it is not usually possible to promise a time ahead. Neither the secretary nor the doctor knows the order of priorities and in any case new and more urgent calls may come in later. The secretary should answer such queries by saying that he will come as soon as he is able. When the person making the call says that she has to go out at a certain time, the secretary should make a note of this fact. If the doctor is told that 'Mrs Jones will be out between 3.30 p.m. and 4.00 p.m. but she will leave the back door unlocked', this can save a lot of irritation.

The doctor will develop a system of carrying the cards with him on his visits. They may simply be held with a rubber band, together with the list and carried in the glove pocket of the car, or some more elaborate system of a wallet or folder may be used. This latter has the advantage in that the cards are securely held, they can be conveniently carried to the bedside, the folder gives a surface to write on and it may have space in it to take continuation cards (forms FP 7 and 8), prescription pads or FP 1 forms.

The importance of the clinical note made at the bedside has been established by clinicians over hundreds of years and it is the secretary's duty to see that they are available for the doctor. A difficulty may arise when branch surgeries are used. The patient's record card may be kept at Surgery A, where the patient is usually seen, and the request for the visit may be received at Surgery B. Under these circumstances it may not be possible for the doctor to take the medical record envelope (form FP 5 or 6) with him but it is always possible for the secretary to ensure that he has a continuation card (FP 7 or 8) with the patient's name and address filled in. This can be inserted in the patient's notes at a later date. The same routine should be followed when a call comes in to see a new patient or one whose record envelope has not yet been received from the FPC.

There are times when emergency calls come in after the doctor has left on his rounds. At such times it is often possible for the secretary to contact the doctor. Some doctors, particularly those with scattered country practices, have radio-telephones in their cars. At other times the secretary can leave telephone messages in houses that are on his list asking him to ring her as soon as he gets there.

It is worth remembering that ambulance personnel are all highly trained in first-aid and emergency resuscitation and that the equipment required for prolonged resuscitation is often present only in hospital. In certain emergency cases, therefore, it may be quicker and much safer to have the patient transported rapidly to hospital than to wait until the doctor is available. The secretary may continue to try to contact the doctor after having sent for the ambulance and the doctor will then be able to check with ambulance headquarters whether his presence is required. In any case, on all occasions when the secretary cannot contact the doctor she should resort to the standing arrangement she has made with him to cover emergencies under these circumstances.

THE VISITING BOOK

This is an important piece of surgery equipment (Fig. 31.4) and to be satisfactory it must:
1 be durable enough to stand up to frequent handling.
2 allow a day's visiting list to be made up quickly.
3 allow names to be carried on from month to month.

A loose-leaf book is more satisfactory than one with fixed leaves; it enables visits several months ahead to be 'booked' and several months behind to be

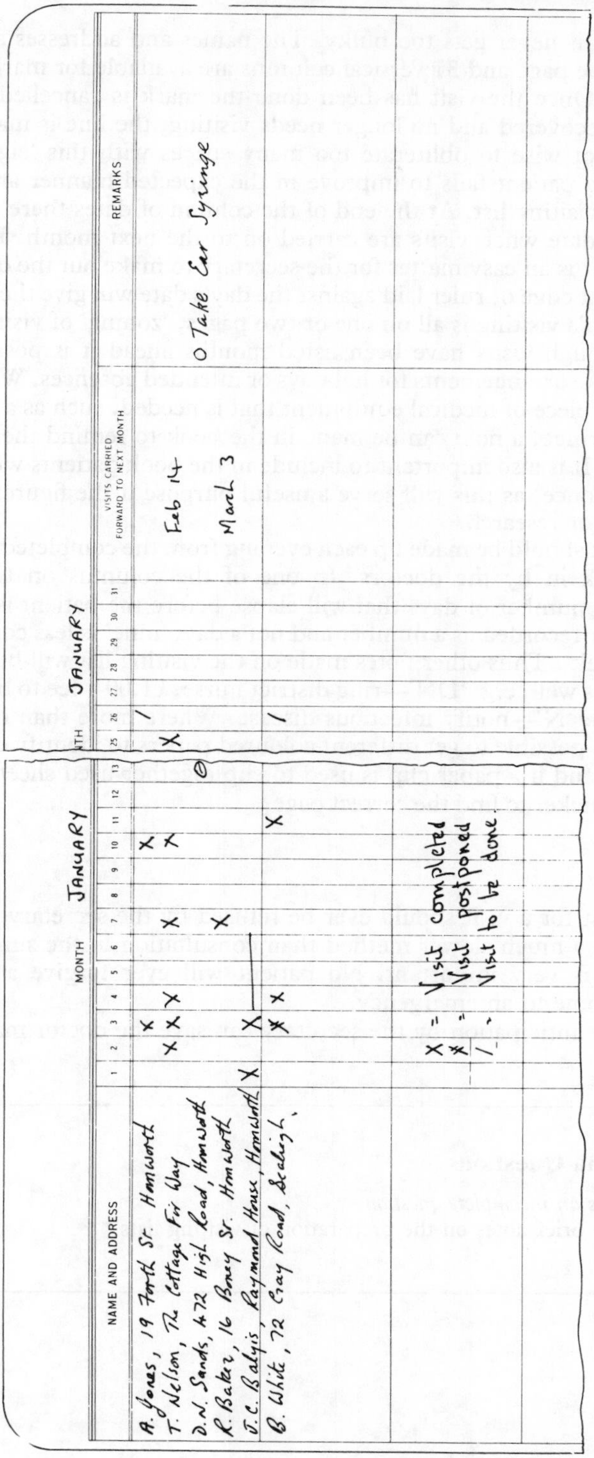

NAME AND ADDRESS	MONTH JANUARY													MONTH JANUARY								VISITS CARRIED FORWARD TO NEXT MONTH	REMARKS
	1	2	3	4	5	6	7	8	9	10	11	12	13	25	26	27	28	29	30	31		
A. Jones, 19 Forth St. Henworth		X	X				X			X	X			X								
T. Nelson, The Cottage Fir Way		X	X	X			X			X					1						Feb 14	O Take Ear Syringe
D.N. Sands, 472 High Road, Henworth			X			X	X														March 3	
R. Baker, 16 Bonny Sr. Henworth	X																					
J.C. Balyis, Raymond House, Henworth		X	X							X			O		1							
B. White, 72 Gray Road, Bealizjh		X	X								X											

X = Visit completed
X̶ = Visit postponed
I = Visit to be done

Fig. 31.4 The visiting book.

retained, but it never gets too bulky. The names and addresses are listed on one side of the page and 31 vertical columns are available for marking when a visit is due. Once the visit has been done the mark is cancelled. When the patient has recovered and no longer needs visiting, the line is marked with a dash. It is not wise to obliterate too many spaces with this 'signing off' as occasionally a patient fails to improve in the expected manner and has to go back on the visiting list. At the end of the column of dates there is a space to write in the date when visits are carried on to the next month. By means of such a book it is an easy matter for the secretary to make out the day's visiting list. A straight edge or ruler laid against the day's date will give the day's visits. As the month's visiting is all on one or two pages, 'zoning' of visits is possible and even though visits have been listed months ahead it is possible for the doctor to make arrangements for holidays or intended absences. Where there is some special piece of medical equipment that is needed, such as a proctoscope or special syringe, a note can be made in the book to remind the secretary to put it ready. It is also important to include in the book patients who have only been visited once, as this will serve a useful purpose if the figures are needed for statistics or research.

The book should be made up each evening from the completed visiting lists brought back in by the doctors. In one of the columns on these will be recorded the number of days that will elapse before the patient is seen again. This is better recorded as a number and not a day; 'nine' is less confusing than 'Monday week'. Thus other notes made on the visiting list will be attended to at this time as well, e.g. 'DN'—ring district nurse, £1.00—fee to be entered on account card, 'N'—notify infectious disease. Where more than one doctor is involved it is possible to get different coloured papers to identify each doctor's visiting list, and if a paper clip is used to clip together used sheets it makes it easier and quicker to find the correct page.

Summary

1 No request for a visit should ever be refused by the secretary.
2 Visiting is a much slower method than consultation in the surgery.
3 Accuracy is very important. No patient will ever forgive a doctor who 'forgot' to come to an emergency.
4 Intelligent anticipation by the secretary can save the doctor many a wasted hour.

Diploma Questions

*Denotes an incomplete question
1 Write brief notes on the preparation of visiting lists.*

32

Midwifery and Contraception in General Practice

Midwifery is the foundation of complete general practice. The relationships that are made during the period of antenatal care and confinement are ones that the doctor finds the most satisfying of all. This is a time when preventive medicine can really be practised. In most other medical conditions the doctor is consulted by a patient who is either ill or believes he is ill. In midwifery he is consulted usually by a patient who is well, and all his efforts are devoted to keeping her well. Furthermore, with the arrival of a new baby, the doctor has an opportunity to educate and help a mother in the ways and means by which she can keep her baby healthy. Most of this is done in the surgery and as the standards of antenatal care are raised, so the quantity of work involved increases. Unfortunately, this increase in the medical care is matched by a corresponding increase in the documentation necessary during antenatal and post-natal care. Therefore a considerable degree of organization is needed to keep the maternity work of a busy practice running smoothly.

As we have seen in Chapter 5, the maternity services in this country had developed along the three separate lines: hospital services, local health authority services and general practice. This inevitably led to a lack of coordination and often to a duplication of medical attention. Part of the maternity care in general practice consists of ensuring that cooperation does occur and that nothing that ought to be done is left undone.

The average GP in this country will see about 40 maternity patients a year. The great majority of babies will be born in hospital and only a tiny number in the home. Some of these mothers will be cared for in the hospital by a Consultant Obstetrician and some by the GP but in either case they will probably be seen by both in the antenatal period. This form of 'shared care' requires particularly good organization and record systems. Patients will be seen about 17 times in the antenatal period, sometimes at the hospital and sometimes in the surgery, either in a special antenatal clinic or during routine consultation sessions.

The contract of service that the GP has with the FPC commits him to provide 'general medical services'. He does not contract to provide maternity services. If he wishes, he may enter into contract with an individual patient to provide her with services and may then claim payment from the Committee for the services he has given. The FPC maintains a list of suitably qualified or experienced doctors called the 'obstetric list'. Doctors who are on this list may claim payment at the full rate for care given. Doctors who are not on this list receive payment at a lesser rate. If a doctor decides that he will not do maternity work, his patients, whilst remaining on his list for general medical services, will contract with another doctor for maternity medical services.

The situation is further complicated by the fact that these maternity services may be shared, to a greater or less degree, with the hospital or the local health authority or both.

There is no 'obstetric list' in Scotland.

FIRST ANTENATAL ATTENDANCE

Patients who think they are pregnant often attend the doctor soon after they have missed their first period. Sometimes they do not wish to continue with the pregnancy but in any case they seek confirmation. This is not possible at this early stage by clinical examination but may be confirmed by a urine test.

Once the pregnancy is confirmed an appointment is made for a first antenatal attendance, which should not be hurried. The health of the mother and baby depend upon the activity carried out at this early consultation. There are physical and emotional areas to explore and much health education activity to be carried out. There are a number of complex forms to be completed. If an appointment system is run it may be possible to complete a number of these forms in advance but, in any case, the doctor will need between 10 and 20 minutes. Ideally a special weekly antenatal clinic will be run but there will be expectant mothers who have other children or go out to work and can only attend during evening surgeries. These mothers will have to be fitted in. Special care must be taken to be tactful when dealing with expectant mothers, who may be shy or embarrassed. This refers especially to the unmarried mother.

On first attendance the doctor will wish to talk to the patient and then to examine her. The discussion will include topics such as where the baby is to be born and what antenatal care is needed, as well as advice on smoking, diet, work and exercise. The examination will include:

1 a general medical examination
2 an examination of the breasts and pelvis
3 testing the urine and weighing the patient and, sometimes,
4 taking blood for required tests.

Forms required at first antenatal attendance

On completing the history and making this examination the doctor will wish to make his notes. Some doctors still use the continuation form (FP 8) for this purpose, but more often a special antenatal record card is used. The maternity cooperation record card (form MCW 01, Northern Ireland MMS 2) (Fig. 32.1) is obtained from the FPC and kept in an envelope (MCW 01, Northern Ireland MMS 2A). The patient should be told to keep the card in her handbag at all times so that it is available to the hospital, midwife or GP when shared care is being given. This may be a private one or may be provided by health authority, Royal College of General Practitioners, or other sources. These cards have spaces for the necessary details and fit inside the medical record envelope (FP 6). They are sometimes kept in the surgery between attendances but more often are kept by the patient in a specially designed envelope and

ANTE-NATAL RECORD

FORM M.C.W.01

INVESTIGATIONS	DATE	RESULTS
A.B.O. Blood Group*	7.1.86	O
Rhesus Blood Group*		Rh -ve
Antibodies*	7.1.86	nil
WR KAHN		
X-Ray Chest		
Other Rubella		immune 17.4.85

*IMPORTANT NOTE–In the event of a transfusion this record of the blood grouping should always be checked and cross-matching should always be carried out.

HISTORY
Oedema nil
Headache "
Bowels normal
Micturition "
Discharge nil.
Date of quickening

FIRST EXAMINATION Date 30.12.85 Sig. M.D
Height 1.69
Teeth ✓
Breasts ✓
Heart ✓
Lungs ✓
Varicose veins nil
Pelvis
Cervical smear 17.4.85 – Gd. II
Special observations

EXAMINATION 35/37 week
Date
Head/Brim relationship
Pelvic capacity
Sig.

This patient is fit for inhalation analgesia
Date
Signature of Doctor

DATE	WEEKS	WEIGHT	URINE ALB. SUGAR	B.P.	HEIGHT FUNDUS	PRESENTATION AND POSITION	RELATION OF P.P. TO BRIM	F.H.	OEDEMA	Hb	NEXT VISIT	SIG	NOTES e.g. antibodies, other tests, infections, drugs, immunisation, classes attended, etc.
7.1.86	10	68 Kg	nil nil	112/72					0	14.6	1/12	M.D	M.S.U = sterile
5.2.86	14	67.5	nil nil	110/76	14/52				0		1/12	M.D	Utrasound = 14.5 weeks
													α feto protein =
													Apptmt. at hospital. ✓
													for midwife ✓

Dd 8343239 736m 2/83 RB Ltd.

Fig. 32.1 A maternity cooperation record card.

Form FW 8

Part 1   **APPLICATION FOR A CERTIFICATE FOR FREE PRESCRIPTIONS**

(Please read notes below)

SURNAME ....
(Block capitals)
OTHER NAMES ....
(Block capitals)

....

ADDRESS ....

....

TOWN ....

COUNTY ....
(including postcode)

Former
or any
other
surname ....
Address shown on your medical card if different
from your present one

....

....

My NHS number is
(as on my medical card)

My date
of birth

My NHS General Practitioner's name and address (if none write NONE) ....

....

I wish to apply for a certificate entitling me to free prescriptions

Date ....   Signed ....

NOTE: An exemption certificate issued by an FPC (Health Board in Scotland) entitles you to free prescriptions (regardless of income) during pregnancy and for a year after the date of confinement.

To apply for a certificate, complete and detach **THIS PART** of the form and send it in a stamped envelope to your NHS Family Practitioner Committee (or Health Board if you live in Scotland) **AT THE ADDRESS OVERLEAF.** If no address is shown, ask at your main Post Office or Public Library.

If you have to pay for any prescriptions before you receive your exemption certificate, ask the chemist at the time for a receipt form FP 57 (EC 57 in Scotland), and claim a refund at the Post Office when your certificate arrives.

Part 2   **FREE MILK AND VITAMINS**

Many expectant mothers and young children can get a free pint of milk a day (or dried milk for a bottle fed baby) and free vitamins.

IF YOU GET SUPPLEMENTARY BENEFIT OR FAMILY INCOME SUPPLEMENT

If your family is getting Supplementary Benefit or Family Income Supplement you are automatically entitled to free milk and vitamins for yourself during your pregnancy in addition to free milk and vitamins for any child under age 5. Write to your local social security office if you are getting supplementary benefit, or to the FIS Unit if you are getting FIS, quoting your Supplementary Benefit reference number or FIS order book number. Give your name and address and the date your baby is due. You can get a stamped addressed envelope from your local Post Office.

IF YOU ARE ON A LOW INCOME

If your family's income is low you may be entitled to free milk and vitamins for yourself during pregnancy and for any child under age 5. Full details are provided in leaflet MV.11, obtainable from your social security office, Post Offices or maternity and child health clinic. If, after reading the leaflet, you think you may qualify, fill in the form attached to the leaflet and send it to your social security office. You can get the address from the local Post Office, who will also provide a stamped addressed envelope.

If children in your family already get free milk and vitamins simply write to your social security office telling them the date your baby is due.

Printed in the UK for HMSO Dd 8810689 3/84 550m 20841

Fig. 32.2 Form FW 8.

only returned to the doctor for inclusion in FP 6 when attendances finish. This is particularly useful when antenatal care is being shared by different authorities, for it is then that it really becomes a 'cooperation card'. This card will be used at each attendance and will record significant features in the medical history. It will also record the previous obstetrical history, the mother being referred to as a primiparous woman or primigravida until after the birth of her first baby, and thereafter as a multigravida. The LMP (first day of the last menstrual period) and the EDD (estimated date of delivery) will be completed.

As soon as the doctor is certain that the patient is pregnant he will want these forms to be made out as completely as possible by the secretary. Some details and the signing of the form will have to be completed by him. (In Scotland for FP read GP.)

1 *Form FP 24 or 24A (Northern Ireland MMS 1).* These are issued in book form and are perforated so that they can be detached when the doctor's payment claim is submitted to the FPC. FP 24 refers to doctors who are on the obstetric list and FP 24A to those who are not. FP 24 is in three parts. Part I is signed by the doctor and handed to the patient. It is an acceptance of the application of the patient to be looked after by the doctor. Part II must be signed by the patient. This is the application for maternity services. Part IIB is the certificate and claim form for payment and is not completed until the post-natal examination has been made.

2 *Form FW 8 (rev.) (Northern Ireland UFW [rev.])* Fig. 32.2). This is filled in by the secretary and then signed by the doctor. The mother completes the reverse side and sends it or takes it to her local FPC. This form entitles the mother to free prescriptions and dental treatment, and if the family income is low she may also be entitled to free vitamins and concessionary milk. It is explained in the booklet *Medical Evidence for Social Security Purposes, Guidance for GPs.*

3 *Blood test forms.* These vary from hospital area to hospital area but will usually include tests for percentage of haemoglobin, blood group, rhesus factor, rubella immunization status and WR and Kahn test. If the mother is not immune to rubella a note will have to be made so that immunization is carried out in the immediate post-natal period.

4 *Forms and bottles for a midstream urine test.* This is carried out early in pregnancy to detect an abnormal number of bacteria in the urine, which requires treatment to prevent subsequent kidney infection.

5 *Ultrasound screening.* Procedures have been developed for detecting a number of conditions from which the foetus may suffer which depend upon blood tests or upon tests performed on the fluid surrounding the foetus in the uterus. The accuracy of these may depend upon very accurate dating of the pregnancy, which can be done by taking an ultrasound 'film' of the baby. This can also help by detecting other conditions such as multiple pregnancy or an unusual situation of the placenta. Special forms are required by the X-ray department and for subsequent blood tests for, say, alpha-fetoprotein blood levels.

6 *Prescription (FP 10).* A prescription for iron and folic acid tablets is sometimes issued routinely during pregnancy.

7 *Appointment form for a Consultant Obstetrician's opinion.* As care is usually shared between the obstetrician and the GP early consultation is desirable.

These are the usual forms that are used at the first antenatal consultation. The secretary should ensure that the doctor has on his desk the patient's record envelope (FP 6) and all the papers with the patient's name, address and date of birth correctly filled in before the consultation begins. A further appointment will be made before the patient leaves.

FURTHER ANTENATAL ATTENDANCES

Where an appointment system is used the appointment will be entered in the book and either written on the back of the cooperation card or on a separate card (Fig. 32.3). As well as this appointment a separate register of midwifery attendances is usually kept. There are three reasons for this register.
1 Reminders can be issued to patients who have failed to attend.
2 The doctor can plan his work so that he is prepared for the time when babies are due.
3 Where maternity work is shared it is necessary to fill in FP 24, Part IIB with the dates on which the patient has been seen.

Antenatal Appointments Card
Please bring this card with you at every appointment, together with a sample of your urine, in a bottle clearly labelled with your name and the date.

Patient's name

Address

Tel. No.

Doctor's name

Address

Tel. No.

Fig. 32.3 Antenatal appointments card.

This register can be kept in a book or in a card-index system. Whichever method is used the book and page of the FP 24 should be identified by a number which is put on the cooperation card and in the register. If the card-index system is used each card should be made out with the patient's name, LMP and EDD and the number on the FP 24. A guide-index marker is used for each month of the year and the index cards are filed in the alphabetical order of the patient's name in the month in which the baby is due. In this case

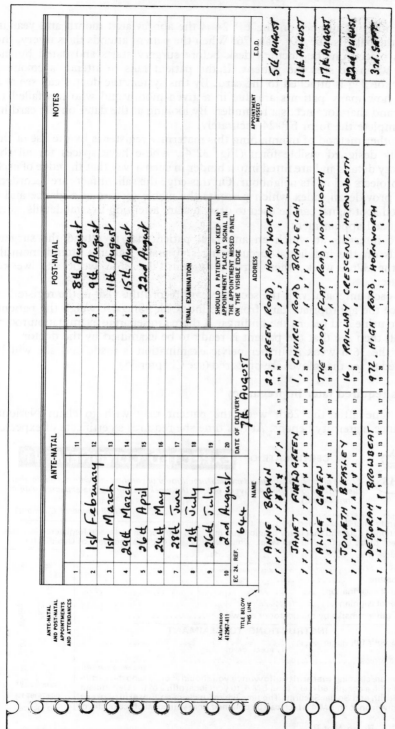

Fig. 32.4 An obstetric case records card.

the identifying number on the FP 24 is the abbreviated month and year in which the baby is due, e.g. Jan. 76. When the patient attends the surgery, the card is placed on the doctor's desk before surgery starts and dated by the doctor when he sees the patient. If the patient fails to attend, a coloured 'tickler' or flag is attached to the card. By this system the doctor can see at a glance how many patients are due in a given month and who has failed to attend and therefore needs a reminder. By looking at the dates on the card he can complete the form FP 24 accurately.

Another method of maintaining this maternity register is by the use of the specially designed visible form (Fig. 32.4). These have spaces for all the necessary details and are fitted into a binder in such a way that the edge of each sheet projects below its neighbour. On this edge the salient facts are recorded. These provide an index which presents the whole picture at a glance and a coloured spot signal can be used to draw instant attention to vital details, such as a missed appointment.

The intervals at which an antenatal patient has to attend the surgery depends on the individual circumstances. Usually patients attend monthly until the 32nd week, then fortnightly until the 36th week and weekly thereafter.

At each antenatal visit the secretary will record the visit in the register, or produce the appropriate card from the index-file. She will weigh the patient, test the urine and record the findings. If there are separate examination rooms she will then see that the patient is ready to be examined by the doctor.

At the 36th week a further pelvic examination is made and she will be required to see that gloves are prepared (see Chapter 35).

Forms required later in pregnancy

Some time after the 26th week the patient may wish to claim National Insurance maternity benefit. At this time she requires a certificate of expected

CERTIFICATE OF **EXPECTED CONFINEMENT**

(*To be given by a registered medical practitioner or certified midwife not earlier than the beginning of the 14th week before the week containing the expected date of confinement.*)

To..(*Full Name of Claimant*)

I certify that I examined you on the under-mentioned date and that in my opinion you may expect to be confined in the week which will

include the................................day

of..................19...... (*Here insert the expected date of confinement*)

Signature ....

Date of examination............................

Date of signing ....

Any other remarks by the doctor or midwife............................

If certified midwife, add Registered Number or Address and Date of Qualification

....

....

....

....

....

INSTRUCTIONS TO CLAIMANT

Give your full name .... (*in* BLOCK CAPITALS)

and address................................ (*including postcode*)

If you are claiming **maternity allowance** you should at once send this certificate with a completed claim form BM 4, to your local office of the Department of Health and Social Security. The time limits for claiming **maternity grant** are given on form BM 4 which can be obtained from your local office or clinic.

Form Mat B1

Dd.576985 150M
2/78 D.Ltd.
T.52 1308(2b)

Fig. 32.5 Form Mat B1.

confinement (form Mat B 1) (Fig. 32.5). This has to be signed by the doctor or by a registered midwife and sent with a completed claim form (BM 4) to the local DHSS office. Form BM 4 can be obtained from this office, or the local health authority antenatal clinic or be supplied to the doctor by the FPC.

Further blood tests will be required during the pregnancy.

The secretary's responsibilities

Important points to be observed during antenatal work by the secretary are:
1 Always inform the doctor personally if any abnormality or unusual feature is detected in urine-testing or weighing (see Chapter 36).
2 Always inform the doctor personally if a patient fails to keep an antenatal or post-natal appointment.
3 Always ensure that the patient makes a further appointment before leaving the surgery.

When an expectant mother goes into labour during the day-time the call may be received during the surgery hours. In this case it is wise to pass the call through to the doctor. The message requesting a visit may come through at a time when the doctor is out and it is in such circumstances that the secretary will feel the full weight of responsibility resting upon her. She will not, of course, be expected to give advice but to take a clear message and pass it quickly on. Most of these details are dealt with under the section on 'telephone technique' but the points that are peculiarly relevant are dealt with below.
1 Not all midwifery 'calls' are urgent, but the secretary is wise to treat all as urgent unless proved otherwise.
2 Apart from normal details of name and address there are other important points that will help in assessing the problem.
  (a) Has the baby been born?
  (b) Is the midwife present?
  (c) Is the case booked for home delivery or hospital?

3 If the message has been sent by a midwife she may use technical terms to indicate the state of progress. The labour may be described as first, second or third stage; membranes may be intact or ruptured. The cervix may be described as two fingers dilated or half, three-quarters or fully dilated. The foetal heart rate may be given or the quantity of haemorrhage may be measured in ounces. If this information is given it must be clearly recorded.

The secretary should arrange with the doctor a clear policy to be adopted in the event of her being unable to contact him for an emergency call, and she should leave the caller in no doubt that she is now in charge. If the call requires a visit from the doctor this will be a good point at which to look out the 'midder bag' and give it a final check.

If the patient is booked for delivery in hospital, and no emergency has arisen, arrangements can be made directly with the hospital by the patient's husband, but the secretary will help in any way possible.

POST-NATAL VISITS

This aspect of maternity work is also dependent upon the relationship between the three branches of the maternity services. The doctor will be involved when the delivery took place at home, or when delivery took place in hospital and the patient was discharged early. Discharge of maternity patients, who have had the full 'lying-in' period in hospital, occurs between the 10th and 14th day after delivery. Patients may, however, be discharged at any time from the first 24 hours onwards. In these circumstances they will require visiting by both the midwife and the doctor. It is the hospital's responsibility to notify doctor and midwife and this is done either by telephone or by letter. When the doctor is notified he will arrange to visit the patient and will probably see her at home, at least until the 14th day. The secretary should draw his attention to early maternity discharges and should note on the register or index card the date on which the visit is done. If the mother and child are in normal health by the end of the visiting period of two weeks, the patient will not be seen again until the post-natal examination is made.

POST-NATAL EXAMINATION

This examination is made in the surgery or at the hospital six weeks after the baby is born. It is an important medical examination which is designed to check that no physical abnormality due to the pregnancy is left undiagnosed. At the same time it is important because advice about the new baby is given and because this is an occasion when the mother may seek advice about 'family planning'. From the secretarial point of view there are three details to be attended to apart from the preparation for the medical examination. These are:
1 completion of form FP 24 or 24A (Northern Ireland MMS 1)
2 registration of baby by form FP 58 (Northern Ireland HS 123)
3 arranging appointments for first immunization of baby
4 completion of forms relating to contraception
5 completion of forms for cervical cytology where needed

Forms required in the post-natal period

Completion of form FP 24 or 24A. This form has to be submitted to the FPC within six months of the completion of services. The secretary should check that Part II was signed by the patient at her first antenatal visit. She should then present to the doctor at the time of post-natal examinations:
1 the antenatal cooperation card.
2 form FP 24 or 24A.
3 the register or card-index of attendances.
4 forms for blood tests (haemoglobin and level of antibodies if a Rhesus-negative (Rh −ve) mother).
5 forms relating to contraception (FP 1001, Scotland GP 102).
6 forms for cervical cytology test.

If the doctor has provided complete maternity medical services then he will tick the appropriate box on the form. If only partial services have been provided the secretary will fill in the dates of these services before presenting the form. The date of every attendance up to the 14th day after delivery must be entered but the full post-natal visit claim is only payable up to the 12th week after delivery. When Part IIB of the form has been signed by the doctor it is put in the envelope that is sent periodically (once or twice a week) to the FPC. The antenatal cooperation card will then be placed in the medical record envelope, and the register of attendances will be kept so that the maternity fees paid can be checked off against it. The scale of fees paid is to be found printed on the cover of the book of forms FP 24 and 24A. It is not included here as it is subject to periodical revision.

Registration of baby. If form FP 58 was not received earlier it should be completed at this stage as it is important to ensure that a medical record envelope containing a form FP 7A or FP 8A is present when the baby attends for his first immunization. If the mother has lost the FP 8 form, FP 1 (Northern Ireland HS 22X) should be used.

Appointment for first immunization. This should be made at the time of the post-natal examination. If the post-natal examination has been done at the hospital a note should be made by the secretary so that an appointment can be sent to the mother when the first immunization is due.

Form Mat B2. Certificate of confinement (see page 262).

Forms relating to contraception

Family planning is part of general practice and advice is sought by men and women during the whole of the period of a woman's fertility. A fee is now paid to the doctor for contraceptive advice to women and although it may relate to many other periods than the post-natal time it is convenient to consider the documentation here.

Claims are made on forms which consist of three parts:
1 identification particulars—completed by the secretary
2 a claim form signed by the doctor
3 a declaration signed by the patient.

Form FP 1001 (Scotland GP 102) (Fig. 32.6). This refers to all contraceptive advice given to registered patients excepting intrauterine contraceptive devices.

Form FP 1002 (Scotland GP 103) (Fig. 32.7). This form relates to insertion of intrauterine devices.

Form FP 1003 (Scotland GP 104). This relates to all forms of contraceptive advice given to a temporary resident (if other general medical services are given an FP 19 should be completed as well).

The first two of these forms are valid for one year from the date of completion but must be renewed from the 11th to the 18th month after completion.

The secretary should keep a monthly contraceptive index up-to-date so that fees are not lost. When patients attend, or telephone, for repeat prescriptions for oral contraceptives a check should be made to ensure that a claim form has been submitted. Claim forms should be submitted weekly.

**NATIONAL HEALTH SERVICE
CONTRACEPTIVE SERVICES
PART I**
(to be detached and given to the patient)

Patient's name ....

You have been accepted for contraceptive services by Dr ....
for the 12 months ending on .... 198 ....

Please bring this slip with you the first time you visit the doctor for contraceptive services
after that date. If you change to another doctor for contraceptive services please take this
slip with you
Form FP 1001

**NATIONAL HEALTH SERVICE
PART II
APPLICATION FOR CONTRACEPTIVE SERVICES**
(to be completed by the patient)

To Dr ....

NAME (surname first) AND ADDRESS	(Name in BLOCK LETTERS please)

Date of birth	NHS Number (if known)

Former name(s) (if applicable)	

I apply to be accepted for contraceptive services for 12 months

Have you received contraceptive services from another doctor in the last 12 months?
YES/NO

If YES, please give the doctor's name and address
Name: Dr ....
Address: ....
....

Signed: .... Date ....

*Delete whichever does not apply
Form FP 1001

PART III
(to be retained by the doctor)
CONTRACEPTIVE SERVICES

NAME (surname first) AND ADDRESS	Date accepted	
	Date claim sent to FPC	
	Renewal date	

Form FP 1001

Fig. 32.6 Form FP 1001.

NATIONAL HEALTH SERVICE   CONTRACEPTIVE SERVICES

PART I

(to be detached and given to the patient)

Patient's name ....

You have been accepted for contraceptive services by Dr. ....

for the 12 months ending on .... 198 ....

Please bring this slip with you the first time you visit the doctor for contraceptive services after that date. If you change to another doctor for contraceptive services please take this slip with you.

Form FP 1002

NATIONAL HEALTH SERVICE
PART II
FITTING OF INTRA-UTERINE DEVICE

(to be completed by the patient)

To Dr. ....

NAME (surname first) AND ADDRESS   (Name in BLOCK LETTERS please)

Date of birth	N.H.S. Number (if known)

Former name(s) (if applicable)

I have been advised to be fitted with an intra-uterine device.

Have you received contraceptive services from another doctor in the last 12 months?   *YES/NO*

If YES, please give the doctors's name and address

Name: Dr. ....

Address: ....

....

Signed: , ...   Date ....

*Delete whichever does not apply   Form FP 1002

PART III
(to be retained by the doctor)
FITTING OF INTRA-UTERINE DEVICE

NAME (surname first) AND ADDRESS		
	Date IUD fitted	
	Date claim sent to FPC	
	Renewal date	

Form FP 1002

Fig. 32.7 Form FP 1002.

Forms for cervical cytology

(see Chapter 36)

A cervical cytology examination is recommended for all women at the age of 35 and every three years thereafter or after a third pregnancy has been confirmed in a woman of any age. However, in an attempt to lessen the number of women who develop cancer of the cervix most doctors now are advising a first smear in all women soon after they start sexual activity or opportunistically at post-natal examination.

One other form is occasionally required relating to pregnancy and that is an abortion certificate (form HSA 1). This is not part of maternity services and the form is usually either initiated by the gynaecologist and sent to the GP for completion or sent by the GP to the gynaecologist with a referral letter. If the need for an abortion arises after the patient has been accepted for maternity services then form FP 24 must be submitted to the FPC as a claim for 'miscarriage'.

Diploma Questions

*Denotes an incomplete question

1 How would you, in general practice, deal with a telephone call from an expectant mother in labour?*

2 Write notes on the filing of obstetric records.*

3 State the documentation, office and general procedures necessary when patients attend general practice for contraceptive services.*

33

Infectious Diseases in General Practice

Immunity is the process by which living organisms acquire a protection against infections from bacteria or viruses by virtue of having come into contact with the bacteria or virus in question. When a child recovers from an attack of measles it has an immunity to measles and is therefore unlikely to acquire the infection again even though the organism causing it is no longer present. Immunity is not necessarily long-lasting. A common cold virus will leave man with an immunity for one or two weeks, whereas other infections may produce an immunity that is life-long. Furthermore immunity may be only relative and the development of an infection depends upon the balance between the degree of immunity of the host and the strength, or virulence of the infecting organism. This immunity depends upon the production in the host of certain substances which will attack further organisms or poisons and 'neutralize' them, and once the host has had an infection then further exposure to the infecting agent will produce a rapid rise in the quantity of these 'neutralizing' substances that are present. There are a wide range of these substances varying in type. Some are called antibodies and some antitoxins, but the details of the mechanisms are too complicated to be described here.

Some species of animals have a natural immunity to certain types of infection; man does not suffer from distemper and dogs do not suffer from measles. Infants acquire an immunity to some infections from their mothers, but this immunity usually passes off during the first year of life. It is also known that some external factors will affect the degree of immunity that a person has. Malnutrition or the absence of substances such as vitamin A in the diet will increase the susceptibility to certain infections, as will injury or exposure to cold. Changes in weather conditions will also cause a lowering in the degree of protection in some infections.

Man has paid particular attention to those infections which give a long-lasting immunity, because an artificially produced immunity to those infections will be equally long-lasting. One of the ways in which preventive medicine can play a part is by the artificial production of immunity in a person. This artificial immunity can be produced in two ways.

Active immunization is performed by the administration of the living organism which causes the disease, after it has been weakened in some way. *Passive immunization* consists of the administration of the dead organism or its altered poison, in sufficient quantity to produce immunity. Immunization or vaccination in the UK falls into two groups:

1 The protection of the community, resident in the UK, from diseases which are present in the UK or may be introduced.

2 The protection of individuals, who are travelling abroad, from conditions which are normally only present in other countries.

IMMUNIZATION FOR THE PROTECTION OF RESIDENTS

For the protection of residents in the UK active immunization is practised because this lasts for months or years, whereas passive immunization is normally only very temporary. The first person to practise active immunization in the UK was *Jenner (1749–1823)*. He was an English physician who recognized that the virus of cowpox would protect people from attacks of smallpox.

Routine immunization

The diseases for which routine immunization is advocated in the UK are diphtheria, whooping cough, tetanus, poliomyelitis, tuberculosis and measles. Immunization is performed by injection by hypodermic syringe or by pressure gun, by 'scratching' the substance through the surface of the skin (vaccination), or by taking it by mouth. The route of administration depends upon the substance being given. Where injection is concerned it is possible to give a number of different substances together, e.g. diphtheria, whooping cough and tetanus. The number of injections used and their spacing affects the degree of immunity produced, and it is up to the individual doctor to decide which method and routine he will use. The Secretary of State is advised on this matter by a standing medical committee, and they have advised a schedule of immunization which is followed by most doctors (see Table 33.1).

Table 33.1 Schedule of immunization.

Age of child	Vaccine	Dose and route
3–12 months	Three administrations: DTP[1] + OPV[2] 6–8 week interval DTP + OPV 4–6 month interval DTP + OPV	DTP injection OPV—3 drops orally
12–14 months	Measles immunization	Injection
First year at school	DT[3] + OPV booster	DT injection OPV—3 drops
10–13 years	BCG[4] for the tuberculin negative	Injection
Girls: 11–13 years	Rubella immunization	Injection
15–19 years or on leaving school	TT[5] + OPV	TT injection OPV—3 drops orally

1, DTP: diphtheria/tetanus/pertussis (whooping cough)—Triple vaccine; 2, OPV: oral poliomyelitis vaccine; 3, DT: diphtheria/tetanus vaccine; 4, BCG: tuberculosis vaccine (Bacille Calmette Guérin); 5, TT: tetanus toxoid

These schedules may be modified in a number of different ways. Sometimes the order in which the vaccines are given is varied and occasionally certain of the vaccines may be omitted on medical grounds, such as any patient with a temperature, active immunization during pregnancy, or some patients with a history of allergy or convulsions.

Routine immunizations are done by:

(a) the patient's family doctor or attached nurse or health visitor.

(b) the health authority through the child welfare clinic or the school health service (BCG is always, and rubella usually, given by the school health service).

Where these services are given by the family doctor the secretary will have a number of duties.

These will consist of:

1 the arrangement of appointments
2 ordering and storing the vaccines
3 preparing the necessary documents
4 sending records to the FPC.

The arrangement of appointments

These immunization procedures may be done in the course of the normal surgery or may be done at special 'mother and baby' sessions. Although the procedures are normally done very quickly it is important to allow sufficient time for them. They are often an opportunity for the mother of a new baby to ask questions about many other problems, and they also give the doctor a chance to check that the baby is developing normally. As well as noticing that the baby is well fed and contented he will observe whether the baby can see and hear normally, when it can lift its head, sit up, stand, etc.

When making the appointment it is a good policy to make a note in the appointment book indicating the procedure to be carried out. This will enable the secretary to check that the appropriate forms are ready when she gets out the medical records.

Vaccination and immunization procedures are not compulsory in the UK and it often requires positive action from doctor and secretary to ensure that they are done. A good time to do this is when the mother attends for her final post-natal examination or when the baby is first registered with form FP 1. This is usually carried out at about six weeks after the birth of the baby and it is then often convenient to make the appointment for the first immunization procedure. Sometimes this examination is carried out at the hospital and where this is the case some method may be adopted by which a 'reminder' card is sent out to the mothers of all new babies registered with the practice if they have not attended for immunization at the appropriate time. This may be done by keeping a small loose-leaf book and entering the names and addresses of all new babies registering with the practice. If they attend for first immunization at 12 weeks the name is crossed out. If they fail to attend a reminder card is sent. In spite of these efforts some babies will not be brought to the surgery and this may be because the parents object to the immunization or because the baby is being immunized by the local baby clinic. The chief disadvantages of this latter course are that the family doctor loses touch, he does not know what has been done and he is no longer seeing his patient regularly. For this reason most doctors endeavour to have the babies brought to the surgery.

In country districts it may be necessary for the doctor to visit in order to immunize and under these circumstances the secretary must see that everything he needs is ready to go with him.

Lastly the secretary must see that the mother does not leave the surgery without the next appointment being made.

Ordering the vaccines

The secretary will not only have to order the vaccines so that a supply is ready for the patient, but she will also have to see that they are properly stored and do not get out of date.

Under Section 26 of the NHS Act these vaccines may be supplied free of charge to the doctor:
1 Diphtheria, tetanus and pertussis vaccines, separately or combined, polio vaccine, measles vaccine and rubella vaccine are all obtained through the District Community Physician services in single ampoules or multi-dose vials.
2 Cholera, typhoid and paratyphoid A and B vaccines supplied separately, combined or combined with tetanus vaccine may be got on prescription for each patient.

Storing the vaccines

All the above vaccines should be stored in a refrigerator at a temperature between 2° and 10°C (36° to 50°F) and should be protected from the light. Poliomyelitis oral vaccine remains potent for six months if kept in the unfrozen state at a temperature of under 10°C. At room temperature, under 25°C, it will keep for two weeks. The expiry dates of triple and combined vaccines are printed on the box and again should only be relied on if the vaccine is kept at a temperature below 10°C. These vaccines should not, therefore, be kept in the 'freezing' compartment and should be dated by the secretary when they are received. The store must be inspected periodically to ensure that none is out of date, and care should be taken to use the oldest stock first.

Documentation

When immunization procedures are carried out it is important they are carefully and accurately recorded. It is often necessary to know the state of protection of a patient and this can only be done when the proper records are kept. Where the routine immunization of babies is concerned, the record envelope should contain either form FP 7A (male) or form FP 8A (female) (Northern Ireland HS 26A and 27A) which can be filled in by the secretary as each immunization is done. Parents may also carry an individual record for their child and this should be completed at each attendance. Where the patient is an adult then an entry will be made on the record card by the doctor. The record of immunization against tetanus is particularly important and in many cases the injection itself is given at a factory, surgery or in the casualty department of a hospital after an accident. The hospital or factory should then notify a doctor when one of his patient's has been immunized in this manner and an appropriate entry will be made on the card. Some doctors like to have a special identification for record envelopes and they may 'tag' them with a piece of coloured sticky tape when tetanus immunization has been completed.

All the vaccinations and immunizations listed under the schedule of immunizations for children (see Table 33.1), and certain others for travel abroad, qualify for a fee to be paid to the doctor by the FPC. A full list of the vaccinations and immunizations covered by these arrangements and sections 27 and 28 of the Statement of Fees and Allowances (SFA). This is periodically revised and should be kept in a convenient place for reference.

Procedures for which FPCs will pay these fees are:

1 Diphtheria, pertussis and tetanus vaccine to pre-school children.
2 Diphtheria and tetanus to pre-school children.
3 Diphtheria for staff in hospitals at risk.
4 Tetanus for children aged 15 to 19 or on or after leaving school.
5 Poliomyelitis to all people under 40 and all travellers to countries outside Europe and North America.
6 Measles to children from 9 months to 15 years.
7 Rubella to girls between their 11th and 14th birthdays.
8 Anthrax to workers at special risk.
9 Typhoid and paratyphoid to hospital staff at special risk and travellers to all countries except North America and North Europe.
10 Rabies to workers at special risk.
11 Cholera to travellers to listed countries.
12 Hepatitis A to travellers to any region with poor standards of food and water hygiene.

Arrangements for sending for children and carrying out documentation are fully computerized in many areas. The computer prepares a list of children and the required immunization procedure. The practice is supplied with a duplicate list and the times of their appointments. This list is marked to show the procedure has been carried out, signed by the doctor and then returned to the computer staff who prepare the next schedule and programme it. In these cases there is no need to complete individual FP 73s and this saves a lot of clerical time and effort. Form FP 73 (Fig. 33.1) has to be returned to the FPC as soon as it is completed, in any case in which an immunization procedure has been carried out under the NHS except where a computerized program is operating.

Immunization against other infectious diseases

Influenza vaccine. This is available for the protection of people who are particularly at risk from an attack of influenza. It is usually confined to those persons who are suffering from a chronic disease and to whom an attack of influenza may prove to be either fatal or a seriously aggravating factor. It is prescribed individually on form FP 10 for each NHS patient and is usually obtained in a disposable syringe containing 0.25 ml. It may be stored at room temperature (below 20°C or 68°F) until the expiry date shown, but must not be frozen. If the doctor immunizes a patient with vaccine that he supplies himself he should submit a prescription to the FPC for that patient and he will receive a fee.

NATIONAL HEALTH SERVICE

Form FP **73** (Rev)

Family Practitioner Committee

VACCINATION AND IMMUNISATION

Part I

Where appropriate both parts of the form should be completed by making "ticks" in the boxes which apply. Both parts should be sent intact to the FPC

Patient's surname (Block Capitals)——————————— Forenames————————

Vaccinated as (a) ☐ a routine measure   and NHS No.————————

(b) ☐ belonging to a group exposed to special risk (as in List of Fees)

(c) ☐ a traveller to————————————(name of country or place)

(d) ☐ recommended by the MOH of the area during an outbreak of disease

I certify that the patient has been vaccinated as indicated in Part II below.

Date———————————— Signature of Doctor————————

Assistant/locum acting on behalf of Doctor————————

For use by FPC			Name and address of doctor or partnership
D P T Polio Smallpox Measles Rubella Other			Drs. Drury, Cowan Blacker & Bax 27, New Road, Bromsgrove, Worcs.

Part II for Local Health Authority

Patient's surname (Block Capitals) ——————— Forenames————————

Address ————————————————————

Home Address if a Temporary Resident ————————————

MALE ☐   FEMALE ☐   School———————— Date of Birth————————

Vaccination		Date of Primary Vaccination	Date of Revaccination	Batch No.	Date of Inspection	
					Successful	Unsuccessful
Smallpox	1st attempt					
	2nd attempt					
	3rd attempt					

Please enter procedure in boxes 1, 2 or 3		Dose	Date	Date of Reinforcing Dose	Batch No.	
	1.	1st				
DPT DTPol DT DP Tet Per Pol(I) Pol(o) Measles Rubella		2nd				Please specify any complication following Smallpox Vaccination
		3rd				
	2.	1st				
		2nd				
		3rd				
	3.	1st				
Other (Please signify as in List of fees)		2nd				
		3rd				

Name and address of Doctor or Partnership

Drs. Drury, Cowan Blacker & Bax
27, New Road,
Bromsgrove, Worcs.

56-5347 B. & S. Ltd.

Fig. 33.1 Form FP 73.

Tetanus vaccine. This is given, either as a 'booster' dose to a person who has already been immunized against tetanus and who needs extra protection as the result of a wound, or as a full course of three injections to an adult who has not previously been immunized. The local health authority does not need to be notified of immunizations with these two vaccines. A fee is claimed on form FP 73. A booster dose is required at between five and ten year intervals.

IMMUNIZATION OF TRAVELLERS

There are five diseases against which it is often necessary to immunize individuals who are travellers abroad. They are immunized, either because there is a particular risk of contracting these infections in certain countries, or because an international certificate (Fig 33.2) indicating that immunization has been done is necessary before entry is allowed.

IMPORTANT: See the Rules and Notes overleaf .

Date	Signature and professional status of vaccinator *Signature et titre du vaccinateur*	Approved stamp *Cachet autorisé*
1 3 January 1986	1 *M. Bryant General Practitioner*	2
2 2 February 1986	2 *M. Bryant General Practitioner*	
3	3	4
4	4	
5	5	6
6	6	
7	7	8
8	8	

Fig. 33.2 Certificate of vaccination against cholera.

Typhoid fever and paratyphoid fever A and B. Immunization against these infections is usually performed with a vaccine (TAB) containing organisms killed by heat. The dose varies, but, for an adult, usually consists of two doses at an interval of four to six weeks followed by a third dose six to twelve months after the second. Where there is a continued risk a reinforcing dose should be given yearly.

Cholera. Two doses are given at an interval of one or two weeks. Immunity is short and lasts only about six months.

Yellow fever. This can only be given at special centres, a list of which is given in the *Notice to Travellers* issued by the DHSS and Department of Health for Scotland. One dose is given and protection lasts for 10 years.

Infectious hepatitis. Immunization is required for all travellers to any region with poor standards of food and water hygiene. This applies particularly to people visiting rural and deprived urban areas of developing countries. The preparations are obtained on prescription, and as protection only lasts five to six months the injection should be given as close to the date of departure as possible.

Documentation

This consists of completion of the international certificates where necessary. These may be obtained by the patient from the shipping or air line, from the travel agent, or the secretary may obtain a stock from the FPC. She should see that the front page of the book or certificate is completed with patient's name, date of birth and sex and signed by the patient before presenting it to the doctor. The doctor is entitled to charge a fee for completing these 'international certificates'.

NOTIFICATION OF INFECTIOUS DISEASE, OR FOOD POISONING

Keeping abreast with the growth of other medical knowledge has been the development of preventive medicine, and for 2000 years man has fought against the great tides of infection which have threatened to overrun him. The plague, the black death, cholera and smallpox have, in turn, forced his attention towards this problem. As long ago as 1518 the first rough attempt at a system of notification of infectious diseases was developed. But it was not until the middle of the nineteenth century that three great waves of cholera in Britain forced legislation upon us. In 1889 the Infectious Disease Notification Act was introduced, and although at first it applied only to a limited number of conditions, it opened the door to the production of proper analysis of the incidence of infection and measures for the control of it. This Act makes it compulsory for the doctor to notify specified diseases to the local Community Physician. Cases of anthrax contracted in a factory must also be notified by the doctor to the Chief Inspector of Factories.

The complete list of notifiable diseases is:

Acute encephalitis	Leptospirosis	Tetanus
Acute meningitis	Malaria	Tuberculosis
Acute poliomyelitis	Marburg disease	Typhoid fever
Anthrax	Measles	Typhus
Cholera	Ophthalmia	Viral haemorrhagic
Diphtheria	neonatorum	diseases
Dysentery (amoebic or	Paratyphoid fever	Whooping cough
bacillary)	Plague	Yellow fever
Infective jaundice	Relapsing fever	Food poisoning or
Lassa fever	Scarlet fever	suspected food poisoning
Leprosy	Smallpox	

The purpose of notification is to allow quick recognition of the type, pattern and spread of an outbreak by the authorities; contact with infection to be traced where necessary and measures for prevention to be adopted. As a result of notification local health authorities publish the figures, and summaries for the British Isles can be published from figures collected centrally.

A doctor is statutorily required to notify any of these diseases and is paid a small fee for doing so. Books of certificates may be obtained from the local District Community Physican and can be partly completed by the secretary. Where the patient has been seen at home the doctor will indicate on his visiting list that a notification has to be made and the secretary can then prepare the form and present it to the doctor together with the patient's notes.

34
Drugs and Dressings

The GP spends a large part of each day talking, listening and writing, but the tools of his trade are the drugs and instruments that he uses in his surgery or carries with him in his bag. Some of these are needed only rarely, others are used many times each day and his secretary should be able to help him with the care and maintenance of them.

DRUGS AND PRESCRIPTIONS

The supply, distribution and storage of drugs are controlled by a series of Acts of Parliament, designed to control their sale and to reduce the danger to life from sale by unqualified people. The general principles of these Acts which may affect the doctor's secretary are as follows:

Medicines Act, 1968. This divides medicinal products into three classes: Prescription only medicines (POM), Pharmacy medicines (P), and General Sale List medicines (GSL). Prescription only medicines are available only on the prescription of a practitioner, i.e. doctor, dentist, veterinary surgeon or veterinary practitioner. Pharmacy medicines may be sold over the counter in pharmacies, under the supervision of a pharmacist, but not from any other retail outlet. General Sale List medicines may be sold from any retail outlet which can be closed so as to exclude the public, or from automatic machines.

The Misuse of Drugs Act, 1971. This came into effect on 1 July 1973. It controls the use and supply of named drugs of addiction or habituation, including certain appetite suppressants. Drugs in this category are termed 'controlled drugs' and the older name 'dangerous drugs' should no longer be used.

Limited list. In 1985 regulations were approved by Parliament to limit the range of drugs prescribed in the NHS. The groups of drugs involved were antacids, cough mixtures, laxatives, analgesics, sleeping tablets and sedatives and vitamins. In each group there is a list of drugs that are prescribable; all others are not. Most of these drugs are identified by their generic or proper 'chemical name' and the proprietary or 'trade' brand is not prescribable.

Prescribing

Prescriptions for controlled drugs or prescription only medicines must be signed by the prescriber and contain his address, the date, and the name, address and age (if under 12) of the person for whose treatment it is given. In addition to this, prescriptions for controlled drugs (except for certain exempt categories of controlled drugs), must contain certain particulars in the prescriber's own handwriting: the date; patient's name and address; dose to be taken; form and strength of the preparation; the total quantity of the preparation or the number of dosage units (which must be written in words as well as figures).

Drugs prescribed under the NHS will be ordered on form FP 10. Prescriptions issued privately for patients on the NHS, or for private patients, are normally written on paper that has the doctor's name and address printed as a heading. It may be asked why NHS patients ever need private prescriptions. There are occasions when this will be necessary and these include:
(a) drugs prescribed by a doctor consulted privately other than the doctor with whom the patient is registered,
(b) medicinal preparations advertised directly to the public,
(c) prescriptions issued for some foodstuffs and certain other preparations.

Prescription charges

Patients provided with pharmaceutical services are liable to pay the chemist (or the doctor in the case of a dispensing doctor) fees in respect of appliances or drugs as set out by the Department of Health from time to time. The back of a prescription form has to be completed in the appropriate section by patients claiming exemption from these payments. These include children under 16 or in full-time education, men aged over 65 and women aged over 60, expectant mothers and mothers of children under one year of age, patients with permanent fistulas, endocrine disease, epilepsy or a continuing physical disability which stops them leaving home without help. Also exempt are any patients holding DHSS exemption certificates such as those on supplementary benefit and patients who have bought a prepayment certificate (FP 96). Where there is doubt about whether a patient should pay or not he can obtain a receipt form (FP 57) which can later be used to obtain a refund if he is entitled to one.

Patients may pay in advance for a three-month or one-year supply of drugs by obtaining a 'season ticket' from the FPC. This may be cheaper than paying for each item on each prescription.

It is possible to direct the chemist, when writing a private prescription, to repeat the prescription a stated number of times. This cannot be done with NHS prescriptions but FP 10 forms may be issued that are dated at intervals when the doctor considers the treatment will last longer than the first supply of medicine. Repeats cannot be ordered on prescriptions for controlled drugs.

Bulk prescribing. When a doctor is responsible for treating at least ten people resident in a school or institution he may issue a prescription for a bulk supply of certain preparations.

The prescription. Prescriptions are issued by the FPC in blocks. Each form is stamped with the name, number and address of the issuing doctor. Complete

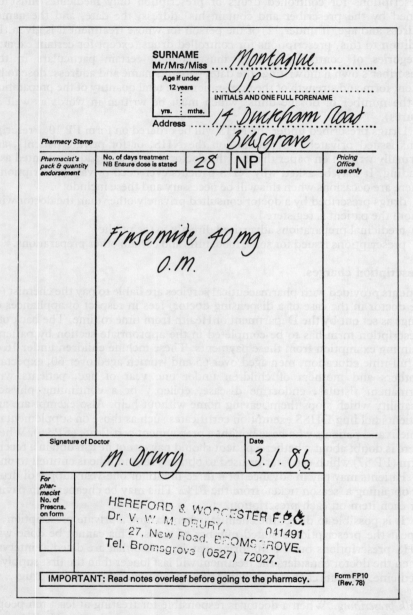

SURNAME
Mr/Mrs/Miss ...... *Montague*

Age if under
12 years ...... *JP*

INITIALS AND ONE FULL FORENAME

yrs. : mths.

Address ...... *14 Duckham Road*

Bromsgrave

Pharmacy Stamp

Pharmacist's
pack & quantity
endorsement

No. of days treatment
NB Ensure dose is stated   28   NP

Pricing
Office
use only

Frusemide 40mg
O.M.

Signature of Doctor

M. Drury

Date

3. 1. 86

For
pharmacist
No. of
Prescns.
on form

HEREFORD & WORCESTER F.P.C.
Dr. V. W. M. DRURY,
27, New Road, BROMSGROVE.
Tel. Bromsgrove (0527) 72027.
041491

IMPORTANT: Read notes overleaf before going to the pharmacy.

Form FP10
(Rev. 78)

Fig. 34.1 Prescription form FP 10.

prescriptions must be carefully looked after to prevent the risk of drugs falling into the wrong hands and blank prescription forms should be guarded equally carefully. They should be kept in a locked cupboard and any loss reported to the police. New prescription forms are ordered from the FPC (or the Health Board in Scotland).

Each prescription has space for the name and address of the patient, the title (Mr, Mrs or Miss indicated by crossing out the inappropriate ones) and the date of birth for children under the age of 12 years. These should be completed accurately. The pharmacist records the recipient's name on the container and will check against the age that a suitable sized dose for that child was prescribed. There are two boxes that should be completed at the top of the form. One records the number of days of treatment required and is useful when several drugs are included on one prescription, and the second should be marked with an 'x' if the doctor does *not* want the name of the medicine written on the container. Each prescription form must be dated, and must be signed by the doctor. Any alterations to the prescription should be initialled by the doctor.

Some practices keep a prescription form with the name and address of the patient inside the medical record envelope for completion at the time of the consultation by the doctor. It may be the secretary's responsibility to ensure that one is present in the notes.

Repeat prescriptions. Many patients are on maintenance treatment and require repeat prescriptions at intervals. These repeat prescriptions make up nearly one-half of all prescriptions issued and their handling takes much time and needs much care.

Some requests come in by telephone, some by the receipt from the patient of a 'repeat prescription card' (Fig. 34.2) and some by a request 'over the counter'. Whichever way they are dealt with it is essential that the details should also be entered on the patient's record card and a system devised that makes it absolutely clear to the secretary or receptionist how many repeat prescriptions may be issued between visits to the doctor.

Telephone requests are numerous, so much so that in some practices an extra telephone line is required. Messages must be recorded accurately in the day book (marked with a 'P' to distinguish them from other calls) and include the full name and address of the patient and the details of the prescription needed. The secretary should extract the medical record envelope and may complete the name and address of the patient and date the prescription ready for the doctor to complete. In some practices staff will be trained to enter the names, dose and quantity of the drugs on the prescription form and in the notes, but it must be done with meticulous accuracy, checked carefully by the doctor and is not allowed in the case of controlled drugs. The patient must be told when the prescription will be ready for him. The secretary should remember that repeat prescriptions are issued to help, not hinder, patients and they must be flexible, especially when patients run out of urgent drugs.

Sometimes a practice keeps a 'repeat prescription register', a list of patients who may have (and how many times) repeat prescriptions. In this case the request must be checked against the register.

Repeat prescription cards are either posted to the practice with a stamped addressed envelope or handed in at the reception desk. They contain a card,

1. Take this card with you if you go to see your doctor at the surgery.

2. Take this card with you if you have to go into hospital and show it to the doctor there.

3. When the card is completely filled up it will go in your records in the surgery.

4. When your medicine needs to be renewed and you do not wish to see your doctor put this card in an unsealed envelope addressed to yourself.

5. Take or send the card and envelope to the surgery.

6. Even if you feel quite well you should arrange to see your doctor by the review date if one has been entered on the card.

7. The prescription for medicine will be ready for you to collect at the surgery the next day. If you put a stamp on the envelope, it will be posted to you.

8. Do not fill in the name of any medicine *yourself*.

9. In an emergency, when you cannot immediately obtain a prescription for a medicine you have run out of and need to take, you should consult a pharmacist. In certain circumstances (particularly if you show him this card) he may be able to supply you with sufficient medicine for up to 5 days' treatment even though you have no prescription. If this happens, you may be asked to pay not just a normal prescription fee, but the full price for any medicines supplied. If you have to obtain such an emergency supply, tell your doctor at your next visit.

WINTHROP
PRACTITIONER SERVICE

Prescription Record Card

Name _____

Address _____

Tel. No. _____

PRESCRIPTION and DOSE	ORDERED BY (Sig. & Stamp)	DATES of FIRST SCRIPT, RENEWAL and AMOUNTS											REVIEW DATE
1 Bendrofluazide 5mg daily 50	M Jones	1-11-85	50	19-12-85	50								Review every
2 Atenolol 100mg daily 50	M. Jones	1-11-85	50	19-12-85	50								third script.
3													
4													
5													

Fig. 34.2 Repeat prescription renewal card.

designed to fit the Post Office Preferred (POP) envelope, bearing the doctor's name and address, instructions on how to use the card, and spaces for the names of the medicines, the dose, the quantity to be supplied and the number of times the prescription can be issued before the patient is seen again by the doctor; the latter must be checked each time. The procedure for dealing with them is the same as for other repeat prescriptions. The medical record envelope is extracted from the file, as much of the prescription is completed by the secretary as the doctor allows, the details are entered on the medical record card and it is then put ready for the doctor to deal with. The repeat prescription card has the added virtue of allowing other doctors concerned, perhaps when the patient is attending hospital, or is on holiday, to know what medication is in use. One of the most popular programs for practice computers deals with repeat prescriptions. Those patients entitled to these are entered and their drugs are printed on to a special prescription form 'FP 10 (comp.)'. Programs have been devised which recall patients at appropriate intervals, can identify patients who are not taking the correct number of tablets and warn when a prescription contains drugs that may interact with each other.

Repeat prescriptions that are being collected at the reception desk must be kept safely and not in a place where patients can help themselves. In the case of private prescriptions a fee is chargeable. Some patients may require help with the completion of the back of the prescription if they claim exemption from prescription charges. Some practices may keep a 'drug card' in the notes showing the current medication of that patient.

The drug cupboard

Every surgery will have a drug cupboard and under the Controlled Drug Regulations all drugs in the custody of an authorized person must be kept in a locked receptacle which can be opened only by him or some other authorized person. (This regulation also applies to the doctor's bag.) In this cupboard may be kept a small stock of drugs such as morphine, pethidine, sleeping tablets, etc., for use by the doctor in emergency when they cannot be obtained in time by prescription.

Controlled drugs register

It is the doctor's duty to keep a register, in a specially provided book, on the same premises as the drugs. In this book are written in ink details showing the quantity of drugs obtained by the doctor, the quantity supplied to any person by the doctor and the names and addresses. The register is inspected periodically, usually by the Regional Medical Officer.

It is the responsibility of the doctor to ensure that the CD (controlled drug) cupboard is locked and that the keys are put safely away. The secretary should see that this has been done.

Emergency medicines

All GPs have to provide drugs or certain appliances that might be needed urgently before a supply can be obtained. These are ordered by the doctor from an appropriate supplier and are checked against the delivery note before being locked away.

The doctor is allowed to claim a fee for any vaccine, anaesthetic or injection that he supplies. This is done by writing out a prescription (FP 10) for each patient, endorsing it with the pack size, and *not* collecting a prescription charge and submitting them each month to the FPC with form FP 34D.

In Scotland the arrangements are slightly different and the doctor is allowed to issue an order (GP 10A for Scotland) for a stock to the chemist and thus keep a small surgery stock of drugs and dressings for immediate treatment.

Drug companies

Many drugs and medicines that the doctor has in the surgery are brought to him as samples by representatives of the manufacturing drug companies. Pharmaceutical firms have three methods of bringing their products to the attention of the doctor. These are:

1 advertisements in medical journals

2 advertising material sent by post
3 visits by representatives

Most large firms send a representative to visit doctors at intervals of a few months. They usually attend during surgery hours and like to talk to the doctor for about five minutes about the products of their firm. If it should be inconvenient for a doctor to see them in the middle of a busy surgery, they are prepared to wait or make an appointment for another occasion. If the doctor is unable to see them they will often leave literature and samples of their products. They can be useful and helpful to the doctor by informing him of new developments in the drug industry, and the secretary should help them to do their job properly. The storage and disposal of the samples they leave is often a problem. These are intended for use by the doctor, either as a trial of a drug new to him, or as an emergency supply of a frequently used preparation. Any dangerous or scheduled drugs left will be locked in the cupboard and other drugs kept in a drawer or cupboard. (All controlled drug samples must be entered in the CD register.) There is a strong tendency for a large collection of unwanted samples to accumulate and these constitute a disposal problem.

The dispensing practice

Every doctor supplies medicines to patients at some time or other, but certain practices dispense all medicines to patients and others only supply medicines required for emergency treatment.

Dispensing practices are situated in rural areas and cover approximately 5% of the population. The doctor may be paid in one of two ways:
(a) as a 'capitation fee' for each patient registered with him
(b) as a 'drug tariff' where he receives a payment for each prescription dispensed.

In the capitation fee system there is also an additional payment for certain drugs and appliances and for prescriptions to certain classes of patients such as temporary residents and maternity patients. In either system the doctor writes a prescription for a patient and dispenses the medicines against it.

Special administrative duties relating to dispensing practices are:
1 A prescription book is kept showing all medicines dispensed. There must be a daily check that an FP 10 has been written for every NHS entry and that private prescriptions are entered on the patient's record.
2 Every prescription must be endorsed with the pack size from which the medicine was dispensed.
3 Each doctor's prescription must be checked, counted and a written record kept before they are sent in a separate bundle to the pricing authority together with a signed form FP 34D.
4 All deliveries of drugs have to be checked against delivery notes, against invoices and against statements.
5 Appropriate prescription charges must be collected for each item or appliance prescribed.
6 There must be an entry book for payments and some safe storage place for money.
7 The dispensary must be kept secure against theft.

Dressings

The quantity and variety of dressings kept in the surgery will vary according to the practice. In a country district, far removed from hospital, a large number of wounds, ulcers and rashes may need to be dressed by the doctor and in other practices very few dressings may be done. Lists of dressings available can be found in the Drug Tariff issued to all doctors and in the back pages of *MIMS*.

It will not be the duty of the secretary to administer drugs and apply dressings unless she has had a special training for this purpose. It will be her job to make sure that there is always a sufficient stock of the various dressings that the doctor commonly uses and that containers in his medical bag, his consulting room or treatment room are kept full. She may also have to buy quantities of dressings from time to time, or, in Scotland, collect these on prescriptions form GP 10A. Generally speaking it is more economical to buy in the larger size packs. The doctor's secretary is often regarded by the general public as a nurse and she is likely to be asked to give advice on a range of problems. A lot of these are often only common sense matters which she will gain experience in whilst doing her job, and many of the simple tasks such as temperature taking and simple dressings can be undertaken after a little training from the doctor. A Red Cross or St John's Ambulance Association course will be of the greatest help and every medical secretary in general practice or in hospital should be encouraged to take one.

Diploma Questions

*Denotes an incomplete question

1 As a medical secretary in a large group practice describe fully the possible procedures to be adopted when dealing with the following: a request for a repeat prescription.*

2 As a senior medical secretary in a busy general practice describe in detail the procedure you would follow to ensure that adequate medical and non-medical supplies are always available.*

35

The Doctor's Equipment

MEDICAL EQUIPMENT USED IN THE SURGERY

The equipment that the doctor uses will depend partly on his own skill and assessment of his duties and responsibilities and partly on the proximity of his practice to hospitals and specialists. It is possible to divide it into two groups.

1 *Equipment needed for diagnosis*. This is an essential part of every doctor's practice and will be used in the surgery and the patient's home: it will be fairly standard from one practice to another.

2 *Equipment needed for treatment*. The type of equipment included here will vary according to the factors mentioned already and only part of it will be carried by the doctor on his visits.

Diagnostic equipment

The diagnostic equipment, such as stethoscope and thermometer will be carried with him in his bag, although duplicate instruments may also be kept in the surgery to save time. Some equipment, diagnostic and otherwise, is bulky and only used on special occasions and where this is so it is kept in the surgery and only taken out when needed.

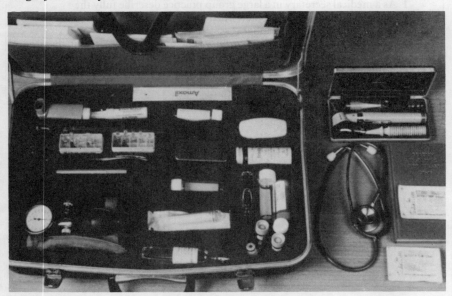

Fig. 35.1 A doctor's bag.

A list of the most commonly used instruments is now given and the more detailed care of them is described later.

Stethoscope
Thermometer
Sphygmomanometer
Torch
Auriscope
Ophthalmoscope
Peak flow gauge
Throat swab
Syringes for taking blood
Hypodermic needles
Sterile bottles — labelled, for
  specimens of urine

Specimen bottles — labelled, for
  blood, sputum, faeces etc.
Tongue depressors
Patella hammer
Tuning fork
Hat pin   } for testing skin
Cotton wool   } sensation
Tape measures
Finger stalls
Gloves
Lubricant for gloves
Urine testing equipment
Cleaning solutions, spirit, cetrimide
  etc.

Equipment for diagnosis or treatment

Bowls and kidney dishes
Proctoscope
Vaginal speculum
Nasal speculum

Trocar and cannula
Head-lamp
Nebulizer and pump

Equipment used for treatment

Ear syringe
Bowls and kidney dishes
Scalpels
Scissors

Forceps
Probes and other minor surgical
  instruments
Suture material

PRINCIPLES OF STERILIZATION

Before dealing with the care of these instruments in detail it is necessary to understand the general principles of sterilization.

In order to diminish the risk of introducing bacterial infection to a patient it is important to ensure that the highest standards of cleanliness and sterility are maintained. Every part of the doctor's consulting rooms must be kept spotlessly clean and attention must be paid to the waiting room as well as the examination room. Similarly, whenever the secretary has touched a patient, or an instrument that has come into contact with a patient, she should wash her hands thoroughly. (This constant washing may produce dry, sore hands and a lotion or cream should be used to prevent this occurring.)

Normal, healthy, human skin is an effective barrier to bacterial infection and instruments that come into contact solely with the patient's skin need to be clean but not sterile. When the skin is broken, i.e. by wound, ulcer or injection, bacteria may be introduced into the bloodstream and cause serious disease, thus any instrument or dressing coming into contact with broken skin should be sterile. Similarly the mouth, eyes, vagina and other orifices of the body present portals for the introduction of infection and any instrument used in these regions should be sterile.

All microorganisms can be killed by exposure to sufficient heat for a period of time. The amount of heat and the length of time necessary will vary according to the type of organisms and the way in which the heat is applied. For example, spores will resist boiling for several hours; steam under pressure is more effective than dry heat, and so on.

Methods of sterilization

There are four methods of sterilization which can be used in the doctor's surgery.
1 Boiling
2 Dry heat
3 Autoclaving
4 Cold sterilization

Boiling. This is the method most commonly used. It is cheap and convenient but has the disadvantages that it will not kill certain spores or viruses and that the steam produced may cause damage to decorations. It is suitable for:
(a) Syringes, other than those used for intravenous injection or the collection of blood samples
(b) Blunt, metal instruments
(c) Enamel or stainless-steel bowls and dishes
(d) Soft rubber goods.

The sterilizer should be half-filled with cold water, brought to the boil, and the instruments should then be boiled for 10 minutes. The instruments should be removed with a pair of sterile forceps and placed in a previously sterilized container. They will remain sterile once they have cooled if they are left exposed to the air.

Unless distilled water is used there will be a gradual accumulation of scale on the inside of the sterilizer and this should be removed weekly by boiling for one hour after the addition of four ounces of vinegar or using a small quantity of descaling fluid.

Dry heat sterilizing. The dry heat sterilizer can be used to sterilize all the items which boiling will sterilize and will deal with sharp instruments without causing blunting by corrosion.

The sterilizer may be pre-set for both time and temperature. Thus soft rubber goods may be sterilized at 100°C and syringes at 160°C. It is possible to sterilize quantities of syringes or instruments together and, by using the time control, at times when the surgery is not in use.

Instruments and syringes can be sterilized at 160°C for 60 minutes, but should be left in the sterilizer during the time it takes for the oven to heat up and cool down. Syringes treated in this manner will be suitable for intravenous injection.

Autoclaving. The autoclave is a steam pressure-cooker and is the most efficient method of sterilization. Contents should be sterilized by autoclaving for 10 minutes at 120°C. The material to be sterilized must be loosely wrapped in porous material such as surgical towels or special crêpe-paper packs. It may be left as individual packs or put in a small drum or tin and autoclaved inside this. The lid or air-vents of any metal container must be open during autoclaving to allow steam to enter, and closed when autoclaving is completed.

Cold sterilization. This depends upon the immersion of the instrument in a chemical solution inside an airtight container. A number of germicidal solutions are available and the manufacturer's instructions must be accurately followed.

This method is suitable for sterilizing small metal instruments and hard rubber materials.

CARE AND USE OF INSTRUMENTS AND EQUIPMENT

Diagnostic equipment

Stethoscope

This instrument is used for listening to the heart and breath sounds, to the pulse whilst the blood pressure is being taken and to the foetal heart. No special care is needed apart from checking that the doctor is not without one when he leaves the surgery.

Thermometer

The thermometer is graduated in degrees centigrade. The average normal temperature is 37°C. Fractions of degrees are indicated by small lines and whole degrees by longer lines. There is now available a thermometer connected to a dial which works on the principle of a thermocouple and can register the temperature in about five seconds.

The temperature may be taken in the mouth (oral temperature), in the armpit (axillary temperature) or in the rectum (rectal temperature).

The oral method is used for adults and older children unless they are unable to breathe through their nose. The thermometer should be placed under the patient's tongue, at the side of the mouth with the lips closed, and left in place for three minutes. The oral method should not be used if the patient has recently had a hot drink.

The axillary method is used for smaller children. The thermometer is placed in the armpit and the arm crossed over the chest. The thermometer should be left in place for five minutes.

The rectal method is used for infants or unconscious patients and should only be performed by trained nurses.

Reading the thermometer. The light should be behind the person reading the thermometer, who holds it between right thumb and fore-finger by the end opposite to the mercury bulb. When the thermometer is slowly rotated back and forth the head of the mercury column can be seen and the point at which it lies on the scale can be noted.

The thermometer will then be shaken down to 36°C by wrist movements and then rinsed under a cold tap and wiped before being replaced in its container. Never wash a thermometer under a hot tap. The disinfectant should be wiped off on a pledget of clean cotton wool before the thermometer is placed in the patient's mouth.

The doctor will always carry a thermometer with him on his rounds and this may be in a spirit-proof case which needs refilling from time to time. In the surgery thermometers are often kept in small jars or tubes containing suitable germicides such as Lysol, spirit, cetrimide or chlorhexidine. There must be sufficient of this to cover the part which has been in the patient's mouth and these jars will need periodical 'topping up'. A rectal thermometer should be labelled with adhesive tape and a supply of spare thermometers should always be kept in the surgery.

Taking the pulse. The pulse is the distension felt in an artery produced by the wave of blood pressure caused by the heart beat. It is normally felt at the wrist. It should be located with the first two or three fingers (not the thumb) on the inside of the wrist just above the thumb. The second hand of a watch should be looked at for half a minute and the pulse beats counted. The number of beats is then multiplied by 2 to give the pulse rate. This is normally between 60 and 80 in an adult. In children it is normally higher.

Taking the respiration rate. This is the number of breaths taken in one minute. It should be observed without the patient being aware. It is normally 15 to 20 in an adult and faster in children.

Sphygmomanometer

This instrument is used for measuring the blood pressure. It consists of a rubber bag enclosed in a cuff. The bag is inflated either by pressure on a rubber bulb or electrically by a pump. In the former the pressure is recorded either by the height of a column of mercury (manometer) or by a needle and dial (anaeroid). The electronic sphygmomanometer registers the pressure digitally and may print it out. The secretary may be trained to take a patient's blood pressure. Considerable practice is necessary in order to become familiar with the sounds heard, but the basic principles are as follows:

The blood pressure of a patient is normally taken in the sitting or standing position.

1 The cuff is wound firmly around the upper arm above the elbow joint and secured by tucking the end in or using the hook provided. Care is taken to ensure that there is no clothing underneath the cuff and none that is tight around the arm above.

2 The chest piece of the stethoscope is then laid on the front aspect of the elbow joint and the cuff inflated with the valve on the bulb closed. As the pressure rises a thumping sound is heard which disappears as the inflation occurs. At this point the artery underneath the chest-piece of the stethoscope is fully compressed.

3 The valve is then slowly opened and the pressure gradually reduced. At a certain point, known as the systolic pressure point, the sound reappears. A note is made of the figure at which this appears.

4 The pressure continues to fall and the sound will gradually disappear. The

point just before the complete disappearance of sound is known as the diastolic pressure.

5 The bag is deflated and the cuff removed from the patient's arm.

The blood pressure is expressed as

$$\frac{\text{systolic pressure in mm of mercury}}{\text{diastolic pressure in mm of mercury}} \quad \text{e.g.} \quad \frac{120}{70}$$

Sphygmomanometers are cleaned with a duster or damp cloth, they require to be maintained carefully if they are to remain accurate. Dirt gets into the mercury manometer and sticks to the inside of the glass tube, so the spring-loaded cap holding down the top of the tube should be lifted and the tube taken out and cleaned with a long pipe-cleaner. A sticky label with the date on should be stuck to the machine when it is cleaned so that this procedure can be repeated at yearly intervals.

Obviously, the electronic sphygmomanometer 'listens' to the sounds and records the results automatically. Extra long cuffs are required for patients with fat arms in whom the standard cuff may give erroneous results, and small cuffs are used for children.

Torch

A torch is an essential piece of the doctor's equipment. It will be used to examine the patient's mouth and throat, to illuminate skin lesions and to test the reflexes of the pupils. A supply of appropriate sizes of batteries and bulbs must be kept in store. The doctor will often have a heavy hand lamp that he takes with him at night to read street names and numbers. This may also be used to provide a source of light for midwifery work.

Auriscope and ophthalmoscope

These instruments are used for the examination of the ear and eye. They may work off torch batteries in which case a supply of spares is necessary. It is possible to obtain batteries for torches, auriscopes, etc., that are rechargeable. There are other combined torches and auriscopes now available which have disposable ear-specula and plastic tongue depressors.

Peak flow gauge

This instrument is used in the diagnosis of respiratory disease, especially asthma. It is, essentially, a tube that is blown into and measures the flow-rate in litres of air per minute. Sometimes it is used to measure the response to drugs. A special version of the gauge is used for children.

Tongue depressors

These may be disposable wooden ones, or made of metal or plastic. The former are thrown away after use, but the latter require cleaning and sterilizing. Translucent plastic spatulas are made and include a variety which fit on to the end of a torch and transmit the light into the throat. These must be cleaned after use and will withstand boiling. In the house, the handle of a spoon or fork will serve as an excellent spatula, although a lot of time may be wasted while relatives hunt for the best spoon.

The patella hammer, tuning fork, hat pin and cotton wool

These are kept together as a part of the equipment used for testing the nervous system.

Tape measure

This is used for measuring the expansion of the chest when breathing and for recording differences in the circumference and length of limbs. The circumference of the infant's head may be measured to detect abnormalities.

Throat swab

This consists of a small pledget of cotton-wool twisted onto a carrying stick and contained in a glass, plastic or cardboard tube. It has been previously sterilized and is used to collect moist material from throat, ears, wounds, etc., for bacteriological examination. The wool should not be handled as this will introduce contamination and may give false results. The tube should be labelled with the patient's name.

Hypodermic syringe

The care and maintenance of syringes is an important duty that the secretary will have to perform. Syringes are of two types.

Disposable syringes. These are made of synthetic fibres and have several great advantages. There is no time wasted on cleaning and preparing them and the sterility is ensured. They come in a number of different sizes and may be fitted with a wide variety of disposable hypodermic needles. They are excellent for taking blood or giving intravenous injections, for here a very high degree of sterility is required in order to guard against the transmission of infection. Five sizes of syringe, 1, 2, 5, 10 and 20 ml, and three sizes of needle, 5/8, 1 and 1½ in (25, 23 and 21 gauge), may be obtained from the FPC on an order form signed by the doctor. Cartons of a hundred needles or 2 ml syringes and 25 10 ml syringes are supplied. It is also possible to obtain them already charged with the medicine to be injected, e.g. influenza vaccine.

Glass syringes. These syringes are now only used by diabetic patients requiring daily injections or for special purposes such as the injection of haemorrhoids with specially designed syringes. They may be sterilized by placing in cold water and then raising to boiling point for 10 minutes. The barrel and the plunger must be separated before they are put in the water. If the plunger is metal it will certainly break the barrel if this is not done. After boiling the syringes may be stored in airtight containers, or in surgical spirit, cetrimide or chlorhexidine. They may also be sterilized by dry heat in an oven. This is a more efficient method of sterilization and if they are 'cooked' for 60 minutes at 160°C this will kill spores. All glass syringes can be sterilized with needles already on in suitable tins with screw caps. After cooling in the oven the caps can be tightened and they will then remain sterile for several days. Syringes sterilized in hot air should have the barrels lubricated with a special silicone liquid after cleaning to prevent sticking.

When sterilizing by boiling or dry heat remember that it is more economical to do a large batch at one session and then store enough sterile syringes to last until the next session. If a time switch is used for dry heat they can be sterilized during the night and will be cooled for use in the morning.

Sometimes the plunger of a syringe will get stuck in the barrel. When this has happened it can often be freed by soaking in ether for about 30 minutes. If this method fails to release the plunger the syringe should be boiled in a 25% solution of glycerine and the plunger twisted whilst still hot.

Hypodermic needle

Disposable needles with plastic hubs are used in the surgery by doctors and nurses. Non-disposable needles may be obtained on prescription by patients needing daily injections. Their size is indicated by a number relating to the standard wire gauge (SWG).

Needles stuck on syringes may be removed by grasping the hub in a pair of forceps and twisting. It is of the utmost importance to ensure that used syringes and needles are disposed of safely. There are two hazards, firstly that refuse collection men may be injured by needles and secondly that usable syringes can fall into the hands of drug addicts. Syringes can be burnt or have their hubs cut off. Needles can be broken off the hub or be collected and disposed of in sealed boxes or tins so that they are safe to refuse collectors.

Sterile containers for urine, blood, sputum and faeces

In many areas a pathology service is now provided for GPs. Blood may be collected at home by the doctor or the patient may attend the laboratory with the appropriate form. Where this service is available:

1 Ensure that ample supplies of the different bottles are in stock. It is advisable to keep a list near at hand showing which sort of bottle is required for each test.

2 See that every patient who is taking a specimen bottle to the laboratory has his name on the bottle and has the appropriate request form completely filled in.

3 Find out the correct time for the patient to attend the laboratory and notify him.

4 Tell the patient when the result will be returned and make an appointment for him.

When a specimen of urine is required it is usual to send a midstream specimen (MSU) (see Chapter 36). When a culture of the urine is required it may also be necessary to send a 'dipinocculum' bottle containing a special 'spoon' that has been dipped in the MSU bottle.

Finger-stalls

Single finger-stalls are made of thin polythene and are used for rectal examinations or palpating lumps in the mouth. They should be kept in small tins or jars near the examination couch. A tube of lubricant is necessary. The doctor will also carry them in his bag and the container must be refilled periodically. They are thrown away after use.

Gloves

Two types of glove may be used in general practice:
1 disposable polythene gloves
2 disposable rubber gloves

Disposable polythene gloves come in four sizes, petite, small, medium and large. They will fit either hand, and are sold in boxes of fifty. They are normally unsterile, but sterile goves in sealed envelopes can be obtained at greater cost. Disposable rubber gloves are also supplied sterile or unsterile. They are more expensive but can be used for minor operations.

Whichever variety of glove is used, stocks are kept and a small supply put on a tray in each examination room. This tray may also contain the finger-stalls and lubricant and be covered with a small white cotton towel.

Lubricant for gloves. This is necessary for both rectal and vaginal examination. Vaseline, tubes of surgical lubricant or chloroxylenol (Dettol) cream are all suitable. Pledglets of cotton-wool should be kept on the tray that is laid for rectal or vaginal examinations.

Urine testing equipment

(see Chapter 36)

Cleansing solutions

Industrial methylated spirit and 1% cetrimide or chlorhexidine are usually kept in glass-stoppered bottles where needed. A small bottle of each is kept filled in the doctor's bag.

EQUIPMENT FOR DIAGNOSIS OR TREATMENT

Stainless steel instruments such as metal spatulas, the proctoscope, vaginal speculum, bowls and kidney dishes will need to be sterilized after use. They should be washed in hot, soapy water and a nylon-bristled brush used for cleaning. They can then be boiled or put into the dry-heat sterilizer for 10 minutes at 160°C. In the surgery they are normally required to be clean but not sterile and if they are needed urgently they can be cooled under the cold tap. If bowls are needed for minor surgery or dressings they must be removed from the sterilizer with sterile forceps and placed on the dressing tray. If they are not required immediately they can be wrapped in a sterile towel. They should be polished periodically and proprietary window cleaners are excellent for this purpose. Cracked or chipped enamel bowls should not be used as sterile containers.

The proctoscope is used for rectal examination and minor rectal surgery such as the injection of haemorrhoids. It needs to be cleaned and sterilized after use.

There are a number of different varieties of the vaginal speculum in use. Stainless steel varieties include bi-valve, Ferguson's or Sims'. Hardened glass or translucent plastic types are also available. Careful washing and sterilizing after use is important.

Both proctoscope and vaginal speculum need a powerful light to be efficient. This may consist of a 12-volt battery connected to a bulb and carrier that clip to the instrument, or a mains supply run through a small transformer. A *head-lamp* provides excellent illumination. Care must be taken not to leave the light on for an unduly long time as the bulb burns out easily. The mirror of a head-lamp should be kept clean and polished.

Nasal speculum, and trocar and cannula need no special treatment.

Nebulizer and pump. This is used to deliver a 'mist' of medication, it helps patients with an attack of asthma, for example, to breathe. It consists of a pump which is either driven by electricity or by foot pressure and a delivery system directing the jet of air through the liquid, thus producing the mist.

EQUIPMENT USED FOR TREATMENT

With the exception of the ear syringe all the surgical instruments needed under this heading should be sterile before use. They include:
- needles and needle holders
- sharp-pointed scissors
- scalpel handles and blades
- forceps — toothed, dissecting, plain and splinter
- Spencer Wells forceps
- suture material — this is now usually provided in sterilized sachets which can be opened when required. The needle is sealed to the ligature.
- sinus probe
- eye spud
- the ear syringe may be a rubber bulb syringe or three-ring metal syringe.

The removal of wax is one of the commonest procedures adopted in general practice. The equipment necessary is the ear syringe, a tank or jug containing water at a temperature of 38°C (100°F) (higher or lower temperatures than this may cause the patient to become giddy), a kidney dish or Noot's ear-tank to catch the returned wax and water, and an auriscope to inspect the canal. The secretary may be expected to have the patient seated with a towel around the neck, and the equipment ready. Regular checks must be made to ensure that all of this equipment is in good working order when it is needed. It is pointless to suggest any sort of routine method of doing this, but the secretary and the doctor should get together at an early opportunity and work out a system by which she will know what is needed. One of the greatest time wasters is the practice of running to and fro from patient to consulting room, or even from surgery to house and back because the right piece of equipment is not where it should be or is not working properly. An hour or two spent working out a method at the beginning may save both doctor and secretary many hours later and a check list should be written out for all procedures.

THE DOCTOR'S BAG

The same rules apply to drugs, equipment, dressings, and forms in the doctor's bag. A plan must be devised and a check list made so that a constant supply can be kept in the proper place.

Some group practices have an arrangement whereby similar doctor's bags are used by each partner. Where this is done a spare bag may be kept at the surgery and each bag exchanged at intervals. The bag itself needs some attention. The outside can be sponged and polished and the inside emptied and wiped with a damp cloth. The contents are then replaced and fresh supplies of spirit, cotton-wool swabs, syringes, forms, spatulas, etc. may be introduced.

If the bag contains dangerous drugs it must be locked in order to comply with the Controlled Drugs Regulations.

A typical check list might include the following:

Instruments

1 Stethoscope
2 Sphygmomanometer
3 Torch
4 Thermometer
5 Auriscope
6 Ophthalmoscope
7 Patella hammer
8 Tuning fork
9 Hypodermic syringe
10 Hypodermic needles
11 Tape measure
12 Scissors
13 Tongue depressors
14 Finger cots
15 Gloves
16 Lubricant
17 Cotton-wool swabs
18 Surgical spirit

Drugs

1 Morphine ampoules
2 Pethidine ampoules
3 Adrenaline HCl
4 Ergometrine
5 Aminophylline
6 Diazepam
7 Hydrocortisone
8 Piriton injection
9 Frusemide
10 Penicillin injection
11 Antibiotic tablets

Accessories

1 Clinistix and Albustix, or Uristix
2 Sterile bottles for blood, urine and sputum specimens.
3 Sterile dressings
4 Bandages
5 Safety pins
6 Adhesive plaster
7 Fountain pen

Forms

1 Prescription pad
2 FPC forms (FP 1, 7 and 8)
3 National Insurance forms (Med 3 and Med 5)
4 Request forms for X-ray or pathology examination

The check list should be made out in consultation with the doctor and referred to whenever the bag is checked; this should be done at not more than weekly intervals.

Where separate dressing, accident or midwifery bags are kept a similar procedure should be followed for these.

LINEN AND LAUNDRY

It will be the job of the secretary to care for the linen in the surgery. (The secretary working for the Consultant in private practice may also have the same duty.) The regularly laundered items will include:
1 towels
2 pillow cases
3 sheets

Towels. These consist of hand towels by every wash-basin, and also cotton squares that are used to cover instruments, trays, etc. These squares may be laid over pillows on examination couches so that a fresh pillow case is needed less frequently. There is an increasing use of disposable paper sheets and towels which are quite soft and comfortable.

Sheets. Two sheets are needed for each couch. An undersheet which overhangs the sides of the couch and an oversheet which is kept neatly folded. A blanket is often provided and there may be an electric blanket beneath the undersheet. A patient who is warm and relaxed is very much easier to examine.

Spare linen will be kept in a cupboard or drawer and a sufficient stock of clean linen must be kept. Arrangements will be made for laundry to be collected and returned and the bill to be checked. Paper sheets supplied singly or in rolls are now available.

Uniform. The question of whether the secretary will wear uniform or not is something which she will have to discuss with her employer. Generally speaking a clean overall looks smart and efficient and will protect her own clothing. Overalls may be made of cotton or synthetic fabrics and plain coloured or white nylon overalls can look attractive.

Removal of stains

However careful the secretary is, there are a number of liquids in the doctor's surgery or the Consultant's rooms which will stain materials. Here are a few hints for removing those that commonly occur. Whenever possible try to remove the stain immediately. An old stain is much more difficult to remove than a fresh one.

1 *Blood.* Wash immediately in cold water until the stain is removed. If there is any residual stain left it can be sponged with hydrogen peroxide and then washed in soap flakes.

2 *Ink.* Soak the stain in milk. The residual stain can usually be removed by washing or dry-cleaning. Old stains can be treated with dilute oxalic acid, three quarters of an ounce to half a pint of water, but this may bleach colour out of the material. Ball-point ink is soluble in methylated spirit.

3 *Grease.* This can be removed with a commercial cleaning fluid or by washing in hot water and detergent.

4 *Iodine*. Soap and water washing will remove fresh stains, and industrial methylated spirit will remove old stains.

5 *Silver nitrate*. Stains can be removed by soaking in salt water and then by the application of iodine. This can then be removed as described above.

6 *Gentian violet*. This can be removed with alcohol.

36

Laboratory Procedures and Other Tests in General Practice

There are two main groups of laboratory tests performed in general practice: tests on urine and tests on/for blood. Other procedures carried out include cervical smears and tests on the heart and lungs.

URINE TESTING

Nearly every secretary in general practice will be expected to know how to test the urine for sugar and albumin, to measure the specific gravity and to test for acidity or alkalinity. Other more detailed tests may also be done

Albumin is a protein which is present in the urine when there is disease of some part of the urinary tract. This disease may be secondary to a condition in another organ such as in heart disease or toxaemia of pregnancy, or primary, due to infection or disease in the kidney or bladder.

The urine may be collected by catheter or may be a midstream specimen. The collection of a catheter specimen of urine (CSU) must be done in a proper aseptic manner; for normal purposes the midstream urine test is sufficient. When bacteriological examination is required the first morning specimen passed is most suitable as this is likely to contain the highest number of bacteria.

A midstream specimen of urine (MSU) is collected after the external genitalia have been swabbed with 1% cetrimide or chlorhexidine. The first small quantity of urine is discarded and the remainder passed into a sterile container. This may be either the bottle provided by the laboratory or a previously boiled cup which has been allowed to cool. The urine is then transferred to the bottle which is sealed and labelled.

Specimens of urine from infants can be collected in small disposable plastic bags which have a circle of adhesive material so that they may be stuck around the external genitalia. When the said bag contains urine, the mother removes it and cuts off one corner over a sterile urine bottle.

Albumin in the urine

Albustix test. This relies on a colour change when one end of a strip of absorbent paper impregnated with chemicals is dipped into the urine. The strip is immediately removed and compared with a colour scale on the side of the bottle. This gives a reasonably accurate indication of the amount of albumin present. It is important to keep the bottle tightly closed and not to touch the test end of the strip.

Every specimen of urine is tested for albumin and this includes tests at every antenatal examination.

Sugar in urine

One of three tests are commonly used to demonstrate sugar in the urine. The urine must be in a clean container or false results may be obtained from any of the tests.

1 *Clinitest.* This simple test is carried out without boiling. A small outfit contains all the equipment. With the special dropper provided, five drops of urine and ten drops of water are added to a test tube and a special Clinitest tablet is added. The mixture boils by means of reagents in the tablet and the percentage of sugar present can be determined by comparison with a colour scale.

2 *Clinistix.* The test end of a strip of absorbent paper impregnated with chemicals is dipped in the urine. A positive result is indicated if the end turns blue within one minute. Ignore a colour appearing after a minute. The strips must be kept in a cool, dry and dark place, tightly stoppered and the test end must not be handled. If the unused strips are brown they should be discarded.

3 *Diastix.* A plastic dip stick.

A reagent strip is available which will test for albumin and glucose.

Specific gravity

The specific gravity of urine is measured by means of an instrument known as an urinometer. This consists of a glass float with a scale upon the upper half. A sufficient quantity of urine at room temperature is placed in a container. The urinometer is then placed in the urine and allowed to float freely without touching the sides. The cylinder is then placed so that the lower end of the miniscus is at eye level and the level at which this would cross the scale is read off.

Generally there is a considerable variation in the specific gravity of urine specimens passed during 24 hours, anything between 1015 and 1025 being normal. Reading above or below these levels may indicate disease, as may fixed recordings around 1010.

Reaction—acid or alkaline

If a piece of blue litmus paper turns red when dipped in the urine the reaction is acid. If there is no change a piece of red litmus should be dipped in the urine, and will turn blue in alkaline urine. If both change colour it is due to the presence of acid and alkaline phosphates and if neither changes the reaction is neutral.

Other tests of the urine which may be performed are as follows.

Acetone in urine (ketonuria)

An *Acetest tablet* is placed on a piece of white paper. One drop of urine is put on the tablet and the colour compared with a scale after 30 seconds. If acetone is present the tablet changes to a colour varying from lavender to deep purple.

Blood in urine (haematuria)

1 This may be seen on a slide under a microscope. One drop of well-mixed urine is placed on a clean slide and covered by a clean cover-slip. Red cells may be seen under the low-power objective.

2 *Occultest reagent tablets*. One drop of urine is placed in the centre of one of the special test papers and a tablet placed in the centre of the moist area. Two drops of water are allowed to flow over the tablet and if blood is present a blue colour appears on the test paper after two minutes. The speed of development and the intensity of the colour are roughly in proportion to the concentration of blood.

This test can be used to determine the presence of blood in the faeces, in which case a thin smear of faeces is placed on the test paper instead of the drop of urine and the same procedure is repeated.

Bilirubin in urine

Bilirubin in the urine is an indication that jaundice is present. Large amounts of bilirubin may be detected by shaking the urine. The froth of normal urine is white, but in the presence of bilirubin may become yellow or greenish.

Ictotest reagent tablets. These provide a simple and accurate method of detecting the presence of bilirubin. Five drops of urine are placed on a square of the special test mat provided and one Ictotest tablet put in the centre of the moistened area. Two drops of water are allowed to flow over the tablet and, if bilirubin is present, the mat around the tablet will turn a bluish-purple colour. The speed of appearance and intensity of the colour is in proportion to the amount of bilirubin in the specimen.

Phenylketonuria

The presence of phenylketones in the urine of an infant has been shown to be associated with one form of mental illness. These substances can be detected by dipping a test strip in the urine or by moistening the end between the folds of a wet napkin. A positive result is indicated by the end of the strip turning green within 30 seconds.

Combination strips

Combination strips for a variety of urine tests are now available:

1 *Uristix* test for glucose and protein.
2 *Labstix* test for pH, glucose, protein, ketones and blood.
3 *Keto-diastix* test semi-quantitatively for glucose and for urinary ketones.
4 *n-Labstix* include all the tests of Lanstix and have an area that tests for the presence of nitrites, which indicate bacteriuria.

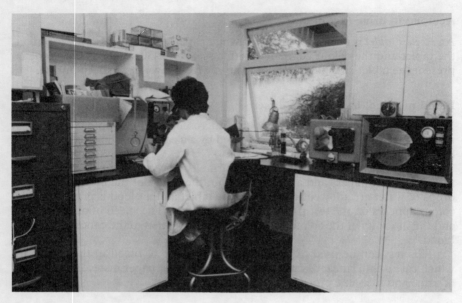

Fig. 36.1 Laboratory work in the surgery.

TESTS ON/FOR BLOOD

Blood glucose

Capillary blood can be obtained from a finger prick and the blood glucose
measured by either a *Dextrostix* or a *Reflotest* test patch. Other methods involve
using a blood glucose meter for reading a colour change or, most recently,
glucose reagent sticks that can be read without the use of a meter.

Occult blood

Certain diseases of the bowel may first be detected by the presence of small
quantities of blood in the faeces. This may be invisible to the naked eye, but
can be detected by a simple test using *hematest tablets*.

A thin smear of faeces is made on the filter paper provided, and a tablet
placed across the edge of the smear. One drop of water is placed on top of the
tablet, and 5 to 10 seconds later a second drop is placed that flows down the
tablet on to the paper.

Exactly two minutes later the filter paper around the tablet is observed. A
blue colour indicates the presence of blood.

Erythrocyte sedimentation rate (ESR)

If a tube of blood containing an anticoagulant is allowed to stand, the red cells
will sink slowly to the bottom. The rate at which they fall is measured and
provides evidence of the presence or absence of certain diseases. This is a test

which can be conveniently and simply carried out in the surgery. The Westergren method is as follows:

1.6 ml of blood is mixed with 0.4 ml of 3.8% sodium citrate. The mixture is drawn up into a tube calibrated in millimetres. This tube is then stood upright with one end pressed firmly into a piece of soft rubber and the other end held with a spring clip. The rate of fall of the red cells is measured in millimetres per one hour. If the test is being conducted in the surgery a bell-timer may be used to indicate the time at which the test should be read. The tube should be thoroughly washed out after use.

The haemoglobin level

There are three methods commonly used in general practice of estimating the haemoglobin level.

1 *The Sahli method.* A graduated tube is filled to the mark 10 with decinormal hydrochloric acid. Blood (20 mm^3) is drawn up into a pipette and then thoroughly mixed with the acid. The mixture is then allowed to stand for 10 minutes and at the end of this time distilled water is added until the colour of the fluid exactly matches the standard. The haemoglobin percentage is then read from the graduated tube. The normal range in an adult is between 85 and 105%.

2 *The AO Spencer Hb-Meter.* This uses a definite thickness of haemolysed blood in a special chamber and compares the light coming through it with a special glass wedge. An answer is provided in about three minutes. The technique of using it is simply learnt.

3 *The MRC Grey-wedge Photometer.* This is one of the simplest and most reliable of all methods. It works on the same principle as the AO Hb-Meter but is believed to be more reliable. It can be used for other biochemical determinations, including blood sugar and blood urea.

CERVICAL SMEAR

This test is used for diagnosing a pre-cancerous condition of the cervix, i.e. one which left untreated could later develop into a cancerous lesion. It depends on the fact that cells from such a cervix, when suitably stained, can be identified by an expert as possessing certain characteristics.

In an attempt to lower the incidence of cancer of the cervix, a campaign to screen women in a priority group was launched in 1966. At present this group includes all women over the age of 35 and women under that age who have had three or more pregnancies.

Outside this group it is also recommended that cervical smear is a routine part of antenatal and post-natal care and family planning advice.

The medical secretary will certainly be involved in preparing the equipment and documentation for this and might in some circumstances be trained by the doctor to take the smear. Equipment required consists of:

1 suitable speculum with light
2 wooden speculum with light
3 glass microscope slide
4 pencil and ball-point pen

5 fixing solution
6 container for slide

The documentation required consists of:
1 form FP 74
2 cervical cytology form

Method. The patient is placed in the left lateral position and the speculum, warmed and moistened with water (a lubricant may affect the smear), is inserted into the vagina. After the cervix has been visualized, the surface of the

---

NATIONAL HEALTH SERVICE   FP74

To the Administrator of ....

CERVICAL CYTOLOGY CERTIFICATE

PART I (To be completed by the patient)

Surname of patient ....,.. **Mrs/Miss**

Forename(s) ....

Address ....

....

Date of Birth .... **NHS No.** ....

I wish to apply for a cervical cytology test.

Delete lines that are not appropriate
{
I have not had such a test before

I had a similar test in............................. *(month and year)*

I have had 3 pregnancies and my third pregnancy was confirmed in .... *(month and year)*

My present pregnancy confirmed in .... is my third   *(month and year)*
}

Date ....
                                                      (Signature of patient)

PART II (To be completed by the doctor)

I have taken a cervical smear from the above patient and have arranged for it to be examined at a hospital pathology laboratory.

I claim the appropriate fee.

Date ....
                                                      (Signature of doctor)

Assistant/locum acting on behalf of

Dr. ....

PART III (For use by paying authority)

Name and address of doctor or partnership

89073   Dd 576850   820M   4/78   StS

Fig. 36.2 Cervical cytology certificate (FP 74).

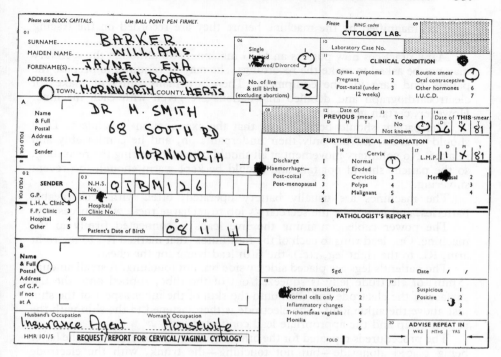

Fig. 36.3 Request form for cervical cytology.

cervix, including the os, is firmly scraped with the wooden spatula. (A little bleeding is of no consequence.) The spatula is then drawn several times along the surface of the slide, on the ground glass end of which the patient's surname has been written in pencil. The slide is then flooded with the fixing material and left to dry. When it has dried, it can be placed in the container for dispatch to the laboratory. The procedure is virtually painless.

Form FP 74 (Fig. 36.2) is a claim for the fee that is paid to the doctor and must be signed by the patient and the doctor. The cervical cytology form (Fig 36.3) is carbonized and produces three further copies. It requires very careful completion and, as some information has to be obtained from the patient, should be completed when she signs her FP 74. Completion is essential so that the national recall system can send for each woman who has had a smear every five years.

A fee is payable for a test after the third pregnancy is confirmed or if the patient is aged over 35, then for every test at five yearly intervals. A further fee is payable if the laboratory requests a repeat for an unsatisfactory smear.

ELECTROCARDIOGRAPH EXAMINATION

The ECG machine measures and records the very small changes in electrical voltage which occur with the heart beat. These changes are so small that they must be magnified by the machine before they are recorded on the tracing paper.

Many practices now possess an ECG machine, and although the secretary may not be asked to make the recordings, she may be required to prepare the patient and care for the equipment. There are many different makes of electrocardiograph and detailed instructions are given with each machine. However, certain general rules apply.

The patient should be reassured that the examination is painless. They should undress, leaving only their underpants on, and lie comfortably and relaxed. No voluntary movement at all should take place during the recording, so the patient should not talk and should be kept warm enough to prevent shivering.

The machines are usually battery operated, often with rechargeable batteries, and it may be the secretary's job to recharge these when necessary.

The power cable containing the five leads is connected firmly to the machine. One lead runs to each of the four limbs (that marked RA to the right arm, RL to the right leg, etc.), the fifth lead being for the chest.

The patient's legs are placed side by side but not touching. A small amount (5 mm) of electrode jelly is squeezed out of the tube, rubbed onto the flat surface of the electrode and then onto the skin of the inner aspect of the shin just above the ankle joint. The electrode is then fastened to the shin with the rubber strap and the appropriate lead connected to it.

The procedure is repeated for the other leg and then for each arm, the latter being placed alongside—but not touching—the trunk, with the electrode fastened to the inner aspect of the forearm just above the wrist. The patient is then covered with a sheet or blanket until the doctor is ready.

After the recordings have been made, the patient is disconnected from the electrodes and the jelly wiped off the arms and legs with a paper tissue.

All traces of the jelly are then carefully removed from the electrodes and rubber bands, and they and the leads are replaced in their case.

The recording will appear as one long paper strip. This will be numbered by the doctor, who will indicate which sections he requires mounted. These are usually stuck on a thin card using a glue pen, and the number written on the card beneath each section as it appears on the tracing. Finally the patient's name and address is put on the card. The secretary should see that spare tracing-paper is available.

WRIGHT PEAK-FLOW METER

This small machine is designed to measure the efficiency of the lungs. It is used on patients with suspected lung disease such as emphysema or chronic bronchitis. The patient blows through a disposable cardboard tube, which is connected to the dial. A recording is read off the dial in litres per minute. The patient stands or sits up straight and the instrument is held with the dial vertical. The patient inhales deeply and on the command, 'Blow!' he blows out as hard as possible in a short blast. After the reading has been taken, the dial is reset by pressing a button and the test repeated three or four times so that an average can be obtained.

Diploma Questions on a Broader Basis

1 Describe the procedures and documents involved from the time the patient sees his GP in the surgery until he is discharged from hospital after an operation.

2 Outline the ways in which the medical secretary may assist in the field of preventive medicine, giving examples from general practice, hospitals and local authorities.

3 You are responsible for the training of a student secretary in your general practice. Draft notes for her guidance on the main procedures which are carried out and the forms with which she will have to become familiar.

4 Mention administrative problems which might occur from time to time in general practice and how you, as a medical secretary, would deal with them.

5 Compare the organization of the office work in a single-handed general practice with that in a health centre.

6 State the possible duties which a busy GP might undertake in the course of a working day and how you, as a medical secretary, might be expected to assist.

7 As a medical secretary in the absence of the practice administrator in a large group practice, you have been asked to organize field-work for trainee medical secretaries. Prepare a schedule for an induction period of five days.

V

Appendixes and Index

Rapid Revision

HOSPITAL

1 List the main categories of staff employed in a hospital.
2 Put the medical staff in order of seniority.
3 Give three of the medical records officer's responsibilities.
4 How may medical secretarial services be organized?
5 What is the diagnostic index?
6 On what is its coding based?
7 Describe briefly methods of keeping the index.
8 What is HAA?
9 Name two kinds of information involved in HAA.
10 What is HIPE?
11 Name the four main sections of the case notes.
12 Give four examples of what you would expect to find in each section.
13 Using terminal digit filing, how would case notes with the following numbers be treated: 687534 and 89213?
14 Give two advantages and two disadvantages of microfilming.
15 What is COM?
16 Define the term 'on line'.
17 What information does the personal medical secretary keep in her case notes record book?
18 Why do all non-alphabetical filing systems require a master index?
19 What information would you expect to find on a hospital master index card?
20 For what purpose may 'mechanical' labels be used?
21 Explain the term 'pre-registration'.
22 Name three reasons for the existence of the out-patient department.
23 How do patients reach the out-patient department?
24 Are there any exceptions?
25 How is the casualty card filed?
26 Describe the organization of the X-ray department?
27 By what methods may X-ray films be filed?
28 What is the points system pertaining to X-ray films?
29 What happens to the two copies of the radiography report?
30 For what is the Consultant Pathologist responsible?
31 Basically, there are two kinds of surgery performed in the operating theatre; what are they?
32 There is, however, a third type. What is it?
33 What information is contained on the operations list?
34 To whom is the operation list circulated?
35 From where does the secretary obtain the details necessary for the typing of the list?
36 What must she do if the information is incomplete in some way?
37 What is the cooperation card?
38 List the duties of the surgical appliances officer.
39 Give the information required by the transport officer.

40 How much notice does he require when transport is booked?
41 What are bed states?
42 What is the bed board?
43 Explain the initials 'EBS'.
44 List the main types of admission.
45 What is the 'A and D' book?
46 Outline the information that appears on an admission card.
47 How can the admissions officer produce, at a moment's notice, the running total of admissions?
48 What is a domiciliary visit?
49 How can the waiting list be kept?
50 List the information it contains.
51 What is particularly important about the Mental Health Act, 1959?
52 What are Sections 25, 26 and 29 about?
53 Name the two main classes of patient to which the Act applies.
54 To what places may patients be discharged?
55 What happens when a patient discharges himself against medical advice?
56 Why is a discharge pro forma sent to the GP?
57 Explain why one version of the bed states return dispenses with the need to send a discharge note to the medical records department.
58 What is a consent form and who is, ultimately, responsible for its completion?
59 How might an electronic jotting-pad be useful in hospital?
60 Define the 'bleep'.
61 In terms of office equipment, what is a text editor?
62 The HASAW Act, 1974 is an 'enabling' Act; explain this.
63 On whom does the Act place responsibility?
64 Name some flammable liquids the secretary uses.
65 How can she render them safe?
66 Briefly describe a method of lifting heavy objects without placing undue stress on the spine.
67 Name two private medical insurance schemes.
68 When patients are being treated under such schemes, what must the secretary do?
69 Give three points to consider in the event of a bomb scare.
70 Explain the word 'interface'.
71 What do the letters BASIC represent when referring to computer language?
72 Briefly, what purpose does the follow-up department serve?

GENERAL PRACTICE

1 What types of premises are doctors' surgeries usually found in? Give three examples.
2 Give a list of six rooms to be found in a doctor's surgery.
3 Medical record envelopes may be filed vertically or laterally, in filing cabinets, on shelves or attached to a rotary drum. In what order may they be filed?
4 A male medical record envelope is an FP.....
5 A female medical record envelope is an FP.....
6 Continuation cards for male and female patients respectively are forms FP.....
7 FP 7A's and 8A's are.....
8 FP 9A's and 9B's are.....
9 What is an FP 19?
10 Under what circumstances is this issued?
11 What other documents are filed in general practice? Give three examples.
12 Very briefly describe three methods by which patients may change from one doctor to another.

13 A medical card is an FP......

14 What form does a parent use to register his child with a doctor for the first time?

15 What form is used for an adopted child?

16 What is an FP 13 used for?

17 What should the receptionist ask all patients to do when they first enter the waiting room?

18 Give three principles regarding the management of a waiting room.

19 Define 'surgery flow'.

20 What may the receptionist do or what can be used in the surgery to facilitate the steady flow of patients?

21 What is a prescription form—FP.....?

22 Give four examples of those entitled to exemption from prescription charges.

23 What form is used when claiming a night visit fee—FP.....

24 What form is used when claiming an emergency treatment fee?

25 When is a doctor entitled to claim a night visit fee?

26 What is an FP 30?

27 What is an FP 3?

28 What is the FP number of the cervical cytology certificate and claim form?

29 How may patients be notified of the introduction of an appointments system?

30 Give five advantages for doctors of appointment systems.

31 Give five advantages for patients of appointment systems.

32 Give three disadvantages for patients of appointment systems.

33 Give three disadvantages for doctors of appointment systems.

34 A doctor with qualifying employment or diploma may be included in the O.......... L..... and offer maternity services to all those requesting it—i.e. not necessarily his own patients.

35 The form used throughout maternity care, from the acceptance of a patient by a doctor to claiming of fees, is an FP.... for those on the O.L and an FP.... for those who are not.

36 What is a Mat B1?

37 What is a Mat B2?

38 What major record is kept throughout maternity care?

39 Name three other forms which are used during the maternity care.

40 What information is a patient normally requested to give when requesting a visit?

41 In what book is the message originally recorded?

42 What other messages are recorded in this book?

43 Define: ophthalmic medical practitioner
ophthalmic optician
dispensing optician

44 What is an FP 81 used for?

45 The doctor receives allowances for the staff that he employs—what forms are used?

46 What forms are completed in order to obtain the allowances available for the practice premises?

47 What is an FP 31 used for?

48 For what purpose are FP 69 and FP 69B's issued?

49 What is an FP 10D?

50 What is an FP 10HP?

51 What is an FP 10A?

52 What statistical records are kept in a general practice?

53 What do the abbreviations EDD and LMP stand for?

Examination Syllabus
Association of Medical Secretaries, Practice Administrators and Receptionists

SYLLABUS II. MEDICAL SECRETARIAL PRACTICE AND OFFICE PROCEDURES

General

Candidates will not be expected to have a detailed specialist knowledge of any topic, but to have a broad understanding of the topics in each section of the syllabus.

Fieldwork plays an important part in the course work and this should be evidenced, where appropriate, in the candidates' examination answers.

The examination will offer *thirteen* questions each carrying the same number of possible marks. There will be two sections (A and B). Question 1 (multiple choice) will be *compulsory*. Candidates will be required to answer an additional *two* from section A and a further *three* from section B—a total of *six*. Some questions may cover only the general aspects of office practice, others the medical aspect; some will require an integrated knowledge of both medical and general secretarial/office procedures.

While candidates will not be marked specifically on their standard of English, this will be taken into account together with the overall presentation and legibility of their answers. There is a small mark allocation for this purpose.

Aims

1 To develop an understanding of secretarial practice and office procedures as practised generally and in the medical sphere.
2 To understand and appreciate the relationships created in the personnel and client/patient context.
3 To enable candidates to become fully aware of the theoretical and, as far as possible, the practical aspect of the syllabus which will enable them within the minimum amount of time to become competent medical secretaries in hospitals, general and private practice and health clinics/centres and so on, thereby easing the administrative work of the medical personnel in these areas.

Learning objective At the end of the course students should be able to:	**Behavioural objectives** At the end of the unit students should be able to:

1 Background to Medical Secretarial Work

1.1 know and understand that in the medical field office workers are closely concerned with patient care; to appreciate where the medical staff are fulfilling management functions rather than medical functions;

1.1.1 identify these 'managerial' functions, and state clearly and factually how the medical secretary can assist;

2 The Office

2.1 understand the importance of the office to the smooth running of any organization;

2.1.1 recognize that documentation is essential to record the action which has been and must be taken;

2.1.2 identify the connection between such documentation and the departments from which they emanate.

3 Inter-relationship between Departments and/or Personnel

3.1 appreciate the importance of the interrelationship between departments and/or personnel for the smooth running of the organization and for a high standard of patient care;

3.1.1 identify the nature of the interrelationship so that the best possible service will be given to the patient.

4 The Function of the Medical Secretary
The purpose and scope of secretarial assistance;
4.1 understand the scope of the secretary's role;

4.1.1 identify the supportive role of the secretary in relation to the employer;

4.1.2 identify the day-to-day work and routine;

Technical skills and abilities
4.2 know what the secretary must be capable of;

4.2.1 identify the technical skills and knowledge required;

Personal qualities
4.3 appreciate the range of qualities desirable in a secretary;

4.3.1 describe the importance of courtesy, tact and diplomacy as well as loyalty, reliability and initiative;

4.3.2 describe the importance of deportment and appearance;

Possible career structures
4.4 understand the career possibilities and limitations;

4.4.1 compare the likely responsibilities of the:
(a) receptionist/clerk
(b) junior typist/secretary
(c) secretary
(d) personal assistant
(e) senior medical secretary
(f) practice administrator.

Learning objective	Behavioural objectives
At the end of the course students should be able to:	At the end of the unit students should be able to:

5 The Medical Secretary in Hospital

5.1 know the special duties of the medical secretary in hospitals; duties relating to in/out patients; pre-registration; appointments systems; admissions and discharges; follow-up systems; waiting lists;

5.1.1 describe the duties of a medical secretary in relation to the care of in/out patients in hospital.

6 The Medical Secretary in General Practice

6.1 know the special duties of the medical secretary in general practice—single-handed, group and health centre practices, including dispensing practices;

6.1.1 identify the difference between the role of the medical secretary in the different types of practice;

6.2 appointment systems, visiting lists;

6.2.1 maintain appointments systems and prepare visiting lists;

6.3 know the forms issued by FPC, health authorities and DHSS or equivalent authority;

6.3.1 identify forms in general use, their purpose and necessity for accurate completion;

6.4 know insurance reports; employment medical forms, and so on;

6.5 understand rota systems and locum services;

6.5.1 devise a rota system and know how to help locum;

6.6 understand stock control;

6.6.1 be capable of operating a simple system of stock control;

6.7 understand the need for care and maintenance of surgery premises and equipment;

6.8 appreciate how the medical secretary can assist the practice manager.

7 Organizing and Planning Work

7.1 understand the need to organize and plan work;

7.1.1 describe the needs of the employer in given situations;

7.1.2 identify and order priorities;

Use of internal services and facilities

7.2 know of the internal services and facilities;

7.2.1 select and justify methods, services and facilities to maximize efficiency.

8 Working Relations

Relations and interpersonal behaviour; modes of address, tone and words

8.1 be aware of the importance of good relations;

8.1.1 describe appropriate interpersonal behaviour in given situations;

8.2 be aware of the impressions created by manner, tone and language;

With the chief

8.3 appreciate the need to adapt to the chief's personality to achieve a professional yet personal working relationship;

Learning objective	**Behavioural objectives**
At the end of the course students should be able to:	At the end of the unit students should be able to:

With seniors

8.4 appreciate the significance of difference in position as well as personality;

With peers

8.5 understand the link they provide with other departments and other personnel;

With juniors

8.6 appreciate their inexperience; their need for induction training; their need for reassurance when placed under work pressure; their career hopes and their potential;

With patients, relatives or others when they call or telephone

8.7 understand the importance of dealing with all callers with kindness, tact, efficiency and discretion; care in speech.

9 Office Communications

Oral—the telephone; communication by internal and external telephone

9.1 understand that the telephone is an important and possibly expensive means of communication;	**9.1.1** present efficiently information communicated by telephone for action or onward transmission;
9.2 be aware of the telephone services available through the British Telecom both by direct dialling and the operator;	**9.2.1** select the most appropriate service in given situations;

Written—letters, memos, invitations and reports

9.3 appreciate and understand the importance of matching English style to the given situation;	**9.3.1** compose from notes supplied, written correspondence appropriate to situations and topics within the syllabus.

10 Record Keeping and Retrieval

Importance: principles of classification and arrangements for safe retention and easy recall

10.1 understand the importance of medical records and the general principles underlying any record keeping;	**10.1.1** describe where different methods would be appropriate;

Diaries: the correlation of doctors' and secretary's; nature of entries

10.2 understand the purpose of the diary as a forecasting and record-keeping document;	**10.2.1** describe how efficient record keeping is achieved;
10.3 know the secretary's and the doctors' diaries must correlate;	**10.3.1** make diary entries; prepare an appointment sheet from the diary and from given information.

Learning objective At the end of the course students should be able to:	Behavioural objectives At the end of the unit students should be able to:

Filing and indexing: methods of storage—vertical, lateral, horizontal, rotary, strip and visible card

10.4 understand that efficient filing underpins the efficiency of the hospital, practice or organization;

    10.4.1 identify and compare different methods of storage and indexing for all types of documents, including computer print-out and X-rays;

Microfilming

10.5 understand the purpose of such a method of filing;

    10.5.1 identify the equipment and processing required;

    10.5.2 identify problems and benefits of the system.

Classification: alphabetical, subject, numerical, geographic and chronological

10.6 understand the necessity for different classifications;

    10.6.1 identify problems and benefits of classification.

Procedures: absent files, release for filing, cross-referencing, follow-up systems

10.7 understand the importance of these procedures;

    10.7.1 identify suitable procedures for recording absent files;

    10.7.2 distinguish when documents have been released for filing;

    10.7.3 identify the need for cross-referencing;

    10.7.4 select follow-up systems for given situations.

11 Office Equipment, including Word Processors, Electronic Typewriters

    11.1 be aware of the application of such equipment and machines to medical secretarial work, medical office procedures and general office work;

    11.1.1 describe the chief capabilities of such equipment; keep abreast of new developments;

    11.1.2 understand the terminology;

    11.1.3 describe the range of equipment which is currently available. (Technical knowledge is not required.)

12 Reprography

Ink stencilling, offset lithography, spirit duplicating, facsimile transmission

    12.1 appreciate the relative advantages and disadvantages within an organization;

    12.1.1 identify each method;

    12.1.2 compare the characteristics of the methods;

    12.2 know the equipment involved and the method of transmission; services available from outside agencies;

    12.2.1 select on given criteria including speed, quality, cost, availability and quantity required, the method best suited to a given situation.

13 Sources of Information

    13.1 be aware of procedures for finding any information that may be required;

    13.1.1 describe what sources are available for given types of information.

14 Travel and Accommodation

Planning and booking procedures for journeys and entertainment, including the use of agencies, money arrangements, insurance, passports

    14.1 know of sources of information on accommodation and travel by road/ rail/sea/air;

    14.1.1 plan journeys and entertainment using appropriate guides and outside agencies;

Learning objective At the end of the course students should be able to:	**Behavioural objectives** At the end of the unit students should be able to:
14.2 know the services provided by travel agencies;	14.2.1 state the steps necessary: (a) to obtain a passport/visa (b) arrange credit facilities (c) effect insurance cover;

Procedures to be adopted prior to and during the absence of doctor/chief

14.3 understand the need to inform all concerned in advance and to arrange for the delegation of his/her duties;

    14.3.1 describe procedures for informing those concerned during his/her absence;

    14.3.2 describe how to deal with a problem and when to forward it to another person.

14.4 know means available for contacting him/her, forwarding documents;

    14.4.1 state means available for contacting him/her whilst absent.

15 The Mail—external and internal

15.1 know and understand the daily routine;

    15.1.1 describe how to use the daily routine procedure for reception and despatch of mail.

Handling incoming and outgoing mail

15.2 appreciate the need for communication and to observe any special instructions.

Registered, recorded, first/second class, express services, etc.

15.3 know the functions of each service and the appropriate circumstances for its use;

    15.3.1 identify need for use of special postal services.

The Post Office Guide—inland and overseas post

15.4 be able to use it;

    15.4.1 extract accurate information which is up-to-date from the Post Office Guide.

16 Elementary Statistics and Collection of Data

Visual presentation of data: graphs, charts, control boards and so on

16.1 understand the methods of data presentation;

    16.1.1 extract information from data given and present it in graph and chart form.

Computers

16.2 appreciate the importance of computers (including microcomputers) in medical and general office practice;

    16.2.1 describe the main computer terms;

    16.2.2 understand the capabilities of computers for medical and commercial office practice applications;

16.3 understand the need for statistics in medical office practice;

    16.3.1 prepare and understand simple graphs, histograms, tabulations, etc.;

    16.3.2 describe the chief statistical records kept in hospitals, in general practice and elsewhere in the medical field.

17 Meetings

17.1 understand that the function of a meeting (formal or informal) is to provide a means of communication and decision making;

    17.1.1 know about different types of meetings;

Learning objective At the end of the course students should be able to:	Behavioural objectives At the end of the unit students should be able to:
The personnel: chairman, secretary, treasurer, members **17.2** appreciate their role and responsibilities;	17.2.1 identify and specify the roles and responsibilities of officers before, during and after the meeting; 17.2.2 draft notice, agenda, chairman's agenda and minutes from given information;
17.3 know the differences between minuting and reporting.	
Terminology **17.4** the meaning of the terms and their significance in the conduct of meetings;	17.4.1 define the common terms used.
18 Business Documents **18.1** understand the purposes of common business documents, such as invoice, credit note, statement;	18.1.1 check the accuracy of business documents; 18.1.2 appreciate the purpose of each.
19 Book-keeping and Banking Services *Receipts and payments: bank current account facilities—paying into an account, payment by cheque, cashing cheques, etc.* **19.1** know the procedures for each;	19.1.1 select and prepare documents, such as bank reconciliation statements.
Accountability for cash **19.2** understand the importance of accountability when handling cash;	19.2.1 devise a simple system; to record receipts and payments.
Accounts **19.3** understand the necessity of accounts for private patients, the records required, the rendering of accounts; **19.4** understand income and expenditure accounts and petty cash accounts;	19.3.1 know how to deal with such accounts; 19.4.1 know how to deal with income and expenditure accounts; 19.4.2 prepare a specimen petty cash analysis account from given data.
PAYE and wage records **19.5** understand the compilation of payroll and the forms and procedures required by inland revenue for PAYE and National Insurance; **19.6** know the different methods of payment, such as cash, cheque and credit transfer;	19.5.1 prepare wages records and make the appropriate deductions; 19.6.1 appreciate the advantages and disadvantages of each method both to employee and employer.
20 Preparation of Material for Publication **20.1** understand the requirements of printers and publishers for scientific material;	20.1.1 prepare material for presentation to printers and to correct proofs received from the printer.

From the Association of Medical Secretaries, Practice Administrators and Receptionists 1982, with permission.

Units and Statistics

All quantities on prescriptions must be given in metric measurements.

Centigrade and Fahrenheit equivalents

°C	°F	°C	°F
36	96.8	39	102.2
36.5	97.7	39.5	103.1
37	98.6	40	104
37.5	99.5	40.5	104.9
38	100.4	41	105.8
38.5	101.3	42	107.6

To convert centigrade degrees to Fahrenheit degrees, multiply the centigrade figure by 1.8 and add 32 to the result.

To convert Fahrenheit degrees to centigrade degrees, subtract 32 from the Fahrenheit figure and multiply the result by 0.55.

Metric to imperial

g	lb oz
1000 (1 kg)	2 lb 3¼ oz
500	1 lb 1⅝ oz
100	3½ oz
25	⅞ oz
10	⅓ oz

Obstetrical Table

This date is calculated from the first day of the last menstrual period.

Jan	Oct	Feb	Nov	Mar	Dec	Apr	Jan	May	Feb	June	Mar	July	Apr	Aug	May	Sept	June	Oct	July	Nov	Aug	Dec	Sept
1	8	1	8	1	6	1	6	1	5	1	8	1	7	1	8	1	8	1	8	1	8	1	7
2	9	2	9	2	7	2	7	2	6	2	9	2	8	2	9	2	9	2	9	2	9	2	8
3	10	3	10	3	8	3	8	3	7	3	10	3	9	3	10	3	10	3	10	3	10	3	9
4	11	4	11	4	9	4	9	4	8	4	11	4	10	4	11	4	11	4	11	4	11	4	10
5	12	5	12	5	10	5	10	5	9	5	12	5	11	5	12	5	12	5	12	5	12	5	11
6	13	6	13	6	11	6	11	6	10	6	13	6	12	6	13	6	13	6	13	6	13	6	12
7	14	7	14	7	12	7	12	7	11	7	14	7	13	7	14	7	14	7	14	7	14	7	13
8	15	8	15	8	13	8	13	8	12	8	15	8	14	8	15	8	15	8	15	8	15	8	14
9	16	9	16	9	14	9	14	9	13	9	16	9	15	9	16	9	16	9	16	9	16	9	15
10	17	10	17	10	15	10	15	10	14	10	17	10	16	10	17	10	17	10	17	10	17	10	16
11	18	11	18	11	16	11	16	11	15	11	18	11	17	11	18	11	18	11	18	11	18	11	17
12	19	12	19	12	17	12	17	12	16	12	19	12	18	12	19	12	19	12	19	12	19	12	18
13	20	13	20	13	18	13	18	13	17	13	20	13	19	13	20	13	20	13	20	13	20	13	19
14	21	14	21	14	19	14	19	14	18	14	21	14	20	14	21	14	21	14	21	14	21	14	20
15	22	15	22	15	20	15	20	15	19	15	22	15	21	15	22	15	22	15	22	15	22	15	21
16	23	16	23	16	21	16	21	16	20	16	23	16	22	16	23	16	23	16	23	16	23	16	22
17	24	17	24	17	22	17	22	17	21	17	24	17	23	17	24	17	24	17	24	17	24	17	23
18	25	18	25	18	23	18	23	18	22	18	25	18	24	18	25	18	25	18	25	18	25	18	24
19	26	19	26	19	24	19	24	19	23	19	26	19	25	19	26	19	26	19	26	19	26	19	25
20	27	20	27	20	25	20	25	20	24	20	27	20	26	20	27	20	27	20	27	20	27	20	26
21	28	21	28	21	26	21	26	21	25	21	28	21	27	21	28	21	28	21	28	21	28	21	27
22	29	22	29	22	27	22	27	22	26	22	29	22	28	22	29	22	29	22	29	22	29	22	28
23	30	23	30	23	28	23	28	23	27	23	30	23	29	23	30	23	30	23	30	23	30	23	29
24	31	24	1	24	29	24	29	24	28	24	31	24	30	24	31	24	1	24	31	24	31	24	30
25	1	25	2	25	30	25	30	25	1	25	1	25	1	25	1	25	2	25	1	25	1	25	1
26	2	26	3	26	31	26	31	26	2	26	2	26	2	26	2	26	3	26	2	26	2	26	2
27	3	27	4	27	1	27	1	27	3	27	3	27	3	27	3	27	4	27	3	27	3	27	3
28	4	28	5	28	2	28	2	28	4	28	4	28	4	28	4	28	5	28	4	28	4	28	4
29	5			29	3	29	3	29	5	29	5	29	5	29	5	29	6	29	5	29	5	29	5
30	6			30	4	30	4	30	6	30	6	30	6	30	6	30	7	30	6	30	6	30	6
31	7			31	5			31	7			31	7	31	7			31	7			31	7
Jan	Nov	Feb	Dec	Mar	Jan	Apr	Feb	May	Mar	Jun	Apr	July	May	Aug	Jun	Sept	July	Oct	Aug	Nov	Sept	Dec	Oct

Degrees, Terminology and Abbreviations

ABBREVIATIONS OF QUALIFYING DEGREES AND FURTHER QUALIFICATIONS

BAO Bachelor of the Art of Obstetrics
BC, BCh, BChir Bachelor of Surgery
BHyg Bachelor of Hygiene
BM Bachelor of Medicine
BS, ChB Bachelor of Surgery
BSc Bachelor of Science
CM, ChM Master of Surgery
CPH Certificate in Public Health
DA Diploma in Anaesthetics
DCH Diploma in Child Health
DCh Doctor of Surgery
DCP Diploma in Clinical Pathology
DDO Diploma in Dental Orthopaedics
DDS Doctor of Dental Surgery
DGO Diploma in Gynaecology and Obstetrics
DHyg Doctor of Hygiene
DIH Diploma in Industrial Health
DLO Diploma in Laryngology and Otology
DM Doctor of Medicine
DMD Doctor of Dental Medicine
DMR Diploma in Medical Radiology
DMRE Diploma in Medical Radiology and Electrology
DO Diploma in Ophthalmology
DObstRCOG Diploma in Obstetrics of the Royal College of Obstetricians and Gynaecologists
DOMS Diploma in Ophthalmological Medicine and Surgery
DPA Diploma in Public Administration
DPD Diploma in Public Dentistry
DPhysMed Diploma in Physical Medicine
DPH Diploma in Public Health
DPM Diploma in Psychological Medicine
DR Diploma in Radiology
DSc Doctor of Science
DSSc Diploma in Sanitary Science
DTH Diploma in Tropical Hygiene
DTM Diploma in Tropical Medicine
FACP Fellow of American College of Physicians
FACS Fellow of American College of Surgeons

357

FBPsS   Fellow of British Psychological Society
FDS   Fellow of Dental Surgery
FFA   Fellow of Faculty of Anaesthetists
FFHom   Fellow of Faculty of Homeopathy
FFR   Fellow of Faculty of Radiologists
FLS   Fellow of Linnean Society
FRACP   Fellow of Royal Australian College of Physicians
FRACS   Fellow of Royal Australian College of Surgeons
FRCGP   Fellow of Royal College of General Practitioners
FRCOG   Fellow of Royal College of Obstetricians and Gynaecologists
FRCP   Fellow of Royal College of Physicians of London
FRCPE★   Fellow of Royal College of Physicians of Edinburgh
FRCPS   Fellow of Royal College of Physicians and Surgeons
FRCPath   Fellow of Royal College of Pathologists
FRCPsych   Fellow of the Royal College of Psychiatrists
FRCS   Fellow of Royal College of Surgeons of England
FRCSE   Fellow of Royal College of Surgeons of Edinburgh
FRES   Fellow of Royal Entomological Society
FRIPHH   Fellow of Royal Institute of Public Health and Hygiene
FRS   Fellow of Royal Society
FRSanI   Fellow of Royal Sanitary Institute
FSS   Fellow of Royal Statistical Society
HVCert   Health Visitors Certificate
LAH   Licentiate of Apothecaries Hall, Dublin
LDS   Licentiate in Dental Surgery
LDSc   Licentiate in Dental Science
LM   Licentiate in Midwifery
LMS   Licentiate in Medicine and Surgery
LMSSA   Licentiate in Medicine and Surgery, Society of Apothecaries
LRCP   Licentiate of Royal College of Physicians
LRFPS   Licentiate of Royal Faculty of Physicians and Surgeons
LSA   Licentiate of Society of Apothecaries
LSSc   Licentiate of Sanitary Science
MAO   Master of the Art of Obstetrics
MB   Bachelor of Medicine
M-C   Medico-Chirurgical
MC, MCh, MChir   Master of Surgery
MChD   Master of Dental Surgery
MChOrth   Master of Orthopaedic Surgery
MCPath   Member of College of Pathology
MCPS   Member of College of Physicians and Surgeons
MD   Doctor of Medicine
MDentSc   Master of Dental Science
MDS   Master of Dental Surgery
MFCP   Member of the Faculty of Community Physicians
MFHom   Member of the Faculty of Homeopathy
MHyg   Master of Hygiene
MMSA   Master of Midwifery of Society of Apothecaries
MPH   Master of Public Health
MRCGP   Member of Royal College of General Practitioners
MRCOG   Member of Royal College of Obstetricians and Gynaecologists
MRCP   Member of Royal College of Physicians of London
MRCPath   Member of Royal College of Pathologists
MRCPsych   Member of the Royal College of Psychiatrists
MRCS   Member of Royal College of Surgeons of England

MS Master of Surgery
MRSanI Member of Royal Sanitary Institute
RGN Registered General Nurse
ScD Doctor of Science
SEN State Enrolled Nurse
SRN State Registered Nurse
TDD Tuberculous Diseases Diploma

*This may be written as FRCPEd, FRCP(Ed), FRCP(Edin), or FRCPE. It is correct to add the appropriate College after the MRCP or FRCS of the Scottish Royal Colleges.

MEDICAL TERMINOLOGY

The development of the English language is a complex and fascinating story. It is a child with many parents. The language of the early Britons was gradually modified by Celtic and Gaelic tongues on its frontiers. Then, during the two hundred and fifty years of Roman occupation, many Latin words were added. Successive invasions of Vikings and Danes further influenced the language and the Norman conquest of 1066 introduced French words to our vocabulary. The language was subjected to pressures from within as well as from without. As men grew old and died, words that they had known died with them and as new commerce, new arts and new sciences were developed, new words were formed to express ideas.

The language of medicine has a less complicated history. It was originally the language of the Greeks; the fathers of medicine itself. When the Romans overcame them a Latinized Greek vocabulary grew up to express the new science. This lasted for four hundred years before being swept away by the obscurantism of the Dark Ages. With the Renaissance this language was rediscovered and has been used ever since. It has been adapted and modified in a simple logical way so that it can be applied to the most modern medical techniques and ideas. It has the great virtue of being understood by doctors of many countries and it is capable of conveying meaning to people to whom the 'dead' languages of Latin and Greek mean nothing at all.

The principle behind this system is that the whole medical vocabulary consists of root words derived from Latin or Greek. To these roots may be added syllabuses that modify the meaning of the root word. Where an addition is made to the front of a root, it is known as a prefix. An addition to the end of a root word is a suffix. To be correct, a Greek word should have only Greek prefixes and suffixes and a Latin root only Latin prefixes and suffixes; for example: bronchus is a root word meaning an air tube leading to the lung, bronchoscopy modifies it to mean looking down a bronchus. Thus the knowledge of a relatively small number of root words, prefixes and suffixes will give a wide knowledge of the medical vocabulary.

Root words

Root word	English	Root word	English
adeno	gland	mast-	breast
aesthesis	feeling	mening-	meninges
angi-	vessel	mensis	menstrual
aorta	aorta	mesenter	mesentery
arteria	artery	metr-	uterus
arthron	joint	mnesis	memory
bacillus	bacterium	my-	muscle
bios	life	myel-	bone-marrow
blepharon	eyelid	myring-	ear drum
brachium	arm	myx-	mucous
bronchus	bronchus	nephron	kidney
bursa	bursa	neur-	nerve
cardium	heart	o or oo-	egg cell
carpus	wrist	odont-	tooth
cephale	head	oesophagus	gullet
chole-	gall	oophar-	ovary
chondro-	cartilage	orch-	testicle
coccyg-	coccyx	orexia-	appetite
colon	colon	osteo	bone
colpo-	vagina	pancreas	pancreas
costa	rib	parot-	parotid gland
cranium	skull	peritoneum	peritoneum
cyte	cell	phagia	swallowing
dacryocyst-	lachrymal sac	phasia	speaking
dactylos	finger	phleb-	vein
derma	skin	phonia	speaking
digitus	finger	phren-	diaphragm
diuresis	micturition	pneuma	lung
emesis	vomit	pnoea	breathing
encephal	brain	pollex	thumb
enter	gut	proct-	rectum
epidym-	epididymis	pyel-	kidney pelvis
epiplo-	omentum	pylorus	pylorus
epithelium	epithelium	rhinos	nose
ganglion	ganglion	salping-	tube
gaster	stomach	sperma	semen
genesis	birth	sphyxia	pulsation
glossa	tongue	splen	spleen
glottis	glottis	spondyl	vertebra
glyc-	sugar	stoma	mouth
haema	blood	tars	eyelid
hallux	great toe	tenon	tendon
hepat-	liver	thorax	chest
hymen	hymen	tox-	poison
hypnos	sleep	trachea	trachea
hyster-	uterus	trich-	hair
ileum	ileum	ureter	ureter
kerat	cornea	urethra	urethra
larynx	larynx	uro-	urine

Prefixes

These root words may be modified by the addition of the following prefixes.

Prefix	Meaning	Example	Literal meaning
a- or an-	without	amnesia	without memory
ab-	away from	abduct	to draw away
ad-	towards	adduct	to draw towards
ambi-	both	ambidextrous	ability to use both hands equally
ante-	before	antenatal	before birth
antero-	in front of	anterolateral	in front of and to one side
anti-	against	antibiotic	against life
atelo-	imperfect	atelectasis	imperfect expansion of lungs
auto-	self	auto-immune	immune against oneself
bi-	twice	binaural	hearing with both ears
brady-	slow	bradycardia	slow heart-beat
carcino-	cancerous	carcinogenesis	creation of cancer
contra-	against	contraception	against birth
dextra-	right	dextracardia	a right-sided heart
dys-	painful/ difficult	dysphagia	painful (or difficulty in) swallowing
endo-	inside	endometrium	inside lining of uterus
extra-	outside	extravascular	outside the vessels
fibro-	fibrous	fibroadenoma	fibrous gland
gyn-	female	gynaecology	study of diseases of female organs
haemo-	relating to blood	haemoptysis	coughing blood
hemi-	half	hemiplegia	paralysis of half the body
hydro-	relating to water	hydrocephalus	a head containing water
hyper-	above normal	hypertension	above normal blood pressure
hypo-	below normal	hyposecretion	below normal secretion
infra-	below	infragastric	below the stomach
inter-	between	intercostal	between the ribs
intra-	in the middle of	intrahepatic	in the liver
leuco-	white	leucocyte	white blood cell
litho-	stone	lithotomy	making an opening for a stone
macro-	large	macrocyte	large cell
mania-	madness	maniac	mad person
mega-	great	megacolon	a great colon
micro-	small	microcyte	a small cell
multi-	many	multilobular	having many lobules
myco-	fungoid	mycosis	fungoid infection
neo-	new	neonate	newborn
ophthalmo-	relating to the eye	ophthalmoscope	instrument for inspecting the eye
ortho-	normal	orthodont	normal teeth
oss-	relating to bone	ossification	turning to bone
oto-	relating to ear	otorrhoea	discharge from ear
pachy-	thick	pachydermatous	thick-skinned
pan-	all	panhysterectomy	removal of all the uterus
per-	through	percutaneous	through the skin
poly-	many or much	polyuria	much urine
pseudo-	false	pseudocyesis	false pregnancy
psycho-	relating to mind	psychopath	with a diseased mind
pyo-	pus	pyonephrosis	pus in the kidney

Prefix	Meaning	Example	Literal meaning
retro-	backward	retroverted	tipped backwards
semi-	half	semiconscious	half conscious
sub-	under	submaxillary	under the maxilla

Suffixes

A suffix is added after the root word. Sometimes a root word has both a suffix and prefix, for example: cardiac—heart, carditis—inflammation of the heart, and endocarditis—inflammation of the inside of the heart. On many occasions the same element may be used as a suffix or prefix, e.g. lithotomy—or phlebolith. Where it has already been used as a prefix it is not included in the list of common suffixes.

Suffix	Meaning	Example	Literal meaning
-ac	relating to	cardiac	relating to the heart
-aemia	relating to the blood	toxaemia	poisoning of the blood
-aesthesia	relating to feeling	hyperaesthesia	above normal feeling
-algia	relating to pain	proctalgia	pain in the rectum
-an	relating to	ovarian	relating to the ovary
-cele	hernia of	enterocele	hernia of gut
-centesis	puncture	paracentesis	puncturing of a body cavity to remove fluid
-cyst	a sac of fluid	enterocyst	sac of fluid attached to gut
-cyte	relating to a cell	leucocyte	white blood cell
-cytosis	having more cells	leucocytosis	having more white blood cells
-dynia	having pain in	pleurodynia	pain in the pleura
-ectomy	removal of	gastrectomy	removal of stomach
-gram	a portrait of	bronchogram	portrait (X-ray) of a bronchus
-ist	a practitioner	physiotherapist	one who practises physiotherapy
-itis	inflammation of	appendicitis	inflammation of the appendix
-lysis	loosening	adhesolysis	dividing adhesions
-oid	like	fibroid	like fibrous tissue
-ology	relating to the science	bacteriology	relating to the study of bacteria
-opia	relating to the eye	myopia	short-sighted
-orrhaphy	sewing up	herniorrhaphy	sewing up a hernia
-orrhoea	flowing	leucorrhoea	a white discharge
-oscopy	looking into	cystoscopy	looking into the bladder
-ostomy	making an opening	colostomy	making an opening into the colon
-otomy	cutting into	gastrotomy	cutting the stomach
-pathy	disease of	adenopathy	disease of glands
-pexy	fixing	nephropexy	fixing the kidney
-plasty	repair of	hernioplasty	repair of a hernia
-plegia	paralysed	hemiplegia	half the body paralysed
-rhythmia	relating to rhythm	arrhythmia	without normal rhythm
-uria	relating to urine	anuria	without normal urine flow

MEDICAL ABBREVIATIONS

When typing medical reports and letters the secretary will use a large number of words whose meaning can be deduced by a knowledge of these root words and the suffixes and prefixes listed above. However, the secretary will also need to have a good medical dictionary and to become familiar with its use.

The use of abbreviations is a practice forced upon doctors by the necessity to be brief and quick when writing notes or instructions. Abbreviations are so easy to misinterpret that great care should be exercised in their use. The problem is that there is only a little standardization and therefore the list contains only those that are generally and widely used and are not peculiar to one hospital or one doctor. Many medical abbreviations have a Latin origin and when this is the case the Latin words are given in brackets after the abbreviation.

aa (ana) of each
a.c. (ante cibum) before meals
ad to; up to
ad lib. (ad libitum) as much as needed
aet. (aetas) aged
A/G ratio albumin/globulin ratio
AHA Area Health Authority
alb. albumin
alt. dieb. (alternis diebus) every other day
alt. hor. (alternis horis) every other hour
alt. noct. (alternis noctibus) every other night
AN antenatal
ante (ante) before
AP anteroposterior
APH antepartum haemorrhage
APT alum-precipitated toxoid
aq. (aqua) water
aq.-dist. (aqua distillata) distilled water
ARM artificial rupture of membranes
Ba.E barium enema
Ba.M barium meal
BBA born before arrival
BCG Bacille Calmette-Guérin
b.d. or **b.i.d. (bis in die)** twice daily
BI bone injury
bib. (bibe) drink
BID brought in dead
BMR basal metabolic rate
BNF British National Formulary (with date)
BO bowels opened
BP blood pressure or British Pharmacopoeia (with date)
BPC British Pharmaceutical Codex (with date)
BS breath sounds
C (centum gradus) centigrade
c. (circa) about
c. (cum) with
Ca. carcinoma
caps (capsula) capsule
CCF congestive cardiac failure
cf. compare
circ. circumcision
CF cystic fibrosis

cm centimetre
CNS central nervous system
c.o. complains of
Crem (cremor) cream
CSF cerebrospinal fluid
CSOM chronic suppurative otitis media
CSU catheter specimen of urine
CVS cardiovascular system
Cx cervix
D&C dilatation and curettage
DDA Dangerous Drugs Act
dil. (dilutus) dilute
DMC District Medical Committee
DMT District Management Team
DNA did not attend
DT delirium tremens
D and V diarrhoea and vomiting
DU duodenal ulcer
DXR deep X-ray
ECG electrocardiogram
ECT electroconvulsive therapy
EDC expected date of confinement
EDD expected date of delivery
EEG electroencephalogram
ENT ear, nose and throat
e.s. (enema saponis) soap enema
ESN educationally subnormal
ESR erythrocyte sedimentation rate
EUA examination under anaesthesia
ext. (extractum) extract
F Fahrenheit
FB foreign body
FH fetal heart or family history
FHH fetal heart heard
FHNH fetal heart not heard
Fib. fibula
fl. (fluidum) fluid
FMF fetal movements felt
FPC Family Practitioner Committee
ft. (fiat) let there be made
FTM fractional test meal
g gram
GA general anaesthetic
G and O gas and oxygen
GB gall-bladder

GC   gonorrhoea
GCFT   gonorrhoea complement fixation test
GI   gastrointestinal
GP   general practitioner
GPI   general paralysis of insane
GTT   glucose tolerance test
GU   gastric ulcer
gt. (gutta)   drop (eye-drops)
Gyn.   gynaecology
h. (hora)   hour
Hb   haemoglobin
HMC   Hospital Management Committee
HP   house physician
HS   house surgeon
h.s. (hora somni)   at bedtime
HV   health visitor
id. (idem)   the same
i.e. (id est)   that is
in d. (in dies)   daily
IP   inpatient
IQ   intelligence quotient
ISQ (in statu quo)   without change
IV   intravenous
IVP   intravenous pyelogram
IZS   insulin zinc suspension
KJ   knee jerk
KP   keratitis punctata
l   litre (should be written in full)
LA   local anaesthetic or local authority
Lab.   laboratory
LE cells   lupus erythematosus cells
LHA   Local Health Authority
LIF   left iliac fossa
LIH   left inguinal hernia
liq. (liquor)   a solution in water
LMC   Local Medical Committee
LMP   last menstrual period
LOA   left occipitoanterior
LOP   left occipitoposterior
LSCS   lower segment caesarean section
LV   left ventricle
M. (misce)   mix
m.   minim
mCi   millicurie
MCD   mean corpuscular diameter
MCH   mean corpuscular haemoglobin
MCHC   mean corpuscular haemoglobin concentration
MCV   mean corpuscular volume
mEq   milliequivalent
mist. (mistura)   mixture
mm.   millimetre
mmHg   millimetres of mercury
MMR   mass miniature radiography
MO   Medical Officer
MOH   Medical Officer of Health
MRC   Medical Research Council
MS   multiple sclerosis
MSU   midstream urine
MSW   medical social worker (almoner)
NAD   no abnormality detected

NBI   no bone injury
neg.   negative
NG   new growth
no. (numero)   number
noct. (nocte)   at night
NOTB   National Ophthalmic Treatment Board
n.p. (nomen proprium)   give proper name
NPU   not passed urine
OA   osteo-arthritis
Ob.   obstetrics
OE   on examination
Omn. hor. (omni hora)   every hour
Omn. noct. (omni nocte)   every night
Op.   operation
OP   outpatient
PA   pernicious anaemia
Path.   pathology
PBI   protein bound iodine
p.c. (post cibum)   after meals
PCO   patient complains of
PID   prolapsed intervertebral disc
PMH   previous medical history
PN   post-natal
POP   plaster of Paris
PP   private patients
PPH   post-partum haemorrhage
p.r. (per rectum)   rectal examination or by the rectum
p.r.n. (pro re nata)   whenever necessary
PSW   psychiatric social worker
PY   physiotherapy
PU   passed urine
PUO   pyrexia of unknown origin
p.v. (per vaginam)   vaginal examination or by the vagina
PZI   protamine zinc insulin
q. (quaque)   every
q.h. (quaque hora)   every hour
q.i.d. (quater in die)   four times a day
quotid. (quotidie)   daily
q.s. (quantum sufficiat)   sufficient quantity
Rx *(recipe)*   take
RA   rheumatoid arthritis
RBC   red blood corpuscle
Rh.   rhesus factor
RHA   Regional Health Authority
RIF   right iliac fossa
RIH   right inguinal hernia
RLL   right lower lobe
RMO   Resident Medical Officer
ROA   right occipitoanterior
ROL   right occipitolateral
ROP   right occipitoposterior
RS   respiratory system
RSO   Resident Surgical Officer
s̄. (sine)   without
SB   stillborn
SG   specific gravity
sig. (signetur)   let it be labelled
SMR   submucous resection

sol. (solutis) solution
s.o.s. (si opus sit) if necessary
sp. gr. specific gravity
ss. (semis) half
stat. (statim) at once
SWD short wave diathermy
syr. (syrupus) syrup
T and A tonsils and adenoids
TAB typhoid and paratyphoid A and B
TB tuberculosis
TCA to come again
TCI to come in
t.i.d. (ter in die) three times a day

TPR temperature, pulse and respiration
tr. (tinctura) tincture
Ung. (unguentum) ointment
VD venereal disease
vi (virgo intacta) virgin
Vin. (vinum) wine
VV varicose vein
Vx vertex
WBC white blood corpuscle
WR Wassermann reaction
wt weight
XR X-ray
YOB year of birth

Symbols that are commonly used include: ♂ male; ♀ female; # fracture; −ve negative; +ve positive; △ diagnosis

Useful Addresses

ORGANIZATIONS

Association of Medical Secretaries Tavistock House South, Tavistock Square, London WC1.

British Diabetic Association 10 Queen Anne Street, London W1M 0BD.

British Epilepsy Association 3 Alfred Place, London WC1.

British Medical Association BMA House, Tavistock Square, London WC1.

British Rheumatism and Arthritis Association 6 Grosvenor Crescent, London SW1.

British United Provident Association 24/27 Essex Street, London WC2.

Committee on Safety of Drugs Finsbury Square House, 33/37a Finsbury Square, London EC2.

Family Planning Association Margaret Pyke House, 27–35 Mortimer Street, London W1.

General Medical Council 44 Hallam Street, London W1.

General Register Office Somerset House, Strand, London WC2.

Health Visitors' Association 36 Eccleston Square, London SW1.

Imperial Cancer Research Fund Lincoln's Inn Fields, London WC2.

Medical Defence Union Ltd 3 Devonshire Place, London W1.

Medical Protection Society Ltd 50 Hallam Street, London W1.

Medical Research Council 20 Park Crescent, London W1.

Mental After Care Association 110 Jermyn Street, London SW1.

Department of Health and Social Security Alexander Fleming House, Elephant and Castle, London SE1.

Multiple Sclerosis Society 4 Tachbrook Street, London SW1.

Muscular Dystrophy Group 26 Borough High Street, London SE1.

National Council for the Unmarried Mother and her Child 255 Kentish Town Road, London NW5.

National Society for Cancer Relief Michael Sobell House, 30 Dorset Square, London NW1.

National Society for Epileptics Chalfont Centre, Chalfont St Peter, Bucks.

National Society for Mentally Handicapped Children 117 Golder Lane, London EC1.

Nuffield Provincial Hospitals Trust 3 Prince Albert's Road, London NW1.

Royal College of General Practitioners 14 Princes Gate, Hyde Park, London SW7.

Royal College of Obstetricians and Gynaecologists 27 Sussex Place, Regents Park, London NW1.

Royal College of Pathologists 2 Carlton House Terrace, London SW1.

Royal College of Physicians 11 St Andrew's Place, London NW1.

Royal College of Physicians Edinburgh, 9 Queen Street, Edinburgh 2.

Royal College of Physicians and Surgeons of Glasgow 242 St Vincent Street, Glasgow C2.

Royal College of Psychiatrists 17 Belgrave Square, London SW1.

Royal College of Surgeons Nicholson Street, Edinburgh 8.

Royal College of Surgeons of England Lincoln's Inn Fields, London WC1.

Royal National Institute for the Blind 224 Great Portland Street, London W1.

Royal National Institute for the Deaf 105 Gower Street, London WC1.
Royal Society of Medicine 1 Wimpole Street, London W1.
St Andrew's Scottish Ambulance Association Milton Street, Glasgow 4.
Scottish Association for the Deaf 158 West Regent Street, Glasgow C2.
Scottish Council for Health Education 21 Landsdowne Crescent Edinburgh 12.
Scottish Council for the Care of Spastics Rhuemore, Corstorphine Road, Edinburgh 12.
Scottish Council for the Unmarried Mother and her Child 44 Albany Street, Edinburgh 1.
Scottish Epilepsy Association 48 Govan Road, Glasgow 51.
Scottish Home and Health Department St Andrew's House, Edinburgh 1.
Scottish National Federation for the Welfare of the Blind 39 St Andrew's Street, Dundee.
Society of Apothecaries Blackfriars Lane, Queen Victoria Street, London EC4.
Spastics Society 12 Park Crescent, London W1.
Welsh Board of Health Cathays Park, Cardiff.
Women's Royal Voluntary Service 17 Old Park Lane, London W1.
World Health Organization Geneva, Switzerland.

SOME MEDICAL PUBLICATIONS WITH THEIR ADDRESSES

Archives of Disease in Childhood BMA House, Tavistock Square, London WC1.
British Heart Journal BMA House, Tavistock Square, London WC1.
British Journal of Anaesthesia Macmillan Journals Ltd, 4 Little Essex Street, London WC2.
British Journal of Clinical Practice Harvey & Blythe Ltd, 216 Church Road, Hove, Sussex.
British Journal of Hospital Medicine Hospital Medicine Publication Ltd, Northwood House, 93 Goswell Road, London EC1.
British Journal of Surgery John Wright & Sons Ltd, Techno House, Redcliffe Way, Bristol.
British Medical Journal BMA House, Tavistock Square, London WC1.
Journal of Obstetrics and Gynaecology John Wright & Sons Ltd, Techno House, Redcliffe Way, Bristol.
Journal of the Royal College of General Practitioners 8 Queen Street, Edinburgh EH2 1JE.
Lancet 7 Adam Street, Adelphi, London WC2.
Medical World 10 Jamestown Road, London NW1.
Practitioner Morgan-Grampian (Publishers) Ltd, 30 Calderwood Street, London SE18.
Pulse Morgan-Grampian (Professional Press) Ltd, Morgan-Grampian House, 30 Calderwood Street, London SE18.
Update Update Publications Ltd, 33/34 Alfred Place, London WC1.

References and Further Reading

It is important for the secretary to know the sources from which information can be obtained. A list of the principal books likely to be of value is given here.

MEDICAL REFERENCE BOOKS

1 *The Medical Directory*. This is published annually and consists of two volumes containing a directory of all qualified medical practitioners, together with their addresses, qualifications and the posts that they hold. Under each doctor's name a list is given of the more important papers and books that he has published. Information about hospitals is also included. Most secretaries will find that recent copies are kept at their place of employment.
2 *Medical Dictionaries*. Among the smaller dictionaries the secretary will find *Dorland's Pocket Medical Dictionary* and *Baillière's Nurses' Dictionary* very helpful.
3 *The BMA Handbook*. This contains a wealth of detail about medical matters including a schedule of fees. It may be obtained by any doctor who is a member of the BMA.
4 *Guide to the Social Services*. A small handbook published by the Family Welfare Association which provides a comprehensive account of all the social services that are available.
5 *MIMS*. Published monthly and sent to every general practitioner, this contains a list of all proprietary drugs and will be invaluable when checking the spelling of some of these difficult names.
6 *First Aid*. St John or Red Cross First Aid manual.

GENERAL REFERENCE BOOKS

English

1 A good dictionary, such as *The Concise Oxford Dictionary*.
2 *Fowler's Modern English Usage*. A book which will assist with any problem relating to English grammar and modern English usage.
3 *Roget's Thesaurus of English Words and Phrases*. This lists words according to their meaning and will help the secretary to choose the most appropriate one.

Travel

1 The *ABC Railway Guide* will be of help in planning an itinerary, but up-to-date information must often be sought from the railway enquiry office.
2 The *ABC World Airways Guide* gives information about air travel at home and abroad.

368

3 The Royal Automobile Club and the Automobile Association handbooks provide details useful for motorists. Members of these organizations can obtain routes and itineraries on application.

Addresses

1 *Telephone directories*. Separate volumes are published for the large cities and for each country area. Names, addresses, and telephone numbers of subscribers can be obtained from them. The classified telephone directory lists names under the heading of the professions or trades.
2 The *Post Office Directory* gives the name of streets and the occupier of each house or shop. There is also an alphabetical list of residents in which their trades and professions are listed.

General

1 *Whitaker's Almanack*. This book is published annually. It contains information on almost every subject of interest, including:
(a) The calendar year.
(b) Important information about world affairs.
(c) Information about the United Kingdom including the Royal Family, the Peerage, the Government, Parliament, the Law Courts and the Churches.
(d) A wealth of statistical information about populations, housing, crime and divorce, labour, agriculture and fisheries, railways, etc.
(e) Sections dealing with Great Britain and all foreign countries.
(f) Miscellaneous information about books, music, drama, films and poetry of the year. Sport, banking and finance, postal regulations, weights and measures, and many other details are included.
2 *Post Office Guide*. An account of all services and costs. Published annually with amending pamphlets.

FURTHER READING

British Standards Institution. *Copy Preparation and Proof Correction* (Part 1, 1975; Part 2, 1976), BS 5261.
Gartside, L. *English for Business Studies*. Plymouth: Macdonald & Evans.
Harrison, J. *Secretarial Duties*. London: Pitman.
Kerr, J. (1980) *Medical Words and Phrases (Pitman 2000 Shorthand)*. London: Pitman.
Kerr, J. (1979) *Words and Phrases—Medical Shorthand (New Era Shorthand)*. London: Pitman.
Meredith Davies, J.B. (1979) *Community Health, Preventive Medicine and Social Services*, 4th ed. London: Baillière Tindall.
Robertson, R. and Tettmar, M. (1979). *Medical Typing*. London: Pitman.
Rook, J. (1978) *Everyday English*. London: Longman.
West, C. and Lloyd, J. (1984) *You and The Computer*. London: Edward Arnold.

Index